FRANTZ FANON
AND THE
PSYCHOLOGY
OF
OPPRESSION

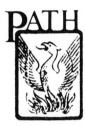

PATH IN PSYCHOLOGY
Published in Cooperation with Publications for the
Advancement of Theory and History in Psychology (PATH)

Series Editors:
David Bakan, *York University*
John Broughton, *Teachers College, Columbia University*
Robert Rieber, *John Jay College, CUNY, and Columbia University*
Howard Gruber, *University of Geneva*

Frantz Fanon AND THE Psychology OF Oppression

Hussein Abdilahi Bulhan

Boston University
Boston, Massachusetts

PLENUM PRESS • NEW YORK AND LONDON

Library of Congress Cataloging in Publication Data

Bulhan, Hussein Abdilahi.
   Frantz Fanon and the psychology of oppression.

CT
2628
F35
B85
1985

(PATH in psychology)
Bibliography: p.
Includes index.
   1. Fanon, Frantz, 1925–1961. 2. Intellectuals—Algeria—Biography. 3. Revolu-
tionists—Algeria—Biography. 4. Psychiatrists—Algeria—Biography. 5. Oppres-
sion (Psychology) 6. Social psychology. I. Title. II. Series.
CT2628.F35B85   1985   322.4′2′0924 [B]   85-19101
ISBN 0-306-41950-5

©1985 Plenum Press, New York
A Division of Plenum Publishing Corporation
233 Spring Street, New York, N.Y. 10013

Printed in the United States of America

FOREWORD

This is a biography of Frantz Fanon. It presents an absorbing and careful account of several impressive themes. First is the review and assessment of Fanon's life. Second is a theory of psychology, by the author, which will augment and prove useful to theorists and practitioners who focus on Third World people. And lastly there is a broad and systematic integration of many areas of scholarship including philosophy, anthropology, political science, history, sociology, mythology, public health, and economics. Bulhan's writing is lucid, creative, and persuasive. It demonstrates that all these scholarly areas must be handled with erudition in order to build a baseline for understanding both Fanon and the psychology of oppression.

Readers of Fanon will be familiar with the psychology of oppression which he presented so forcefully. How life events and experiences led to the formulation of this psychology is the chief emphasis of the author. Yet the book also gives scintillating clinical proof that Fanon made many other significant contributions to his field. He was an outstanding and dedicated physician as well as a philosopher and political activist.

Among the contributions of Fanon was the obligation placed on Western scientists to consider their role in the creation, perpetuation, and consequences of racism and colonialism. Bulhan elaborates this contribution by providing an especially effective and abundant documentation about the excessive pervasiveness, destructiveness, and inequity of racism in all aspects of Western life, including "objective science." It is the weight of this documentation, including the use of many new sources of data, which makes this book so compelling and should make it a standard whenever Fanon is addressed.

Yet Bulhan goes further than mere recitation of facts and interpretation about Fanon's life, the theories he produced, and the impact these theories made on history. For using all of this as background, we are privileged to receive from Bulhan his own theory of psychology. This theory might be termed a psychology of informed militancy. It forces the reevaluation of many orthodox definitions and beliefs basic to how human beings are understood in the Western world.

At minimum, this book will challenge and broaden traditional approaches to the management of oppressed and victimized people. It should stimulate new thinking about the premises of cross-cultural healing. In my opinion,

Fanon would be proud and pleased at Bulhan's sensitive efforts to understand and to extend the legacy that Fanon himself left for all the world.

CHESTER M. PIERCE

Harvard Medical School and
Harvard Graduate School of Education
Cambridge, Massachusetts

PREFACE

People often hurl stones, steel, and insults at one another in order to own, to control, and to secure privileges. In pursuit of these aims, reason is lost sight of, passions run high, and morality is conveniently shelved or proclaimed for self-vindication. Wars are fought, societies disrupted, cultures dislocated, families uprooted, and psyches ruptured.

In reality, few human encounters are exempt from oppression of one kind or another. For by virtue of our race, sex, or class, each of us happens to be a victim and/or perpetrator of oppression. Racism, sexism, and class exploitation are the most salient forms of oppression in the contemporary world. But there also exists oppression on the grounds of religious belief, political affiliation, national origin, age, and physical and mental handicap.

Although we know a great deal about the economics and politics of oppression, the psychology of oppression is neglected and, at best, indirectly broached as a topic. This is not to imply that psychologists—among whom, in the generic sense, I include psychiatrists as did Freud and Fanon—are uninterested bystanders in the history and *status quo* of oppression. On the contrary, establishment psychologists have not only been active participants in social oppression, but also silent beneficiaries of its many privileges. My aim here is to demonstrate this historical complicity, present the Fanonian alternative, and outline the central features in the psychology of oppression. I will focus primarily on racism and, secondarily, on its twin pestilence of sexism and class exploitation.

In particular, this work is on the cycle of violence and captivity in which two races—black and white—are enmeshed. It is also on Frantz Fanon, a revolutionary black psychiatrist, whose insights inform our analysis. The roots of black–white problems no doubt run deep in history and in the collective psyche. Fanon traced them to two related disasters. "The disaster of the man of color" he wrote, "lies in the fact that he was enslaved." But he also added: "the disaster and inhumanity of the white man lie in the fact that somewhere he has killed man."

The following pages examine the various manifestations of black enslavement and white predation from historical and contemporary vantage points. Since this work adopts and hopes to advance a Fanonian perspective, it is necessary to clarify the substance of this perspective and the development of the man who pioneered it. I take issue here with earlier interpretations on Fanon, present new data to shed light on controversial aspects, and bring into the discourse his seminal but neglected insights on the psychology of oppression.

To discuss the psychology of oppression is, of course, also to pose questions about Euro-American psychology and its relationship to oppression. A superficial look at establishment psychology—its diverse theories, profusion of findings, and diverse practices—would suggest that Euro-American psychologists hardly ever speak in one voice and seldom act in concert. But a closer scrutiny, in which the perspective of the oppressed is taken, reveals a remarkable unity of thought and action among these psychologists. We will show that, by and large, their scholarship and practice are unwittingly caught in the same historical violence and captivity as are the psyches they seek to understand and heal.

Every responsible critique offers an alternative solution. The Fanonian perspective elaborated in this work also suggests alternative priorities and orientations to establishment psychology. Having outlined how historical and systemic violence are lived out in interpersonal relations and personal conflicts, I explore directions for social reconstruction and self–reconstitution. The pitfalls of traditional therapies are now widely recognized, but what has yet to be sufficiently appreciated is the difficulty of transforming a systemic violence and sedimented captivity by simply applying or adopting sanctioned theories and techniques. This is so particularly when the sanctioned theories and techniques serve to justify the *status quo* of oppression and are used as instruments of social control.

I must emphasize that this work makes no pretense of dispassionate and detached analysis. Racism has wreaked havoc for generations, forced many to seek refuge in madness, and wrapped the so-called normal majority in a bankrupt culture of silence. To pretend detachment or neutrality in such matters is indeed dishonest and contrary to the Fanonian perspective.

It would surprise me if reading the following chapters does not evoke much that is usually masked by the professional countenance of neutrality and detachment. My hope is nonetheless to provoke thought about our shared predicament of captivity, lay bare repressed but festering wounds, and suggest a direction for change. A project such as this is undoubtedly ambitious and even perilous. But then, I deliberately set out to question, not defend, historical conditions, social boundaries, and sanctioned ideas imposed from without.

ACKNOWLEDGMENTS

To undertake, complete, and improve a project such as this necessarily involves more than one person. I sincerely believe that ideas and all other products of human endeavor are social and collective, that they are advanced through diverse sources, influences, and contributions. I cannot, of course, name all those who, in one way or another, contributed to this work. I will, however, mention a few to whom I am most indebted.

First, I wish to acknowledge my thanks to a network of Fanon scholars who, over the years, shared with me their thoughts and gave a sympathetic hearing to my ideas. Dr. Lewis King and The Fanon Research and Development Center have done a superb job in organizing a series of conferences that brought a number of Fanon scholars together. Thanks also to Hussein M. Adam and Ahmed S. Farah for many fruitful dialogues on Fanon's social and political thoughts.

I am also grateful to the writers who preceded me, particularly Peter Geismar and Professor Irene Gendzier, who first presented the most detailed studies on Fanon. These writers and their invaluable works defined not only what is important in Fanon, but also the terms for subsequent debates on Fanon. Although I take issue with some of their interpretations, I want to acknowledge that they provided essential information without which my inquiry would have been even more incomplete.

I am also deeply indebted to the Fanon family, particularly to Josie Fanon, Joby Fanon, and Félix Fanon. They and Marcel Manville, a close friend of Frantz Fanon and one of the living authorities on him, have been very generous with their time and funds of information. In addition, during my visit to Martinique in 1982, Félix Fanon and his family extended a warm hospitality that I will always remember with gratitude. I also thank them for their patient assistance. During the same visit to Martinique, Linette Lampla was extremely helpful in making necessary contacts, interpreting interviews, and translating documents. Marie Claude Dongar and France-Lyn Rojas-Fanon, two nieces of Frantz Fanon, also helped me in my research and gave me their sense of what it means to live with the legacy of their uncle.

My profound gratitude to Paula Jackson who labored with me on many French documents and spent countless hours translating them. My thanks also to Nouzha Deramche, an Algerian graduate student, who secured some essential documents from Algeria, and to Sandra Dorsainvil, who transcribed a number of taped interviews. Judy Rollins was the first to go through the entire manuscript, pointing out errors, asking helpful questions, and giving encouraging feedback. I am thankful for her help and friendship.

I am also grateful to Professors Francise Grossman, Abby Stewart, and David Winter for reading the manuscript and providing me with helpful comments and to Professor William Mackavey who made departmental facilities, including word processing, readily accessible. Professor Chester M. Pierce offered me a living model of both integrity and commitment. I feel privileged to have his encouragement, support, and friendship.

The manuscript was typed by several individuals, but I especially thank Ms. Shana Greenblatt and Ms. Louise True. The editors of Plenum Press have also been extremely helpful. I am grateful to Eliot Werner for his supportive and prompt responses and to Professor Robert Rieber for his helpful suggestions and fairness in considering views that may be different from his own, to Ms. Carol Miller for her thorough editing of the manuscript, and to Ms. Janice Marie Johnson for her impressive eye for detail, her remarkable patience, and genuine warmth.

Last, but certainly not least, I am deeply grateful to my extended as well as my nuclear family, particularly to my mother and sister who, in spite of my wanderings in distant lands and alien ideas, kept faith with me, and to my wife who gave me the support without which this project would have been indefinitely postponed. I dedicate this work to my two children, Sirad and Hodan, and to the children of the oppressed, wherever they may be.

CONTENTS

I

OVERVIEW OF BIOGRAPHY AND HISTORY

1

QUEST FOR PARADIGM
An Introduction

Oh my body, make of me a man who always questions.
—Fanon, *Black Skin, White Masks*

In 1924, less than a year before Frantz Fanon's birth, Hendrik Frensch Verwoerd was granted a degree as Doctor of Philosophy after completing his dissertation in psychology. Significantly, the title of his thesis was *The Blunting of the Emotions*. On 19 October 1950, a year before Fanon defended his doctoral thesis, Verwoerd became the Minister of Native Affairs, wielding awesome power and absolute control over South Africa's eight and one-half million blacks, nearly four-fifths of the country's total population. Through the Department of Native Affairs and its numerous racial laws, Verwoerd controlled, regulated, and tyrannized blacks—on the farms, in the towns, and on the Reserves. By 1958, Verwoerd was the leader of the ruling Nationalist Party and the Prime Minister of South Africa. Fanon was then 33 years old and a committed revolutionary, fighting against colonialism in Algeria.

The two men—Verwoerd and Fanon—were psychologists who put to practice their profession in ways that made history and affected the lives of millions. Except for their similar interests—the study of and the desire to change human psyches and behaviors—the two men had little in common. In fact, they were as different in social background and skin color as they were diametrically opposed in temperament, ideology, and commitment. Verwoerd was a staunch white supremacist, a Nazi sympathizer, an avowed anti-Semite, and a leading architect of apartheid in South Africa. Fanon, in contrast, was a relentless champion of social justice who, when barely 17 years old, volunteered for the forces attempting the liberation of France from Nazi occupation. After fighting in Europe during World War II, Fanon studied psychiatry to heal tormented psyches. He wrote with passion against oppression and racism, including anti-Semitism. During the last years of his short life, he had fully committed himself to the liberation of Algeria from French colonialism.

3

If Verwoerd and Fanon were thus as different as night and day, they were also products of the same historic currents that led to a Manichean world inhabited by two "species"—whites and blacks, oppressors and oppressed. But just as there can never be a night without a day, these two species locked in combat reside on but two banks of the same river. A historical greed for profit and power, which had long eroded their shared humanity, pitted one group against the other and led to the elaboration of barriers, woven of steel as well as of myths, that obviate genuine contact and reciprocal recognition. The ordering of the material world and the structure of the psyche have both been arranged in ways confirming that one group is "white" and therefore "good" and the other is "black" and therefore "evil." Verwoerd belonged to one camp and he committed himself to fortify it with awesome arms; Fanon was born into the other camp and he sought to change the two camps and their underlying Manichean psychology.

Those interested in the psychology of oppression can learn much from these two psychologists and their application of psychology to different ends. For one thing, both of them unmistakably demonstrate how untenable can be the well-rehearsed claim of professional neutrality and objectivity. For psychologists, as mortal and social beings, do indeed belong to groups, reveal their own share of ethnocentrism, and engage in battles, no less violently or viciously than do others in society. Verwoerd and Fanon present models of psychological practice as they offer summations of a collective experience. Their life histories no doubt reveal obvious contrasts, each with idiosyncracies and unique personal qualities. But more remarkable is how their individual biographies are exemplar summaries, culminations as well as pathos, of collective histories. Even their places of birth and circumstances of death show a telling continuity between individual biographies and collective histories.

Born in the Netherlands and the son of immigrants to South Africa, Verwoerd lived to implement for his generation the mission of domination, exploitation, and self-aggrandizement that for centuries Europe and its descendants had unleashed upon people of color. Fanon, the grandson of a former slave, was born on one of those West Indian islands where plantations and slave labor provided the capital for the Industrial Revolution and whetted Europe's appetite for more profit, more conquest, and more intrusive self-extension.

Verwoerd personified the boundless narcissism, violent pursuit of dominance, and skillful self-exoneration of those long accustomed to being "white" and "masters," readily imposing their will and whim on others. Psychology—its assumptions, theories, and techniques—presented little cognitive dissonance to Verwoerd, his social aims, and actual practice. He thus readily applied psychology to secure and fortify white supremacy. And psychology worked for him and for his constituency with amazing effectiveness. In contrast, Fanon personally experienced the suffering, the gnawing doubts, and the alienation of the oppressed. He delved deep into the social inferno Europe had created for millions, found his destiny inextricably bound to theirs, and sought to build, on the very ashes of that inferno, a world of reciprocal freedom and recognition.

Psychology—particularly its assumptions and theories—presented much dissonance to Fanon and was incongruent with his social aims. In fact, Eurocentric psychology revealed itself more as a part of the problem of domination than as a discipline readily amenable to the resolution of oppression. Unlike Verwoerd and most Euro-American psychologists, Fanon found it necessary to undertake a fundamental reassessment of psychology's basic assumptions, methods, and practice. In the end, Verwoerd's mission was fully accomplished when he died at a ripe, old age; Fanon's had only begun when he died in his mid-30s.

At the height of his power, having effectively established white supremacy in South Africa, Verwoerd was stabbed to death by a white assassin on 6 September 1966, two days before his 65th birthday. His assassin was later found to be apolitical. He was a psychotic man who, while the South African security police searched for a communist plot and accomplices, continued to insist that only a tapeworm with serrated edges made him kill Verwoerd. Another psychotic white man had made an attempt on Verwoerd's life in 1960. This coincidence led Alexander Hepple (1967) to pose an interesting question: "What torment did Verwoerd raise in the disturbed minds of two members of the privileged white community to make them want to kill him?"[1]

Fanon died at a most unlikely time, place, and circumstance. On 6 December 1961 he died in Bethesda, Maryland, at the early age of 36. Some Fanon scholars consider it a "mysterious death," since the CIA had brought the reluctant but desperately ailing Fanon to the United States for treatment for leukemia. The CIA also, according to Geismar (1971, p. 184), had left Fanon in a hotel for eight days without the treatment he urgently needed, forcing him to hire his own private nurse. But if mystery shrouds the circumstances of Fanon's death, there is no doubt about his relentless commitment to the cause of justice and liberty on behalf of the oppressed and the colonized, those he called "the wretched of the earth."

Notwithstanding his short life span and untimely death, Fanon left behind a rich, provocative, and inspiring legacy. It is a legacy full of insights, courage, and committed praxis. Aspects of that legacy, of course, are highly controversial. For Fanon was no ordinary man, neither in ideas nor in practice. One always runs the risk of canonizing or vilifying the man, his ideas and actions, depending largely on one's perspective. Some have called him a "prophet of revolution," an original thinker who "is to Africa what Lenin is to Europe, or Mao to Asia."[2] Others (e.g., Caute, 1970) compared him with Che Guevera and even Karl Marx. Some are convinced he was a "humanist," a "socialist," and a "passionate internationalist," whereas others denounce him as a "nihilist," "an apostle of violence," and a "prisoner of hate" (*Time*, April 30, 1965). His last book, *The Wretched of the Earth*, was compared with Marx and Engels'

---

[1]For a detailed biography of Verwoerd and his role in the development of apartheid, see Alexander Hepple (1967).

[2]See also Cherif Guellal (1971).

The Communist Manifesto and Hitler's *Mein Kampf* *(Time,* April 30, 1965), and called the black man's "Revolutionary Bible" (Geismar, 1971, p. 2).

Various memorials honor Fanon in different cultures and continents. There is, for instance, a Boulevard Frantz Fanon, a Frantz Fanon Hospital, and a Frantz Fanon High School in Algeria; a Frantz Fanon Center in Milan, Italy, and another in Lagos, Nigeria; a Fanon Research and Development Center and a Fanon School in Los Angeles, California; a Fanon Institute of Research and Training in Boston, Massachusetts; and a Frantz Fanon Collection at the Countway Library of Harvard University. During the Ben Bella regime in Algeria, a literary prize was also named for Frantz Fanon.

For the past several years, a series of conferences honoring Fanon have been held in Atlanta, Georgia; Port-of-Spain, Trinidad; Mogadishu, Somalia; and Belaggio, Italy. More recently, when for the first time it became permissible to organize an international memorial of Frantz Fanon in his home island of Martinique following the emergence of a socialist and more tolerant regime in France, the participants included representatives from the Caribbean, Latin America, North America, Africa, Europe, and Asia. A year later, an international conference honoring Fanon was held in Hamburg, West Germany. Such wide recognition of a man who died at so early an age, and well over 20 years ago, underscores the stature of Fanon and the continued relevance of his ideas to a diverse international community.

At least six major books have so far been written on Fanon. Peter Geismar (1969) wrote a highly sympathetic book, the most detailed biography of Fanon to date. David Caute (1970) presented a very concise and informative review of Fanon's intellectual evolution. Jack Woddis (1972) criticized Fanon in a scathing polemic. Irene Gendzier (1973) wrote an interpretative study of Fanon's writings and practice. Renate Zahar (1970) elaborated Fanon's theory of alienation within a Marxist perspective. In addition, two political scientists from Africa, Hussein Adam (1974) and Emmanuel Hansen (1976), wrote extensively on Fanon's social and political thoughts. There are also numerous articles and dissertations on Fanon in English, not to mention the many articles in other languages.

In this extensive literature, however, there is a marked paucity of systematic review in one crucial area: *Fanon's psychological and psychiatric contributions.* Such a paucity is curious indeed. For Fanon was first and foremost a psychiatrist by training and profession. Many of his psychological works, written alone or in collaboration, were published in various psychiatric, medical, and political journals.[3] His translated and better-known books either had psychology as their major point of departure or they incorporated psychological dimensions to complement, illustrate, and concretize the macro-social experiences he sought to unveil and transform. With the exception of Paul Adams (1970), Irene Gendzier (1973, 1976), and myself (Bulhan, 1980a,b,c), much of the literature on Fanon has by and large ignored his psychological contributions.

The reasons for such neglect of his psychological contributions are not

[3]See the bibliography on Fanon's works at the end of this volume.

difficult to surmise. First of all, Fanon wrote at a critical period in the history of the Third World in general and of Africa in particular. His contributions came out of the turbulent years of the 50s and early 60s when many of the former colonies were in the throes of national liberation. His insights into the process of decolonization struck a responsive chord among the oppressed everywhere as his analyses also offered a fresh perspective to Euro-American scholars studying the dynamics of decolonization and social change in the Third World. Given that decolonization was most ostensibly dominated by political content, those who wrote on Fanon tended to emphasize his social and political thoughts to the exclusion of his psychological.

Second, Fanon wrote most of his best-known works when he was a committed revolutionary in the Algerian liberation struggle. He wrote with passion and urgency on the political agenda for liberation. His psychiatric practice nonetheless continued, and his psychological works were published in professional journals. But these contributions remained in the background, untranslated and inaccessible to most readers. It was in fact as a social theorist, polemicist, and roving ambassador that he first won international acclaim. His thesis on political violence, his devastating critique of the colonized bourgeoisie, his conception of the peasantry as most revolutionary—these views that ostensibly were more political than psychological challenged established tenets and generated heated controversy.

Third, those who often wrote on Fanon were political scientists, historians, or sociologists. Naturally, they approached his works according to the priorities, orientation, and concepts of their disciplines. Most of them deliberately de-emphasized his psychological contributions. In fact, Woddis (1972) and Nghe (1963) went so far as to regret the psychological component of his sociopolitical analysis. Having mistakenly reduced his psychology to "existentialism," they used this supposedly negative label to discredit his genuine differences with orthodox Marxism. Others, like Gendzier (1973, 1976), who appreciated the significance of his psychological contributions provided at best descriptive summaries without demonstrating their full implications or relevance to current problems.[4]

Meanwhile Euro-American psychologists, with the narrow definition of their profession, tended to show little interest in oppression. Unlike other disciplines of the human sciences, they traditionally ignored the problems of underdevelopment in the Third World, the dynamics of domination, the reactions of the oppressed, and the patterns of social change. On the occasions they did study people of color, as I shall demonstrate in this work, the result was historically disastrous. In the realm of theory, they universally adopted the legacy of victim-blame. When they worked clinically with the human debris of Europe's historical assaults, they tended to be instruments of social control, extolling the aim of adjustment to the *status quo*, however intolerable and hostile to human needs. Even when they conducted "cross-cultural research"

---

[4]For an earlier critique of Gendzier, see my article on Frantz Fanon: The revolutionary psychiatrist (Bulhan, 1980a).

without the ostensible racism of earlier researchers, their concern has been less in understanding or changing the plight of the oppressed and more in testing hypotheses to advance Euro-American psychology or to settle academic debates at home. This general disinterest, or "mis-placed" priorities of Euro-American psychologists, has limited the diversity and general relevance of psychology.

Black psychologists in the United States, in contrast, continue to show a great deal of interest in Fanon and the problems he studied. This interest has both intellectual and affective roots: The conditions in which they study and practice impose upon them a measure of marginality and alienation. They usually find few ego-syntonic models to emulate during their professional development and in their evolving practice. They study such great pioneers as Freud, Jung, and Skinner only to realize that they have been excluded from the dialogue, that the problems that most concern them hardly figure in the priorities of the discipline, and that they must constantly endeavor to adopt concepts or methods developed for a population other than their own. They sit in lectures as uninvited guests, eavesdropping on discussions and debates relevant to "white psychology." One consequence is that they feel compelled to search for a more resonant and responsive "black psychology," sometimes elaborating their own *reactive* theories to show how whites are genetically inferior to blacks.[5] Involved here is a quest for intellectual relevance and an affirmation of identity—two essential conditions for professional and personal development. Little wonder then that Fanon and his work strike a resonant chord in black psychologists and Third World social scientists.

Unfortunately, however, there is yet no in-depth examination of Fanon's psychological contributions. It is obviously never enough to simply endorse the spirit of his contributions. There must in addition be a careful review of the substance and implications of Fanon's works. But even though his contributions remain seminal and incomplete, there is much we can learn from Fanon's thought and practice. For in his quest for paradigms and identity, Fanon traversed a long and painful course, arriving at results that are instructive as well as inspiring. Yet I am convinced that to leave matters at where destiny stopped him or to occasionally quote him for convenience is simply to eulogize Fanon, burying all the while the man and his ideas. It is more fruitful to build on his works, distill those aspects of his contributions relevant to current problems, and work to further that which he pioneered.

The perspective that we take toward psychology as toward life largely depends on the time and place we inhabit, our social nexus, and our personal and social aims. This happens to be the case even as we assume that there are universals in the human condition, that certain experiences of people are basic and common, irrespective of whether we have in mind experiences in Victorian Europe, contemporary American suburbia, crowded urban ghettoes, or

[5]An example of such reactive theories is the so-called Cress theory of color confrontation, offered by Francis C. Welsing (1974).

forgotten rural Africa. Indeed, Fanon did concede that even a profound comprehension of a single patient can underscore the universal in the human condition.

There are nonetheless two main problems in this regard. First, and still unsettled, is the content of the assumed universals in human psychology, given a multiplicity of cultures and diversities of experiences. It would seem that, to paraphrase Kluckhohn and Murray (1948), every person is in certain respects like all other persons, like some persons, and like no other person. Still unclear, however, is exactly what each of us shares in common with *everyone*, with *some* people, and with *no one*. Second, and more serious from our perspective, there is the historical imposition of Eurocentric "reality" upon those whom Europeans and their descendants rule and dominate. This historical fact of dominance has given rise to a scandal of global dimensions in which, as we shall see, the discipline of psychology remains enmeshed.

Any consideration of Fanon and his contributions brings to the discourse the effects of that historical scandal and the realities of a large population Euro-American psychologists—judging from their theories, the standardization of their instruments, and their usual practices—have completely ignored, actively helped in their conquest, or joined in their mystification. Today, more than ever, there is the rude awakening to the fact that the "human factor" in oppression, as well as plans for national reconstruction, have been neglected far too long with grave consequences. The evident crises in individual identities and collective histories can no longer be ignored. The alarming increase in alcoholism, mental disorders, and personal and state violence in urban ghettoes and developing countries invite the contributions of psychologists.

The last two decades have in fact shown how entrenched old inequities in economics and structure of domination actually are. Dreams of equality and dignity have not come true and old wounds continue to fester, more than ever now as the bankruptcy of an assimilated elite and false symbols, such as a national flag, are understood. The high expectations brought on by promises of "national independence" and "the war on poverty" have faded to be replaced by a generalized demoralization and cynicism, as home-bred demagogues develop little else, but more prisons and armies with which to conquer their own people. Psychological analyses and interventions from the perspective of history and human aggregates have subsequently gained in demand and urgency.

It is by no means insignificant that about 800 million of the world's population, nearly one-fifth of humanity, is so impoverished as to constitute a global "underclass," characterized by malnutrition, disease, and illiteracy, living in squalor. They have the highest rates of mortality at any age, they have chronic health problems and life expectancies of less than 50 years, and they have a reduced capacity for work. This global underclass reflects the extremes of a reality for a large majority of the world population. Unjust distribution of resources, rapid population growth, and increasing degradation of the environment have forced millions more into destitution, disease, and despair. The suffering in a world of improved media is compounded by a recognition of what a "good life" the next-door neighbor or that member of another nationality enjoys. The continuing desertification of land, reducing soil nutrients and arable land, combines with a desertification of values and threatens social disintegration and even "cultural extinction" in parts of the Third World. Urban settlements in the Third World rose from 4% in 1920 to 41% in 1980, with an appalling increase of slums and shantytowns. Political repression and upheavals have also given rise to an ever-increasing number of refugees who are left nothing else but to "vote by their feet."[6]

In reality, most of these problems are manmade. More is obviously involved than a natural disaster when, for instance, over 30% of the world's grain is fed to livestock and poultry each day in order to cater to the appetite and taste of the "haves," whereas only 2% of that grain would eliminate undernutrition among the have-nots. Something is indeed wrong when the international community is unable to raise $40 million a day for clean water for all people, although no less than $1.4 billion a day is spent on weapons, with global spending on weapons research and arms exceeding $500 billion a year (Eckholm, 1982). In short, there are choices to be made, priorities to be redefined, populations to make themselves heard, and a new psychology to find relevance among the dispossessed. It is in considering such problems that Fanon and his work are particularly significant.

This work has three main objectives. First, it seeks to present a comprehensive review of Fanon's psychological contributions. The approach taken to achieve this objective assumes a unifying thread in Fanon's personal experiences, thoughts, and practice. Thus I shall review his personal development, intellectual evolution, and changing practice. Second, this work attempts to demonstrate the historical complicity of Euro-American psychology in global oppression. Such a historical account and critique are necessary because the search for alternatives has meaning and value only when the status quo is clear. The assumption here is that psychology does not exist in a social vacuum and that psychologists are rooted in their society and time. Thus as we find armies fulfilling aims of conquest for their society, so do we discover psychologists justifying domination and conquest. Third, this work attempts to develop a framework for future studies advancing the psychology of oppression. This last objective is necessarily preliminary and exploratory.

These three objectives are interwoven in the various chapters. I present Fanon as I understand him, follow his lead in what seems pertinent, focus on certain aspects of his contributions, address many issues he never addressed, and search for underlying paradigms for the psychology of oppression. Throughout I try to avoid blunting the critical edge of my arguments, even

---

[6]The refugee problem in the world today is both massive and grave. Africa alone harbors no less than 10 million refugees who have been forced to flee their homes because of repressive political states and border conflicts. There is hardly a more tragic contemporary problem than the starkly rapid desertification of lands and of values. The psychosocial consequences of life as a refugee has yet to be assayed, let alone mitigated. Erik Eckholm (1982) provides a harrowing account of the global underclass.

when politeness and diplomacy may have saved my reader and myself some discomfort. We shall see that even politeness and ordinary etiquette are suspect in the psychology of oppression.

Chapters are grouped into four related and overlapping parts. Part I provides a biographical sketch of Fanon and an overview of the historical forces that conditioned the European assault upon the rest of the world. Earlier works on Fanon's childhood and relationship to his family have given rise to interpretations quite at variance with what I found in my interviews with his relatives and friends. I shall present the facts I obtained and show that some of the earlier interpretations are indeed suspect. The chapter following this biographical sketch provides a broad historical overview of the violence Europe unleashed upon the rest of the world and places Eurocentric psychology within this history of conquest and domination. The expansionist trends of burgeoning capitalism, the historical role of gunpowder and alcohol, the transmutation of values and relationships due to a greed for profit—these will be highlighted as the underlying agenda in the nature versus nurture debate and the ethnic content of psychology are reviewed.

Part II presents a critique of Eurocentric psychology and medicine. Basic assumptions, methods, and the experiential foundation of Eurocentric psychology will be evaluated as Fanon's encounters with Sigmund Freud, Carl Jung, and Alfred Adler are discussed. We will see which of their contributions Fanon chose to retain or discard. The ethnocentrism, class bias, and (in Jung's case) outright racism demonstrate that even the great pioneers were very much rooted in their time. Suggested also will be some answers to questions often asked about the oppressed. Why, for instance, do the oppressed manifest high resistance and suspicion when confronted with seemingly innocuous research questions? Why do they fail to take advantage of health services even as they admit a dire need for medical care? How can one explain the high drop-out rate observed among those of them who seek therapy? Why is it often so difficult to arrive at a correct diagnosis regarding maladies of the oppressed? And even when they are correctly diagnosed, why do such patients deliberately subvert the very prescriptions that would restore their health?

Fanon's seminal ideas suggest tantalizing answers to these questions. Chapter 6 is a theoretical discussion on the psychology of oppression in general as well as on slavery and colonialism in particular. I examine three major paradigms of the oppressor–oppressed relationship, including Hegel's master–slave dialectic, Mannoni's colonizer–colonized dynamic, and Fanon's reformulation. It should be clear from this that the oppressors dehumanize others for privilege and power whereas the oppressed forfeit their humanity and freedom out of fear to confront institutionalized violence and internalized prohibitions.

Part III deals with violence and various "forms" of death. Pivotal to oppression and to Fanon's thought, violence requires a careful, in-depth inquiry. I therefore redefine violence, offer a taxonomy amenable to consideration of problems in social oppression, and discuss why Fanon's thesis on violence remains the most controversial aspect of his thought. I review and critically

evaluate that controversy and present data to corroborate aspects of Fanon's
thesis on violence. It is moreover argued that the oppressed suffer multiple
forms of death and that submission to oppression for fear of physical death is
tragically self-defeating thereby ensuring, among other things, higher rates of
physical, psychological, and social death. I further examine psychopathology
from a contextualist perspective in order to underscore that psychopathology
is better defined as the denial of *liberty*.

We will also see that "blackness" and "madness" depend on social definitions and, hence, neither can be understood apart from their socio-historical
context. The concept of alienation that underlies much of Fanon's sociogenetic
perspective to psychopathology will be examined, along with a theory of identity development I find helpful in my work in the psychology of oppression.
Also presented is a discussion of Fanon's views on the psychological sequel of
violence in social liberation and torture. Contrary to his detractors who accuse
him of glorifying violence for its own sake, one can see here the kernel of
Fanon's radical humanism and his fundamental ambivalence toward violence.

Finally in Part IV, I take up the question of clinical and social practice. I
examine Fanon's professional development, his choice of a place for action, his
clinical innovations in Algeria, and his single-handed challenge of the "Algiers
School of Psychiatry." I underscore his little-known impact on French psychiatrists, his thoughts on forensic psychiatry in the context of oppression, and his
explorations in ethnopsychiatry. The state of affairs in Algeria at the time he
committed himself to the struggle against colonialism, his clandestine work
with freedom fighters, and the radical humanism of his clinical work are
discussed. Chapter 12 offers the initial outlines toward a psychology of liberation. In particular, it suggests a change of perspective from individual to the
collective, from fixed instincts to dynamic human needs, and from fostering
adjustment to the practice of empowerment.

Each chapter is preceded by a few introductory remarks intended to emphasize the gist of my argument. Taken together, the chapters present an
intimate look at Fanon, a historical panorama, and diverse data. The discussions deliberately move through different eras and social contexts, all the
while attempting to identify recurrent themes and principles. It is to be hoped
that future work will probe into details and refine suggested formulations. But
for the goals I set for this work, I cannot help but serve a large menu in huge
chunks, offering the only consolation that indigestion is but a minor problem
in oppression.

Before embarking on this menu, however, three caveats should be emphasized. First, this work makes no pretense of evaluating Euro-American psychology in its totality. Rather, it considers only those aspects of a legacy in
psychology that historically contributed to social oppression. To write instead
on what theories and techniques in Euro-American psychology *promise* valuable applications to psychology of oppression or of liberation has not been my
aim here, although I believe a clarification of historical pitfalls as presented in
this work prepares the ground for future endeavors in that direction. I do not

here intend, therefore, a reactive indictment of Euro-American psychology *in toto*, but only a careful critique of certain aspects in order to provoke thought and interest in issues long neglected.

Second, as stated earlier, this work is primarily on racism. Following, in part, Albert Memmi's (1968) cogent definition I use the concept of *racism* to mean the generalization, institutionalization, and assignment of values to real or imaginary differences between people in order to justify a state of privilege, aggression, and/or violence. Involving more than the cognitive or affective content of prejudice, racism is expressed behaviorally, institutionally, and culturally. The ideas or actions of a person, the goals or practices of an institution, and the symbols, myths, or structure of a society are racist if (a) imaginary or real differences of race are accentuated; (b) these differences are assumed absolute and considered in terms of superior and inferior; and (c) these are used to justify inequity, exclusion, or domination.

The focus on racism runs the risk of de-emphasizing the significance of other modes of oppression, notably class oppression and sexism. Much of the data presented here concerns blacks who in reality are working class or belong to the "underclass." It is equally about black women and black men. I consider the debate on race versus class a digression when the black middle class argues for the primacy of "race" to mask its historical complicity with oppression or when traditional Marxists minimize the significance of "race" to underplay the crimes of Europe and its descendants against people of color. One wonders whether such minimization of racial significance also reflects the hidden racism of white radicals.

As this work illustrates, I am of the opinion that only a dialectical consideration offers a fruitful analysis and a program of action. Fanon's point that colonial economic substructure is also a superstructure, that the cause is also the consequence, is yet to be adequately appreciated. The dialectical relations between the substructure and superstructure, mode of production and culture, praxis and psyche will be intimated here with the data available on blacks in the United States and South Africa. The limited data elsewhere in the black world no doubt would impose constraints on validation of theory and proposals for effective intervention.

Finally, but not least, in a world view based on patriarchy, reality is often discussed as if it is always a question of *men* as makers of history and even the sole category of humanity. Male chauvinism is indeed so deeply ingrained in language and thought that we habitually talk of God as "He," humanity as "mankind," and history as "his-story." As the language of this work reveals and in spite of efforts to the contrary, I too—and for that matter Fanon—reveal an unwitting complicity in language if not in substance. As we shall see, we are all enlisted in a history of oppression by virtue of belonging to a given race, class, and sex.

Basic concepts such as freedom, responsibility, violence, madness, and death lose much of their crucial import if not placed in a historical and social context. For to conceive of freedom only as the absence of restraint, responsibility simply as the avoidance of punishment, violence merely as the personal intent to do harm, madness only as the private travails of an individual, or death merely as physical mortality limits our understanding of oppression and serves to narrow our vision of human possibilities. The social and historical foundation of violence, madness, death, and liberty require further psychological consideration.

We must find a way of placing biography in history, the crisis of personal identity in communal uprooting, clinical symptoms in relational systems, and our action (or even inaction) in a social world that is open to intervention not as we wish in our wildest dreams, but in accordance with what historically we must and can. I harbor little illusion as to what the mere act of writing can by itself accomplish. For, in the final analysis, history and society—indeed the development of identity—are realized through human praxis. But since practice without theory is blind, the quest for paradigm remains a worthwhile endeavor. This work will surely have fulfilled its goals if it contributes to a better appreciation of Frantz Fanon and charts a perspective to the psychology of oppression.

2

Fanon's Background and Development

Scientific objectivity was barred to me, for the alienated, the neurotic, was my brother, my sister, my father.

—Fanon, *Black Skin, White Masks*

Nietzsche once remarked: "Man can stretch himself as he may with his knowledge and appear to himself as objective as he may; in the final analysis, he gives nothing but his own biography."[1] It would of course be absurd to label all of Fanon's works only as a disguised personal confession. But it would be equally foolish to assume that his thoughts had emerged out of personal alienation. It is true, however, that Fanon never wrote with the kind of cold detachment and personal distance idealized in establishment behavioral sciences. The objectivity of the narrow positivist was unattainable to him; what is more, he himself made no claim to it. For in a very personal way, Fanon was inextricably bound to the social dialectic he studied and sought to transform.

This chapter first focuses on Fanon's childhood, personality, and family dynamics. These three aspects are of course essential for understanding the man and the forces that conditioned his development. Previous writers have either broached these aspects incidentally or presented selective details marred by puzzling inaccuracies and distortions. Extensive interviews with Fanon's relatives and friends, conducted by this author during the spring of 1982, provide new and corrective data. The chapter then moves beyond the discussion of his childhood and family by relating Fanon's personal development to the evolution of his thought.

Childhood and Family

Peter Geismar (1971) has written the first and most comprehensive biography of Frantz Fanon. Subsequent writers have since heavily relied on Geismar's accounts even when their interpretation of Fanon was less sym-

---

[1] Quoted in Henri Ellenberger (1970, p. 276).

pathetic. Geismar did not, however, elaborate on Fanon's childhood and family. Irene Gendzier (1973) later presented the same sketchy accounts, but arrived at some disparaging conclusions. She regretted Geismar's omission of "personal matters," which, she argued, had an enduring impact on Fanon's personality and politics. It turns out that her selective tidbits of "personal matters" and her interpretation of them are highly suspect. Before outlining some of the data gathered from Fanon's relatives and friends, it is useful to summarize what others, including Gendzier, have written about Frantz's childhood and family.

In reviewing the available literature, we discern the following picture. Frantz was born on 20 July 1925 into a tightly knit black family on the island of Martinique. It was a middle-class family belonging to an emerging black bourgeoisie of small owners and civil servants. His father was a customs inspector whose salary, combined with the mother's earnings as a shopkeeper, managed to keep the family of eight children in relative comfort. The underdeveloped and exploited economy of this Caribbean island permitted little luxury except for the *Békès*, the ruling white aristocracy who controlled the land, business, and politics of this overseas department of France.

The Fanons were by no means spared the tight financial squeeze and insecurity common in this thoroughly colonized island. But the steady and combined income of the parents allowed the Fanon children to enjoy membership in the 4% of blacks whose parents could afford to pay tuition for the *lycée*. Frantz was a middle child, the fifth of eight children and the youngest of four sons. The family is often characterized as quite "conventional," and a high premium was placed on the acquisition of education, French values, and social behavior. The local dialect was discouraged in school and in the family. In short, like other Martiniqueans of their class and color, the Fanons were assimilated into French culture and they reflected the common ambiguities of identity this assimilation entailed.

On these broad sketches, there is agreement among various writers. But major differences emerge on the importance attached to a few personal details and on the interpretation made of them. One of these details concerns the color of Frantz. Another and more important detail involves the temperament of Madame Fanon—Frantz's mother. A third and equally significant detail concerns the relationship of Frantz to his mother. Focusing on these three issues at the very outset is necessary because some writers, Gendzier in particular, interpreted Fanon's background on the basis of some questionable details and drew some unwarranted conclusions.

There are two contradictory descriptions of the mother in the literature. Geismar (1971, pg. 8) described her as a mild-mannered and affectionate person who "likes to smile." He visited her in Martinique in 1969 and found her pleased with the conventional careers of her living children, but proudest of Frantz. She talked with satisfaction about her son as a decorated soldier, doctor, and author. She persistently defended him against those Martiniqueans hateful of Frantz because he had turned against France. At the time Geismar visited Martinique, much of the population had a colonial mentality. But

Madame Fanon prevailed with strength and self-confidence against the hostility and resentment of many who thought that her son betrayed French interests in Algeria. Geismar (1971, p. 9) observed that Frantz's photograph dominated her living room and that she seemed "to share Frantz Fanon's courage if not his convictions." Thus, from Geismar's account, one has the impression that Madame Fanon was a warm, resilient mother, easy to get along with and resourceful, a mother who was proud of her children and particularly of Frantz. Geismar, however, did not use such details in analyzing Frantz.

In contrast, Gendzier (1973, p. 11) characterized the mother as a domineering person, of rather difficult temperament, and not affectionate. She wrote that the mother favored her daughters over her sons and, what is more, that she favored Frantz least because he was the "darkest of the family." Gendzier (1973, p. 11) added that Madame Fanon had already a "surfeit of boys" when Frantz was born and, to make matters worse, the young Frantz was a "junior troublemaker." The impression thus given by Gendzier's account is that of a family burdened by the number of its members, of a mother who dispensed love to her children according to their sex as well as their skin color, and of a young Frantz who, from the start, was perhaps a troubled child. Such a characterization of the Fanon family and of young Frantz no doubt pose important questions from a psychological point of view, particularly since the mother–child relation has a critically formative influence on personality development.

Having thus set the stage for a tantalizing psychoanalytic insight, Gendzier then proceeded to weave an elaborate interpretation of Frantz's life-time engrossment with oppression and "recognition." According to this interpretation, Frantz's *public* struggle against racism and colonialism derived and reflected his enduring *private* struggle to resolve maternal rejection. In other words, Fanon's revolutionary commitment was merely a displacement, a defensive maneuver, to overcome some childhood traumas of which the mother's alleged rejection loomed largest. Even if the Fanon family were in ideal circumstances, unaffected by racism or economic constraints, the mother, we are informed, would still remain a significant problematic for Frantz's development and life. Put tersely and in Gendzier's words (1973, p. 11), "in the best of all worlds, Fanon's mother would have been a formidable challenge."

To support this contention of maternal rejection or at least disfavor, Gendzier cited one incident that allegedly occurred before Frantz departed to study in France. It is said he asked his mother for additional funds to supplement his war scholarship and for "some small things" like handkerchiefs. That request, we are informed, was met with sharp refusal by the mother who at the same time was giving such objects to her daughters. According to Gendzier, Frantz was not only deeply hurt by the refusal, but he also nursed this grudge even in his 30s when his revolutionary credentials were well established.

Gendzier further suggested that this grudge did not remain a private or trivial matter, but that it also served as a critical stimulus for Fanon's life-time engrossment with recognition. Gendzier recounted a conversation Frantz had with Joby, his brother, two months before Frantz's death. While both were reminiscing about their past, Frantz is said to have confided his hopes of being appointed the Algerian ambassador to Cuba. Gendzier (1973, p. 16) reported this conversation with some drama as she brought her psycho-interpretive views to their climax:

> He looked forward to returning home, to Martinique, triumphant as Ambassador, and he described how he imagined being met by the diplomatic corps, with his mother watching the proceedings. As the story was told, it was clear that it had evoked all the mixed feelings in Frantz that the image of a triumphant return of this kind could inspire. In some ways perhaps, Fanon thought that it would have evened the score, forcing mother and officials to recognize him as they had failed to do in the past.

In short, Gendzier faulted Geismar for his omission of "personal matters" and provided little more than tidbits to enhance our understanding of Fanon. The impression thus imparted is that of a Madame Fanon who "in the best of all worlds" would remain problematic and of a Frantz who, obsessed with past grudges, engaged in revolutionary struggle to resolve maternal and official rejection. The remarkable thing in all this is that Gendzier never met Madame Fanon and the two "main authorities"—Joby Fanon and Marcel Manville—on whom she presumably relied for data vehemently dispute her claims in substance as well as interpretation. It was in fact in order to dispel such "untruths" that Joby recently broke his long "silence" on personal matters. The result is an impressive article about the mother's character and the Fanon family in general.[2]

This article by Joby Fanon (1982) and our interviews tend to confirm Geismar's brief characterization of the mother. The recurring impression one gets from this material is of a mother who deeply cared for all her children, including Frantz, and relentlessly worked for family solidarity and pride. Her initiatives to ward off economic distress when her husband's salary fell short of family needs and her persistence to provide the best education for her children, both male and female, are indeed remarkable. She worried intensely about Frantz as a soldier, visited him in France when he was a student and later a doctor, and was immensely proud of his revolutionary accomplishments. Frantz in turn was very much attached to her and, as his correspondence indicates, he wrote to her frequently and movingly. Among the qualities most remembered by her children was her constant attempt to instill family solidarity. Joby (Fanon, 1982, p. 11) remembers that she often said: "My children, it's *unity* alone that saves the family and each of us. As long as you are united, you are strong. That which belongs to one of us belongs to everyone, and through that we are all rich."

Little is written about the father. His surviving children and those who knew the Fanons describe him as one who had worked hard to fulfill his duties as a breadwinner for a large family, a man with the partriarchal authority and distance typical of Martiniquean fathers of his time. He was employed for some years as customs inspector, employment he quit when he found that his salary fell short of his family's needs. A self-educated man who took charge of

---

[2]Issues raised in an article by Joby Fanon (1982) were elaborated on during an interview I conducted with Joby Fanon on April 3, 1982.

the family finances, he stepped in to set limits for the children whenever things got out of hand.

From the accounts of his sons, one gets the impression that he may have been somewhat too distant and sometimes too stern. But they and others who knew him quickly add that his attitude and actions were the norm for Martiniquean fathers. Only Frantz held a highly critical view of him. Writing a letter as a young soldier on the eve of a risky assignment during World War II, Frantz, who thought he would die in that assignment, wrote farewell messages to all members of his family, including the following words to his father (J. Fanon, 1982, p. 10):

> Papa, you were sometimes remiss in your duty as a father. If I allow myself to so judge you, it's because I am no longer of this life. These are the reproaches of one from the Beyond. Mama was sometimes made unhappy because of you. She was already unhappy because of us [children]. . . . If we, your eight children, have become something, it's Mama alone who must be given the glory. . . . I can see the expression you'll make in reading these lines, but it's the truth. Look at yourself, look at all the years gone by; bare your soul and have the courage to say, "I deserted them." Okay, repentant churchgoer, come back to the fold.

Commenting on these words, Joby asserted that Frantz was very hard on their father and harsh in his judgment of him. But then, as Joby argued, Frantz was generally uncompromising and harsh to those he thought had failed in their duties. How much this letter represents a momentary disappointment or an enduring feeling toward the father is hard to say. To be sure, the surviving sons did not share this view of the father. They did, however, admit that, consistent with the "matrifocal" society of Martinique, their mother was the real boss in matters of immediate concern to the children and the home. When her husband's salary proved insufficient, she turned the downstairs livingroom into a boutique and a notions store.

An anecdote that one of her granddaughters told me suggests that the question of paternal distance was a matter of concern to Madame Fanon and that the two parents endeavored to resolve it amicably and with some humor. One day, Madame Fanon posted an announcement she knew her husband alone would notice. The announcement read something like this: "Urgent Notice: A handsome prize shall go to anyone who sees or apprehends a father with eight children!" As expected and planned, Monsieur Fanon saw the announcement and asked where is the prize since *he* had found the father sought. Madame Fanon responded: "You got the prize already since there can be no more a handsome prize than the love of eight children and of their mother!"

As for the questions of skin color and its presumed significance, relatives and friends alike asserted that Frantz was by no means the darkest child in the Fanon family. They asserted not so much that light skin is better, but rather that others had made too much out of this false claim. His two brothers, Félix and Joby, vehemently stated that Frantz was neither the darkest nor rejected by the mother. Marcel Manville, who knew the Fanons well and became a lifetime friend of Frantz, pointed out that Frantz was actually not darker than, for instance, his brother Willy or his sister Gabrielle who, incidentally, had left to study in France in the same year as Frantz did. These individuals add that any complex Fanon may have had derived primarily from exposure to racism in the French army and as a student in France. In short, all of them implicate the prevailing social structure and culture, not the attitude and temperament of Madame Fanon.

As for Frantz's character, the impression given by those who knew him as a child and as an adult is that of a person with unusual courage, of strong will, relentless in play and work, given to practical jokes, but serious in purpose, a born leader who, early in life, took up the theme of freedom and self-sacrifice for others. The stature and ideals of the man are amply demonstrated by how he committed himself to the liberation of France from the German occupation when he was barely 17 years old and how later how he relentlessly worked for the liberation of Algerians from French colonialism when he could have enjoyed the comforts of a life as an accomplished physician. In a word, Frantz not only loved life, he also lived and died for social justice. His oldest brother, Félix, described him as one who believed that "life did not deserve to be lived unless one jumped into it and took it by the horns."[3]

We know very little about Frantz partly because, as Joby emphasized, Frantz hated to talk about himself. "Those who write their memoirs," he often (J. Fanon, 1982, p. 5) told his brother, "are finished men, men who have nothing more to say, who have nothing more to do with their lives." Particularly unavailable is a detailed chronological account of his childhood. There nonetheless exist some anecdotes and indirect information that give some idea of Frantz's childhood and young adulthood. Among the earliest anecdotes his oldest brother, Félix, could recall involved an incident that occurred when Frantz was only eight years old. Félix, then 14 years of age, had a close friend and classmate, called Clébert, who used to play with him and sometimes stay in the Fanon home. One day, Clébert brought along his father's revolver to show and to impress Félix with. When he arrived at the Fanon home, Madame Fanon informed him that Félix was out on an errand and that he could wait for him upstairs where little Frantz was in his room.

Clébert talked with Frantz for a while and began to show off his father's revolver and his skill in handling it. He took off the safety, began to clean it, and, in the process pulled the trigger, unaware that the revolver was loaded. Frantz was nearly killed in this accident. As it turned out, the bullet tore Clébert's index finger slightly. Frantz kept his head. When Madame Fanon, hearing the shot, asked from downstairs what the two boys were doing, Frantz calmly told her that it was a toy backfiring. Meanwhile, he was tearing a sheet and wrapping Clébert's bleeding finger. Shortly after, Frantz told his mother that he was taking a walk with Clébert, but he actually accompanied him to the hospital. Asked whether this indicates the sangfroid of a child, Félix responded in the negative and added: "It was in his nature to be like that. Playing soccer, it was the same thing. He never got too excited; he was always very efficient."[4]

---

[3]Interview I conducted with Félix Fanon in Martinique, April 1, 1982.
[4]Interview I conducted with Félix Fanon in Martinique, April 4, 1982.

If this incident shows Frantz's remarkable courage and efficiency, there are numerous others that demonstrate his love for practical jokes and "irreverence," as one of his brothers called it. For instance, Frantz was eight or nine when he instigated and supervised a practical joke in church. In the midst of the religious service, he and his playmates surreptitiously pinned together the dresses of women sitting next to each other. Frantz and the other children, all the while pretending that they were intently listening to the sermon, calmly waited for the result of their mischief. It was when the women stood up to go to receive communion that the awaited moment came with the spectacle of persons pulling one another in different directions and looking at each other with puzzled amazement.

His brother, Félix, thus remembers the young Frantz as a bold, curious, and irreverent boy who, through his practical jokes, liked to "lead people in circles." He also characterized him as the kind of person who, once he had an idea in mind, kept at it with unusual perseverance and passion. Joby described Frantz as having four main traits: courage, creativity, willpower, and rigidity. As a child, Frantz led youngsters older and bigger than he was. Frantz was two years younger than Joby and three years younger than Manville and Mosole, two intimate friends of Frantz who served with him during World War II. As a child, it was often Frantz who conceived of every mischief or good deed, explained how best to execute it, and often led the way. To illustrate what Joby called the rigidity of Frantz, he cited what the latter told him in young adulthood (J. Fanon, 1982, p. 6): "One must constantly, Joby, put one's life in line with one's ideas. There is no acceptable excuse for not doing so; if you don't, you're nothing but a louse." In Joby's view, the rigidity of Frantz involved his insistence to match *saying* and *doing*. In this respect, at least, what Joby calls rigidity may aptly be considered integrity.

Aside from such anecdotes, which in any case rest on what is only recalled, we lack a detailed account of Frantz's early childhood.[5] More complete and documented accounts are found for his teenage years, beginning when Frantz volunteered to fight to liberate France. Frantz was still in high school when de Gaulle made his broadcast from London calling for the liberation of France from German occupation. These broadcasts "electrified Frantz," who in turn, talked about the battle for liberty with ardor and vehemence. The French administration ruling Martinique at the time collaborated with the Germans and Martiniqueans were not allowed to volunteer for the Free French Army.

Frantz nonetheless tried to escape to Dominica where the Allied forces were recruiting and training volunteers. Boatmen had to be paid and there was always the danger of riding overloaded and ramshackle boats on high seas or of being discovered en route by the collaborationist French navy, which would have sunk these boats without hesitation. Twice Frantz made serious attempts to go to Dominica and failed both times. In the third attempt, which suc-

---

[5]Unfortunately, Madame Fanon, the mother of Frantz, died in the summer of 1981. Geismar, who met and interviewed her, failed to gather the crucial data, which she alone could have provided in detail.

ceeded, the circumstances and the timing jarred all those who learned of his escape, leaving no doubt about his commitment and determination.

His two brothers, Joby and Félix, vividly describe the day the 17-year-old Frantz left the family fold to fight for the liberty of France. Frantz escaped to Dominica on Félix's wedding day. The incongruence and shocking effect of this timing is best described by Joby Fanon (1982, p. 6). On that important day, the Fanon family and no less than 200 guests were in a festive mood. Many preparations had been made days before the event. The shortage and rationing of food in the island increased the anticipation with which everybody waited to fill their stomachs with food and drink. It was a day of pomp and celebration, reuniting old friends and making new friends, of collective laughter and personal joy. On this very day, Frantz took his brother aside to inform him of his imminent departure for Dominica.

Joby was confounded and bewildered by this decision "so entirely out of place, so impudent and indecent," but the stormy discussion that followed failed to have the intended effect of changing Frantz's mind. Joby tried every form of persuasion and argument. He even reminded him of what one of Joby's professor in the *lycée* was telling young Martiniqueans about the futility and foolishness of self-sacrifice for whites. This professor warned his students with unforgettable lucidity and effect (J. Fanon, 1982, p. 6):

> Gentlemen, your friends have left for war without being ordered to do so. Beware, gentlemen! War is a serious thing. Beware, gentlemen—fire burns, war kills. The widows of dead heroes marry living men.
>
> Gentlemen, beware! What is happening today in Europe is not our major problem. It is something else. Be careful that you do not confuse your goals.
>
> Gentlemen, believe me, when white man kills white man, it's a blessing for the Negro.

Yet nothing would change Fanon's mind; his decision was irrevocable, come what may. To be sure, what propelled him toward such self-sacrifice and departure from the family fold, at this tender age, were ideals and convictions, not an aberration of personality or the desire to escape a family pathology. If the professor's warnings to the young Martiniqueans were both wise and prophetic, the response of Frantz to them during the stormy discussion with Joby on that wedding day demonstrates the height of his idealism and his profound regard for human rights. "Joby," retorted Frantz, "each time that liberty is at stake, we are all affected, be we whites, blacks, yellows, or kakos. Your professor is a fool and I swear to you today that no matter where it may be, each time that Freedom is threatened, I'll be there" (J. Fanon, 1982, p. 6).

It was Joby who finally relented, and accepted the unenviable task of informing the family at an appropriate time and in an appropriate manner. What could he tell the family and when? Most of all, how could he face his mother with such news? If he hides it now, how long would it take her to learn the truth and, having lost sight of one son, how would she bear to suffer the complicity and lies of another? As it turned, the first person who saw Joby come to the festivities was none other than Madame Fanon who immediately asked about the whereabouts of Frantz. He told her that Frantz is away to fetch some bread. This evasion worked, but only momentarily. Suspecting that her fears were realized, the mother returned to Joby and said: "Joby, you've lied to me—where is Frantz? Today I've lost two children, Félix who is getting married and Frantz who has left, God only knows where to" (J. Fanon, 1982, p. 7).

After six months of training in Dominica, Frantz returned to Martinique. By then, a recruitment drive for volunteers had started there. Frantz immediately enlisted as did his two closest friends, Manville and Mosole. The time of departure these young men awaited with anticipation and their parents with dread finally arrived. Joby vividly described this day of departure to distant lands and to disquieting risks (J. Fanon, 1982, p. 7):

> It was a mournful procession, almost gloomy, of these young men, encircled by the strong grips of their parents, all of whom were crying, praying, wailing. Here were these children disguised as soldiers, stoic and serious, going all the way with their decision. My mother hung from Frantz's arms, her voice trembling with sadness, and repeating over and over again advice on how to protect himself from the German devils. Then turning toward Marcel Manville, she told him in a voice filled with hope, "You'll watch over Frantz, Marcel. You're older. I entrust him to you." And Marcel, red with embarrassment, replied, "Yes, Madame Fanon, don't worry, I will bring him back to you."

Then came the letters from Frantz in the battlefields of Europe. To read their contents is to take an intimate look at the deep love and bond between Frantz and his mother. Most of the letters to her were written to allay her fears even when Frantz was wounded and recuperating at a hospital in Paris. He often wrote about how he missed the family, joked about his longing for local dishes, admitted that he had made a mistake in fighting for a people who humiliated him, and promised his mother that he would return soon and safely. His mother in turn wrote letters expressing her affection and reporting family news.

One remarkable thing in the mother's letters to Frantz was how she often concluded them. When she wrote letters to her other children, she usually ended with: "Your mother who prays for you." Joby emphasizes that they knew she *did* in fact pray for them. But her letters to Frantz at war usually ended thus: "Your mother who marches with you." Frantz, knowing that she actually meant what she said, therefore took special care of himself so as not to endanger this mother "who marched with him" (J. Fanon, 1982, p. 11). Obviously, such indicators of reciprocal bond, mutual endorsement, and internalization of the other contradict all claims of maternal indifference and rejection.

FROM NEGROHOOD TO NEGRITUDE

The simplistic interpretations of Gendzier aside, the alienating influences in Martiniquean society could not be doubted. The Fanon family was of course not exempt from these influences. And if being one of the darkest of the eight children had any direct bearing on Frantz's preoccupation with recognition,

this could only mean a family reenactment of the more potent racism plaguing
the wider Martiniquean society. As indicated already, the relatives and friends
I interviewed assert that, contrary to Gendzier's claims, Frantz was neither the
darkest child nor was he rejected by his mother. In reality, the emphasis on an
assumed aberration in Frantz's personality and in the family dynamic not only
distorts the facts, but also detracts from the racist social structure. There are
strong indications that Frantz was a highly precocious, empathic child who
grew up in a "normal" family context from the Martiniquean perspective.
Fanon (1967a, p. 142) himself provided a significant clue wherein lies the
pathogenesis: "A normal [black] child, having grown up within a normal family, will become abnormal in the slightest contact with the white world."

The nature of the Martiniquean society was of course such that contact
with the white world was unavoidable. Indeed because of the *Weltanschauung*
that prevailed, contact with the white world was intensely desired by most
Martiniqueans. The motive for this is not hard to discern. Three-quarters of
the island's farms, business, and construction companies were owned and
controlled by a small white aristocracy. Their number was estimated at 1,000,
in an island with a population of 300,000. This affluent white aristocracy also
had the whole colonial machine on its side. The majority of the population
was, in contrast, extremely poor. The black bourgeoisie to which the Fanon
family belonged was therefore situated between a wealthy, powerful white
minority and a poor, powerless black majority. Concomitant with this colonial
social structure was also a hierarchy of values, assigning beauty and virtue
according to class and color.

At home and in school, through songs and folklore, by means of praise or
punishment, and in all aspects of social existence, capitulation to the French
culture and identification with whites were invariably inculcated. *"Je suis
Français"* were the first three words a black child learned to read and write.
Mastery of the French language and internalization of an European outlook
were instilled. As Fanon (1967, p. 147) himself explained, the black schoolboy
in the Antilles read about "our ancestors, the Gauls." He completely identified
with "the explorer, the bringer of civilization, the white man who carries truth
to the savages—an all white truth." Utter contempt was the misfortune of the
middle-class Martiniquean who could not speak "the French of France, the
Frenchman's French, French French" (F. Fanon, 1967a, p. 20). Very early in life,
Fanon learned the lesson well. He knew too well that he must take pains with
his speech, since every Martiniquean was more or less judged by how he spoke.
Not surprisingly, those who personally knew Fanon or read his original works
concur on his impeccable French and his powerful, almost awe-inspiring command of the word.

Among the black bourgeoisie generally, one never spoke Creole except in
orders to servants. Very much desired was association with those who were
lighter, who spoke better French, or who were wealthier. One was white above
a certain level of income. Birth or slippage into a world of Creolism, poverty,
ignorance, and more melanin were viewed as only different sides of the same
curse. The choice of a lover was a particularly risky venture within this rigid

social code. Fanon (1967a, p. 47) discussed this fact with an affective vigor that betrays a personal dilemma:

> Every time I have made up my mind to analyze certain kinds of behavior, I have been unable to avoid consideration of certain nauseating phenomena. The number of sayings, proverbs, petty rules of conduct that govern the choice of a lover in the Antilles is astounding. It is always essential to avoid falling back into the pit of niggerhood, and every women in the Antilles, whether in a casual flirtation or in a serious affair, is determined to select the least black of the men.

With even greater intensity, the Antillean had to go to certain extremes to obliterate vestiges of African descent. For the African was believed to be the savage, the cannibal, the primordial evil, which the Antillean avoided like the plague. The Antillean considered himself a European; in soul and complexion, he thought of himself as a rehabilitated black man, almost a different species than unassimilated African "natives." Fanon explained the psychosocial import of keeping this distinction unmistakable. The West Indian, Fanon explained, was not satisfied to be superior to Africans, a people he completely despised and consciously avoided. The white man allowed himself some liberties in dealing with the African, since the difference between the two was obvious and hence there was no need for a reminder. The West Indian, in contrast, took pains to emphasize his difference from the African and did all he could to keep his distance. If and when a West Indian was mistaken for an African, he suffered this with much indignation and considered it an event of catastrophic proportion.

If the African was generally an object of West Indian contempt, the Senegalese soldier was even more despised and dreaded. Fanon was about 13 years old when he first saw Senegalese soldiers. From stories told by veterans of World War I, he was led to believe that the Senegalese soldier attacked with his bayonet, punched his way through machine-gun fire with his fists, cut off heads, and collected human ears. In school, too, his mathematics teacher used to make Frantz "shiver" with similarly gory stories. Little wonder then that he developed in childhood an uncanny interest in these frightening species of men. Frantz was excited when, for the first time, the occasion had availed itself to take a brief glimpse of those strange beings in flesh (F. Fanon, 1967a, pp. 162–163):

> These Senegalese were in transit in Martinique, on their way from Guiana. I scoured the streets eagerly for a sight of their uniforms, which had been described to me: red scarfs and belts. My father went to the trouble of collecting two of them, whom he brought home and who had the family in raptures.

The influences of these early years of course left deep scars on Fanon's psyche. Their persistence was in fact such that, despite a rude awakening in adulthood, Fanon (1967a, p. 203) in his 20s insisted on a personal identification with the oppressor: "I am a Frenchman. I am interested in French culture, French civilization, the French people. . . . What have I to do with a black empire?" Even as he fathomed with anguish the essential hypocrisy of the oppressor, the remnants of the alienation and depersonalization long suffered remained. Fanon (1967a, p. 191) himself admitted this with characteristic candor: "I am a white man. For unconsciously I distrust what is black in me, that is, the whole of my being."

Yet such psychological "lactification" and instilled negative identity had their countervailing influences. Indications are that, even in childhood, Frantz had felt a vague personal discomfort in the world that was Martinique. During latency, the ego-dystonic quality of the general social milieu heightened, but could not be adequately resolved at this tender age. A conscious awareness of entrenched alienation had to wait a few years. Then came the unexpected moment when a flash of insight crystallized the rudiments of an organizing principle that was to become a life-time preoccupation. Fanon was 14 when he understood the meaning of "cultural imposition." An embarrassing blunder was the occasion of this initial understanding. Fanon, in the presence of an acquaintance, was uttering a disparaging remark about Italians when, suddenly, he realized his listener was himself of Italian extract. The incident underscored for him the force of stereotypes inculcated in him because of France's "cultural imposition" on Martiniqueans.

Aimé Césaire of course had a significant and formative influence on Frantz. A foremost proponent of *negritude* and the man who coined the term, Césaire was also Frantz's teacher in the last year at the *lycée* and his intellectual mentor subsequently. Césaire was known for his vigorous attack on Western civilization in general and French culture in particular. He had, with characteristic eloquence, declared that "a nation which colonizes, that a civilization which justifies colonization—and therefore force—is already a sick civilization, a civilization that is morally diseased. . ." (Césaire, 1972, p. 18). Frantz was only 17 when the first issue of *La Revue Tropique*, edited and directed by Césaire, appeared in 1942. This periodical was crucial in raising the consciousness of young Martiniqueans and in instilling a sense of black identity. It was through this periodical and speeches that Césaire offered what Manville calls the "ideological food" for young Antilleans.

With fierce lucidity, Césaire repudiated assimilation into the French culture and at the same time asserted his African heritage. He preached the inescapable essence of one's blackness: "Paint the trunk white as you will, the roots will remain black."[6] Fanon described the shock with which Césaire's assertions were received by most Antilleans and probably by Frantz Fanon (1967b, p. 21) himself.

> What indeed could be more grotesque than an educated man, a man with a diploma, having in consequence understood a good many things, among others that "it was unfortunate to be a Negro," proclaiming that his skin was beautiful and that the "big black hole" was a source of truth. Neither the mulattoes nor the Negroes understood this delirium. The mulattoes because they had escaped from the night, the Negroes because they aspired to get away from it. Two centuries of white truth proved this man to be wrong. He must be mad, for it was unthinkable that he could be right.

---

[6]Quoted in Fanon (1967c, p. 24).

In his *Black Skin, White Masks* alone, Fanon(1967a, p. 187) invoked the teacher nearly 20 times, imitated his style, and added: "I wish that many black intellectuals would turn to him for their inspiration." Several dramatic developments, both historical and personal, also conditioned Fanon's identification with Césaire and his gradual disillusionment with his identity as a Frenchman. The first was the defeat of France by Germany. Fanon compared this defeat with "the murder of the father." Doubt in the invincibility of the master subsequently set in—never to diminish. The doubt eventually crystallized into a conviction. The second historical event concerned the four-year occupation of Martinique by nearly 5,000 French soldiers and sailors. Fanon was 15 when this occupation took effect and he and other Martiniqueans observed the occupying navy's crude racism, acts of pillage, indiscriminate harassment, and uninhibited sexual assaults. Idealization of the master, at least the modicum of justice attributed to him, gradually eroded. He (F. Fanon, 1967b, p. 23) described it thus: "The West Indian, in the presence of those men who despised him, began to have misgivings as to his values. The West Indian underwent his first metaphysical experience." This rupture in values and metaphysics, more intellectual than affective, was later combined with *personal* humiliations to result in a profound psycho-existential crisis.

For Fanon and his friends, the fact of personal humiliation and disillusionment began in the ships that transported Fanon and other volunteers to North Africa. The Caribbean volunteers were racially discriminated against as they traveled the rough seas to risk their lives for France. Members of the Martiniquean Women's Corps slept with French officers in the ship, leaving many volunteers angered and humiliated. The volunteers in fact made up songs about these women who slept with French officers—songs that, according to Manville, are to this day heard in Martinique and Guadeloupe.

Arriving in North Africa, the volunteers faced a more blatant and hardened expression of bigotry from white settlers, the "Pieds Noir." In the camp at Casablanca, Antillean soldiers suffered the crudest forms of racism, even though they wore a distinguishing beret in the hope of being treated better than the despised African soldiers, all of whom were mistakenly called "Senegalese." But these identifying berets, a symbol only of cultural assimilation, were never a license of equality with whites. The Antilleans found that, without their berets, they were treated as wild savages and, with them, as domesticated servants. In talking about this period, Manville still remembers the experience with obvious anger: "The French subjected us with everyday humiliation in the ranks. Even if we wore the berets, the lesser ranked officers of the French army who were cretans, imbeciles, and fossils . . . *tu-tued* us [addressed us informally] as if we were Senegalese and, for us, to be addressed in such a way was humiliating."[7]

After a period of training in North Africa, the Caribbean and African soldiers were taken to battlefronts in Europe. Fanon, Manville, and Mosole were among those who disembarked at St. Tropez in 1944 with American

---

[7]Interview I conducted with Marcel Manville in Martinique, April 2, 1982.

soldiers. The racism and humiliation Fanon and his friends experienced in the French Army was only exceeded by the abuses that the French populace they came to free poured upon them. When, for instance, these black soldiers disembarked in the port city of Toulon, in central France, they found the residents extremely hostile and racist. During the occupation and subsequent to it, the many Italians and Germans in Toulon fanned racial hatred and white supremacy. Women would not dance with them in discos and residents insulted them in the streets.[8] The experience of crude racism became even more intense as Fanon and the other Antilleans were moved to the Doux region in September 1944.

The assignment of soldiers to different regions and tasks often demonstrated the irrationalities of racism and the dilemma of the Antilleans. Thus, for instance, the African soldiers were mainly kept in areas of warmer climate as winter approached. But since the Antilleans were considered *white* in all respects except skin color, they were moved North and, for the honor of being "white," suffered miserably in the freezing climate of Alsace. At the same time, however, inasmuch as the Antilleans were in fact "black," they enjoyed little exemptions from racism, both crude and subtle. Even in victory, during mass dances or dinners held to welcome French troops, Fanon realized that the blood of black soldiers had been shed in vain. The very Europeans for whose liberation blacks risked their lives now avoided them. Public dances and victory celebrations only added insult to injury. European women found it easier to dance and mingle with Italian war prisoners.

When Fanon returned to Martinique, decorated and a war veteran of almost two years, he brought with him not only memories regarding the horrors of war, but also serious doubts about his identity as a Frenchman. He immediately worked in the election campaign of Césaire, the Communist candidate. Significantly, Fanon(1967a, p. 90) informs us with pride and satisfaction that, many years later, he still could "quote from memory" the following campaign statements of Césaire:

> When I turn on my radio, when I hear that Negroes have been lynched in America, I say that we have been lied to; Hitler is not dead. . . . When, finally I turn on my radio and hear that in Africa forced labor has been inaugurated and legalized, I say we have certainly been lied to: Hitler is not dead.

Any lingering illusions Fanon had about French culture or about his identity as a Frenchman were further undermined during his student days in France. The year 1947 marked a particularly distressing period for Frantz. His father died that year and the family had many financial difficulties. His plans to go abroad for study had therefore to proceed with meager resources. As a decorated veteran of World War II, Frantz won a scholarship to study at a university in France. Drama and politics had a deep personal appeal to him. But devoting his college studies in these fields seemed to him a luxury. He was instead determined to study for a more practical career, which he could apply

[8]Reported by Manville in my interview with him on April 2, 1982.

in his return to his country. Medicine seemed the ideal choice. In his return to Martinique, his home country, the study of medicine would serve him well and provide a needed service. But Fanon felt he had already lost too much time serving in the war. The study of medicine would take him longer than he was willing to accept. Dentistry was an alternative career. Its training was shorter, and at the same time, it would be a very practical and even lucrative profession.

The choice of a career in dentistry was short-lived. Social and financial rewards alone offered no lasting appeals to a man of Fanon's critical intellect and uncompromising temperament. Indeed the very idea of studying dentistry was somebody else's, not Fanon's. Geismar (1969, p. 43) informs us that it was Mansole, a close friend, who suggested dentistry in an effort to help resolve Fanon's agonizing indecision and uncertainty. Fanon was initially convinced, but dentristy soon failed to strike in him the kind of emotional resonance and enduring commitment he sought in a career, and he soon quit dentistry and Paris. The intolerable boredom Fanon experienced at the school of dentistry and the equally intolerable alienation he found among the blacks in Paris are cited as the immediate precipitants for his seemingly sudden action. In fact, Fanon is said to have complained that there were just "too many niggers in Paris" and never in his life had he met "so many idiots" as he did in the school of dentistry (Geismar, 1969, pp. 43–44).

Fanon left Paris for Lyons in order to take the one-year preparatory training in the natural sciences. Soon after completing this training, Fanon enrolled in the medical school at the University of Lyons. Lyons then was a center of radicalism and social unrest. Geismar (1969, p. 45) informs us that on the very month Fanon arrived in Lyons, "there were strikes by the coal miners, the chemical workers, the electrical workers, the beet-sugar growers, train engineers; Peugeot, Simca, Citroen workers; construction workers, concierges, and metro conductors." Fanon did not remain unaffected by this charged political climate. Nor did he stand aloof of the political activism prevalent among the students. He immediately became involved in political debates, left-wing meetings, and workers' strikes—activities he was to continue throughout his student years. It was also during these early years that he experienced a psycho-existential crisis threatening not only his medical studies, but also his sanity. Nowhere is the anguish of those years better reflected than in his first book, *Black Skin, White Masks*.

His daily encounter with racism in France had exacerbated an inner debate. Conflict over his identity subsequently precipitated this crisis. Racism sealed him into "crushing objecthood." His blackness tormented him (F. Fanon, 1967a, pp. 111–112).

> "Look, a Negro!" It was an external stimulus that flicked over me as I passed by. I made a tight smile.
> "Look a Negro!" It was true. It amused me.
> "Look a Negro!" The circle was drawing a bit tighter. I made no secret of my amusement.
> "Mama, see the Negro! I am frightened!"
> Frightened! Frightened!
> I made up my mind to laugh myself to tears, but laughter had become impossible.

Assailed by such frightened stares, bombarded by racial slurs, and cognizant of a disparaging history others had elaborated about his race, Fanon (1967a, p. 117) experienced the kind of intense depersonalization that is now reminiscent of Du Bois' "inaudibility," Ellison's "invisibility," and Baldwin's "namelessness." It was not only a problem of stares and slurs. There also existed a set of rationalizations and logic that were painfully too elusive: "When people like me, they tell me it is in spite of my color. When they dislike me, they point out that it is not because of my color. Either way, I am locked into the infernal circle."

Meanwhile, new publications by black poets and writers were fast appearing. Much of it had *negritude* as a dominant theme. In 1947, the year Fanon arrived as a student in France, the first issue of *Présence Africaine* was published. The earlier teachings of Césaire, his personal encounter with racism, and the influences of negritude poets steered Fanon toward black consciousness and an associated repudiation of assimilation into white society. More personally intense than before, the lesson that the trunk may be painted white but the roots will remain black struck a responsive chord. The encounter with the oppressor in his own land led to a rude awakening previously defended against and postponed: "Subjectively, intellectually, the Antillean conducts himself like a white man. But he is a Negro. That he will learn once he goes to Europe; and when he hears Negroes mentioned he will recognize that the word included himself as well as the Senegalese" (F. Fanon, 1967a, p. 148).

Thus, as a means of defense against the daily onslaught of racism, Fanon conveniently, but with ambivalence adopted negritude. The chapter, "The Fact of Blackness," in *Black Skin, White Masks* is not only a phenomenological description of a psycho-existential crisis. It also portrays Fanon's (1967a, pp. 130–132) temporary intoxication with the reactive maneuvers of negritude.

> I rummaged frenetically through all the antiquity of the black man. What I found took away my breath. . . . The white man was wrong, I was not primitive, not even a half-man, I belonged to a race that had already been working in gold and silver two thousand years ago. . . . I put the white man back into his place; growing bolder, I jostled him and told him point-blank, "get used to me, I am not getting used to anyone." I shouted my laughter to the stars. The white man, I could see, was resentful. His reaction time lagged interminably. . . . I had won. I was jubilant.

Alas! That victory and jubilation turned out to be short-lived and elusive. Indications are that negritude had for him only a fleeting appeal. Even when Fanon adopted it, he did so with a great deal of ambivalence.

FROM NEGRITUDE TO REVOLUTIONARY PRAXIS

Fanon's temporary adoption of negritude as a last refuge coincided with the publication of an anthology edited in 1948 by Leopold Senghor. The book was a significant landmark in the history of negritude. Jean-Paul Sartre wrote its preface, which was markedly sympathetic to the movement. But the preface also contained a devastating evaluation. "Thus negritude," Sartre wrote, "is the root of its own destruction, it is a transition and not a conclusion, a means and not an ultimate end." The suggestion that negritude was merely relative, for that matter only "a minor term" of a dialectical process, struck a final and tormenting blow. This conclusion of Sartre had, Fanon (1967a, p. 132) admitted, robbed him of "a last chance" to find a secure anchorage.

> Thus my unreason was countered with reason, my reason with "real reason."
> Every hand was a losing hand for me. I analyzed my heredity. I made a complete audit
> of my ailment. I wanted to be typically Negro—it was no longer possible. I wanted to
> be white—that was a joke. And, when I tried, on the level of ideas and intellectual
> activity, to reclaim my negritude, it was snatched away from me. Proof was presented
> that my effort was only a term in the dialectic.

Fanon of course angrily resisted. He even tried to retaliate. In the end, however, Fanon conceded his "unreflected position." His latent ambivalence soon crystallized into a definite rejection of negritude. This in turn set the stage for a more decisive swing toward radicalization. Fanon thus parted ways with the proponents of negritude, including Césaire. The final break with Césaire came in 1958 when the latter supported the campaign for total integration with France, instead of commiting himself to the independence of Martinique. The decision of Césaire underscored that negritude, a reactive and racial polemic, was a necessary but not sufficient condition for the liberation of alienated blacks. Fundamentally, it presented neither a total departure from the white world it denounced nor a program of transformative action, objectively transforming oppressive conditions.

That Fanon took Sartre's conclusion so seriously is hardly surprising. Fanon had a deep respect and admiration for Sartre ever since he read his works at the *lycée*. It was in fact the joint influences of Sartre and Cesaire that had for a while steered the young Fanon toward a career in drama. Fanon and Sartre later became close friends. In her *Force of Circumstance*, Simone de Beauvoir (1977, p. 592) described the encounter of Fanon and Sartre in Rome. Fanon was by then a relentless, indefatigable, incendiary revolutionary. She provides us with a vivid and interesting glance of Fanon: "With a razor-sharp intelligence, intensely alive, endowed with a grim sense of humor, he explained things, made jokes, questioned us, gave imitations, told stories; everything he talked about seemed alive again before our eyes."

The two men—Sartre and Fanon—met for lunch and their conversation lasted until two in the morning. When Simone de Beauvoir (1965, p. 592) urged rest and broke off their conversation, Fanon was outraged: "I don't like people who hoard their resources. . . . I would like to give twenty thousand francs a day to be able to talk with Sartre from morning to night for two weeks." Sartre's influence on Fanon is evident in the latter's works. Interestingly, however, the direction of impact is gradually reversed. Thus in the preface that Sartre wrote for Fanon's *The Wretched of the Earth*, it is the latter's influence on Sartre that is the most striking. Nonetheless, indications are that this

reciprocal influence and mutual respect also involved some latent ambivalence and differences on tactics.

If Sartre was a significant formative influence on Fanon's early intellectual
development, the experience of racism as a student in France was also the
occasion for the psycho-existential crisis and profound redefinition of Fanon's
identity. Life in medical school and life in the community of scholars offered
no refuge from racist assaults. The belief that intelligence and personal merit
would overcome prejudice was becoming more untenable. The hope of being
accepted as a Frenchman proved ever elusive. The following examples underscore the point. Fanon and one of his white friends were once cramming for
their finals when the latter remarked that they were really working like "niggers." The two did not speak to each other for months. On another occasion,
the examining professor first inquired about Fanon's country of origin. Upon
learning that he was from Martinique, the professor asked paternalistically:
"What would you like me to ask you about, boy?" Fanon angrily plunged his
hand into the basket, took a question, and answered it with remarkable eloquence and precision. The examiner could no longer get himself to call him *"boy!"*

Soon after defending his medical thesis in November 1951, Fanon left with
his brother Joby for a vacation in Martinique. He worked there briefly as a
general practitioner until his return to France to specialize in psychiatry. In
1952, Fanon was admitted to the residence program at the Hôpital de Saint-
Alban where he worked closely with Professor François Tosquelles. Fanon's
medical thesis was on a neurophysiological disorder with the title: "Troubles
mentaux et syndromes psychiatrique dans l'Hérédo-Dégéneration-Spino-Céré-
belleuse. Un cas de maladie de Friedreich avec delire de possession." What
little information we have of this thesis is indirect and quite sketchy. Geismar
(1969, p. 11) found it to be "the most boring piece of writing Fanon ever
produced." However, it is worth noting that Geismar found little else interesting or significant in Fanon's thesis than to point out a quotation from
Nietzsche's *Thus Spake Zarathustra*—which Fanon used in order to stress the
humanistic orientation of his study. The quote reads "I dedicate myself to living
beings, not to introspective mental processes." Fanon was later to elaborate
the humanistic core of his psychological formulations, as I shall show in subsequent chapters.

It was in the spring of 1953 that Fanon sat for *Le Médicat de hôpitaux
psychiatrique*. This was an intense, grueling series of examinations that included written and oral tests on such areas as pathology, neurology, and forensic medicine. Fanon successfully completed all his examinations by 13 July. It
was then that he wrote to Senghor to inquire about the possibility of working
in Senegal. Senghor never responded. Fanon thus saw no other option but to
accept what was to be a short-lived appointment as *chef de service*, a position
equivalent to a clinical director, in the psychiatric hospital of Pontorson in
Normandy. But when the first opportunity to work in Algeria availed itself, he
immediately hastened to take advantage of it. In November 1953 Fanon arrived
in Algiers and soon undertook his responsibilities as the *chef de service* of the
Blida-Joinville Hospital, the largest psychiatric hospital in Algeria. It was

while working at this hospital that he introduced innovative treatment programs, wrote original articles, and began to articulate new perspectives on indigenous healing practices. For a while Fanon immersed himself in his clinical duties, but a host of problems, many of them endemic to the colonial situation, were never to allow him to fully carry out the treatment innovations to which he was so passionately committed.

Meanwhile the struggle for national liberation was gaining wider support among the Algerian populace. But the French were all the more determined to tighten their grip on their most prized colony. To the escalating challenges from the colonized, they responded with brutal tortures, summary executions, and massive repressions. The practice of psychiatry under these circumstances was proving to be an absurd gamble and an exercise in futility. As I shall discuss in subsequent chapters, Fanon's clinical originality and clandestine political work during this period remain unique in the annals of psychiatry. In the summer of 1956, Fanon resigned. He was by then secretly working for the *Front de Liberation Nationale (FLN)*—the well-known Algerian liberation movement that successfully waged a long and bitter war against French colonialism. In January 1957, Fanon received a "letter of expulsion" and a warning to leave Algeria within 48 hours.

Fanon soon arrived at the FLN headquarters in Tunis to serve in a number of capacities. He became one of the articulate spokesmen for the Algerian liberation movement, an editor of its major paper *El Moudjahid*, a devoted medical doctor in FLN health centers, and a roving ambassador obtaining needed support and resources from other African countries. Fanon also lectured at the University of Tunis, introduced significant reforms at the psychiatric hospital of Manouba, and served at the Charles Nicolle Hospital in Tunis. It was while serving at the latter hospital that Fanon (1967c) took a three-week leave of absence to write his sociological masterpiece, *A Dying Colonialism*. The impact of that book on the French intellectual scene was both timely and momentous. Six months after its publication, the book was banned in France and further printing of it prohibited.

Fanon's stature as a serious intellectual and a committed revolutionary was thus becoming widely appreciated. His earlier book, *Black Skin, White Masks* (1967a) had already aroused interest among many intellectuals and various publishing houses. His psychiatric innovations in Algeria and Tunisia were also attracting foreign interns in search of new approaches to psychiatric care. At the same time, however, this growing fame and his actual role as a key spokesman of the Algerian revolution made him a definite target of assassination plots by right-wing French settlers and made him one of the most wanted persons by the French secret police. Plans to kidnap him or to kill him failed. But during one of his frequent trips to refugee camps near the Algerian border, his jeep was blown up by a land mine (Geismar, 1969, p. 142). Fanon sustained 12 fractured spinal vertebrae and was taken to Rome for treatment. While in a Rome hospital, Fanon one day noticed that an Italian paper had announced his whereabouts and the number of his hospital room. Fanon immediately requested a transfer to another room. Hours later, two masked men entered his previous room and "sprayed the bed with a Browning automatic" (Geismar, 1969, p. 144).

When Fanon recovered, he returned to Tunis to continue to serve the Algerian revolution. He participated in various conferences and traveled widely as the Algerian representative of the Provisional Government. Only revolutionary commitment and profound conviction could have sustained him through his peculiar predicament, confronted as he was with Arab prejudice against his color and with African discomfort in the presence of his white wife. While traveling though Mali to explore new supply routes for the Algerian fighters, Fanon suddenly became ill. It became clear in December 1960 that he was suffering from leukemia and had only a few months to live. He was taken to Moscow and treated for granulocytic leukemia and strongly advised to rest. Fanon instead arranged tours to several psychiatric hospitals in order to observe the psychiatric progress made by the most advanced socialist country. He was, however, quite disappointed by what he found. The straitjackets, barred windows, and barren rooms in these institutions reminded him of Blida-Joinville Hospital when he had first arrived. His observations convinced him that genuine rehabilitation of troubled psyches awaited new discoveries. As for his own treatment, Russian doctors informally advised him to travel to the United States where treatment for leukemia was most advanced.

Fanon returned to Tunis and in 10 weeks completed his last and most controversial book, *The Wretched of the Earth*. He was by then living on borrowed time. Agitation and restlessness dominated his mood and behavior. A treacherous disease, leukemia is characterized by sudden relapses and remissions. Bleeding from the gums, temporary loss of vision, atrocious bruises, marked loss of weight—all these combined with the feeling of hopelessness and helplessness resulting from the knowledge that the disease had little possibility of cure. It was then that his Algerian comrades in struggle urged him to seek treatment in the United States. Geismar reports that the American CIA and the FLN representatives negotiated Fanon's transportation to the United States. Geismar (1969, p. 182), in addition, explains the motivation behind the American gesture of help:

> The black doctor was a nice catch for the intelligence services. . . . Washington would be able to fatten its dossiers on the leftist segment of the FLN; Fanon knew a lot about other African liberation movements. His kind of thinking and activities were a threat to Western interests in the Third World.

Fanon suspected such a peril and for a while resisted the advice of his trusted fellow-revolutionaries. Besides, he loathed the United States, which he called "the nation of lynchers." But, as his condition deteriorated, he was left no choice but to accept the offer. En route to Washington, Fanon had a last encounter with Sartre and de Beauvoir in Rome. His condition had by then worsened. He lay flat on his bed, unable to speak with Sartre. Throughout the interview, he was restless as if to resist the obvious physical disability his illness had imposed.

No sooner did Fanon arrive in Washington than his fears were realized. Simone de Beauvoir (1977, p. 606) reports that he had been "left to rot in his hotel room for ten days, alone and without medical attention." Geismar (1969, p. 184) suggested that more was perhaps involved than bureaucratic inefficiency: "Those who brought him there wanted a chance to grill the sick man without the interference of a hospital routine." The delay of his hospitalization and the frequent inquiries by one of the American agents increased Fanon's suspicions and indignation. His condition was fast deteriorating. In the hospital, Fanon showed symptoms of acute anemia, and after several blood transfusions, he caught double pneumonia. His plans to write on a number of projects, such as the history of the Algerian revolution and the psychology of the death process, were never to be realized.

Fanon died on 6 December 1961 in Bethesda, Maryland. His body was taken to Tunis and then to Algeria to be buried in the soil for which he so relentlessly fought. The Blida-Joinville Psychiatric Hospital was renamed, and today bears his name. His statements in a letter a few days before his death reveal the man's courage and commitment (Geismar, 1969, p. 185):

> What I wanted to tell you is that death is always with us and that what matters is not to know whether we can escape it but whether we have achieved the maximum for the ideas we have made our own. What shocked me here in my bed when I felt my strength ebbing away along with my blood was not the fact of dying as such, but to die of leukemia, in Washington, when three months ago I could have died facing the enemy. . . . We are nothing on earth if we are not in the first place the slaves of a cause, the cause of the peoples, the cause of justice and liberty.

3

The Amnesia of Euro-American Psychology

Leave this Europe where they are never done of talking about men, yet murder everywhere they find them. . . . Look at them today swaying between atomic and spiritual disintegration.

—Fanon, *The Wretched of the Earth*

From the fourteenth century to the present, Europe and its descendants have been embarked on an unprecedented mission of violence and self-aggrandizement throughout the world. Meanwhile, an intellectual debate on the human condition had been raging in academic circles. A discipline called "psychology" emerged by the sixteenth century, when Phillipp Melanchthon, a friend of Luther, coined the term, even though the roots of this new discipline reach back to ancient civilizations. In time, the new discipline flourished and proliferated in various aspects of society. It developed its own concepts, won numerous adherents, evolved its own tradition, won a measure of respectability, and defined a jealously guarded turf. As Europe conquered much of the world, the European imposing as the only honorable model of humanity, the discipline of psychology too emerged as a powerful specialty and a scientific arbiter of human experience.

The discipline of psychology did not of course emerge in a social vacuum unrelated to Europe's history of conquest and violence. From its beginning to the present, the discipline has been enmeshed in that history of conquest and violence. This fact is all too often unappreciated and conveniently avoided. Yet for a discipline known for its commitment to unmask the repressed and for its profusion of studies, such neglect and avoidance of human history and the role of psychologists in that history are curious indeed. The effort of exploring the psychology of oppression requires that we begin by at least sketching the history that determined the nature of social existence, the boundaries of individual biographies, and the direction the discipline of psychology took.

This chapter examines the history and function of Euro-American psychology within the context of Europe's assault upon the rest of the world. First, we review Europe's violent rampage throughout the world and the legacy it bequeathed to the discipline of psychology. Such a panoramic review of history is necessary to correct a prevailing amnesia and the common outlook that psychologists have stood apart, or acted as neutral agents, in the history of oppression. Second, the chapter introduces the *nature versus nurture* debate that has persisted in psychology. We will see that this debate, seemingly academic and abstract, has always had crucial implications for social policy and the *status quo* of oppression. We shall return to this debate in subsequent chapters. Finally, this chapter will outline the ideological and ethnic content of psychology as a background to issues detailed in Chapter 4.

THE VIOLENT LEGACY OF EUROPE

Interdependence of countries and continents is now widely recognized. We know that no country, no continent, can claim true self-sufficiency. This is so in basic commodities, consumer goods, technology, and raw materials. A shift in the price of gas, for instance, sets in motion drastic changes in the mobility and finances of various communities, large and small. A single political unpheaval in one society similarly reverberates in other countries, near and far. Poland, El Salvador, Afghanistan, or the Ogaden are by no means remote arenas embroiled only in internecine, local conflicts. Each is also a pawn to a stubborn superpower conflict that today threatens world peace.

This interdependence in economics and politics also entails an interdependence of psyches. Thus the global problem of war and peace is not merely a question of armaments or economics, but also a problem of psyches confronting, dominating, and influencing each other. More significantly, this global interdependence is based neither on reciprocity nor on equality. It so happens that the wealth of a given set of countries depends on the impoverishment of others. The cultural vigor of some depends on the cultural mummification of others. The brain-gain of certain communities depends on the brain-drain of others. Moreover, the self-objectification and well-being of some depend on the self-obliteration and torment of others. This nonreciprocal, imposed interdependence—in which some gain and others lose, some thrive and others suffer—is not an inevitable, natural order. Tracing the historical genesis of this oppressive pattern in human relations will take us far beyond our purpose. But we can at least sketch some historical antecedents to today's global oppression.[1]

Human oppression has no doubt existed from time immemorial. The exploitation of the weak by the more powerful, the plunder of the poorly equipped by the better equipped, the unjust rule of the less organized majority by the more organized minority—in short, oppression in one form or another has had a persistent human reality. Oppression and the revolt it necessarily entails indeed constitute a primary motive force of history. Human oppression predated and engendered the emergence of human consciousness and civilization. But if oppression was a persistent reality in human existence, its char-

---

[1]For a detailed account, see Williams (1966), Rodney (1974), and Chinweizu (1975).

acter and dimension underwent a drastic transformation with the birth of capitalism. The period 1450–1690 is actually a watershed in the history of Europe and indeed of the world. This period marks the birth of capitalism and the first bourgeois revolution.[2] With the burgeoning of capitalism came drastic changes in the culture, production, technical innovation, and migratory patterns of Europe. Feudal Europe, which immensely benefited from cultural and scientific contributions of societies elsewhere, later imposed its will and greed on these and more distant societies. Thus began the history in which the wealth and development of Europe depended on the ruin and underdevelopment of other societies.

The bourgeois revolution in Europe brought about unprecedented changes in almost all aspects of life (Bernal, 1977, vol. 2). It undermined the feudal order and the dominance of Catholicism. It represented a definite break with the past. At the same time, Europe benefited immensely from the contributions of other eras and non-European societies. With the demise of Hellenic and Roman civilizations, the heritage of Greece returned to non-European societies, whence it had come. Science and culture advanced in Syria, Persia, and China—and these advances were later brought to brilliant synthesis under Islam (Bernal, 1977, vol. 1). The Crusaders of the twelfth and thirteenth centuries brought back much of these cultural and scientific advances to Europe, which had stagnated throughout the Middle Ages, roughly from the late fifth century to about 1350.

Inventions like the horse-collar, the clock, the compass, gunpowder, paper, and printing—all originating in non-European societies—transformed Europe's feudal economy and culture. The contributions of these non-European societies to mathematics, astronomy, medicine, and geography formed the backbone of Europe's Renaissance. The perfection of a number system with place notation and zero, first developed in India and refined by the followers of Islam, simplified computation and made it accessible to the European, adult and child alike. Non-European scientists under the banner of Islam studied eye diseases more prevalent in desert and tropical lands and subsequently improved surgical eye treatment and introduced modern optics (Bernal, 1977, vol. 1). The lens of the eye they studied suggested the idea of crystal or glass lenses and later the telescope. As these contributions extended human sensory apparatus and improved instruments of navigation, reports from Muslim travelers in India, China, Africa, and Russia broadened Europe's narrow conception of the world.

These scientific contributions, the revival of classical culture during the Renaissance, and improved navigation opened new vistas in European outlook and commerce. There was a boom in agriculture. Land and sea travel become safer and more profitable. City and town merchants took on increasing significance in European societies, and social relations previously based on fixed hereditary status were gradually replaced by those based on buying as well as selling commodities and labor. By the fifteenth century, money payments

---

[2]J. D. Bernal (1977) wrote a highly informative, four-volume history on this.

became the dominant means of commodity exchange. As the urban middle class gained ascendancy, first in Holland then in England, money and profit became the measure of all human values. Religion, science, law, and culture served to justify, stimulate, and protect the new greed for money and profit.

The belief took hold that salvation itself lies in more profit and the accumulation of wealth. What mattered was not how one became rich, but rather the fact that one was rich. The old hopes of reconciling man with the world were replaced by the determination to control nature through knowledge of scientific laws. Shipbuilding and commerce boomed. A new quantitative, atomic, and experimental approach to science also emerged. Wealth brought political power to the bourgeoisie. Feudal fetters and old barriers hindering get-rich-quick schemes gave way through political upheaval to a new political order. As paid soldiers replaced the system of feudal levies, wars of expansion and the exercise of might took on a permanent character. The greed for raw materials, new markets, and new wealth intensified. Improved metallurgical procedures, a more sophisticated use of gunpowder, and a more efficient distillation of strong spirits soon provided an effective arsenal for conquest abroad. Christianity and its proselytization too offered rationalizations to numb both the conscience of the predators and the consciousness of the victims. Europe's relation to the rest of the world drastically changed. Slowly but surely, Europe's avid assimilation of the scientific and cultural advances of other societies shifted to a consuming ambition to obtain their lands, labor, and psyches.

By 1492, when Columbus discovered America, Spain and Portugal were the two sea powers of Europe. Portugal initiated Europe's international expansion, but England, France, and Holland soon joined in the rampage to share the loot. The cultivation of sugar, tobacco, and cotton required intensive labor. When white indentured servants and convicts could not meet the demand, Native Americans became the target and victims of slavery. Indeed Wall Street in New York, the noted center of capital speculation, gets its name from the wall built by the Dutch to separate Native American slaves from their relatives (Mannix, 1962, p. 60). Thus in economics as in psychology, the past remarkably survives in the present. Moreover, the ruthless way in which gunpowder, alcohol, and religion were employed to subjugate Native Americans is now a legend. Alcoholism to this day remains the number one health and social problem among the Native American survivors who are left stranded on reservations or in urban centers. Ostensibly denied them are gainful employment, cultural moorings, and spiritual anchors in their own land. Equally appalling is their rate of suicide. It is as if the survivors of genocide, having exhausted all means of self-defense, hasten their ordained extinction.[3]

When Native American slaves could not survive excessive labor, insuffi-

---

[3]In particular, the appalling high rates of suicide and alcoholism among Native Americans underscore the fact of rampant physical, social, and psychological *death* characteristic of oppressed populations—a characteristic we shall illustrate with data on blacks in the United States and South Africa.

cient nutrition, and the white man's veneral diseases, Europe turned to Africa for slaves. That Christianity was once again used to buttress arguments for slavery is hardly surprising. Bartolome de Las Casa, later the Bishop of Chiapa in Mexico, appealed to Charles V and argued that importing African slaves was humane, productive, and consistent with Christian doctrine. The king was convinced by both practical considerations and religious justification. African slavery thus began in earnest and brought immense profit and suffering. The slave trade proper began in 1518 to continue as late as 1880. The greed for capital and the African slave trade had further reduced all human values to those of *profit* and *loss:* "A black man was worth exactly what his flesh would bring to the market" (Mannix, 1962, p. xi). When John Hawkins came back to England with a handsome profit made by capturing and selling African slaves, Queen Elizabeth I quickly set aside her moral disgust with slavery and became a shareholder in Hawkins' subsequent voyages. What is more, she provided Hawkins a ship called *Jesus!*

Even though the psychological impact of the slave trade on Europeans and their descendants is yet to be assayed, we know more about the significant contributions of the trade to the Industrial Revolution. In his classic book, *Capitalism and Slavery*, Eric Williams (1966) documented how the African slave trade financed the Industrial Revolution and made enormous profit for banking concerns as well as insurance companies. Bristol, Liverpool, Manchester, Bordeaux, and Nantes developed as manufacturing centers because of the slave trade. Shipbuilding, the manufacture of cotton goods, sugar refining, rum distillation, the production of chains and padlocks, and the manufacture of guns—these were important features of the triangular trade among these centers of trade and industry. We know, for instance, that James Watts' first steam engine was subsidized with profits from the slave trade. Britain's Great Western Railway was built and funded from the same source. The Barclays and Lloyds, now owners of some of the world's largest banking and insurance concerns, made their initial capital from the slave trade. An early historian of Bristol wrote: "There is not a brick in the city but what is cemented with blood of a slave."[4] A contemporary economist of his who was writing on the unfolding Industrial Revolution also described the slave trade "as the first principle and foundation of all the rest, mainspring of the machine which sets every wheel in motion."[5]

If the impact of this predation on Euro-American psyches is unexplored, the massive hemorrhage inflicted on people of color is well documented. The infamy of slavery and the carnage of the Middle Passage is a legacy of Europe that to this day remains sedimented in the economics, social formation, and psyche of black people. People of color still reel from that hemorrhage and from its second occurrence in colonialism. The Atlantic slave trade represents the largest and most callous mass migration imposed upon a people anywhere in the world. Estimates of Africans forced to be a commodity of the Atlantic

[4]Quoted in Williams (1966, p. 61).
[5]Quoted in Mannix (1962, p. 74).

slave trade range from 15 to 20 million. Recent writers agree that this is a conservative estimate. Some writers now estimate that somewhere between 60 to 150 million Africans were directly involved (Dumont, 1966, p. 33). Africa's population in 1650 was 21.2% of the world population. It was mere 7.7% by 1920. In contrast, Europe's population grew only by 3% between 1650 to 1750. This rose 400% by 1900. By then, Europe's population spilled over to the rest of the world, with 1 million emigrants a year to other continents.[6]

The decline of the African population and the rise of the European population exemplify the simultaneous depletion of African resources, human or material, and the socioeconomic and cultural development of Europe. Great African empires like Ghana, Mali, and Songhay were disintegrating as European states were growing. The recorded history of Ghana goes back to the fifth century A.D. Ghana reached its peak between the ninth and the eleventh centuries; Mali, in the thirteenth and fourteenth centuries (Williams, 1976, pp. 208–222). Historians recognize the high level of culture, the mining of gold and iron, the commerce, and the learning elaborated in these and other African empires. The slave trade and later colonialism prevented the development of indigenous states, technology, and centers of learning. African culture was stripped of its creative reservior and African art hauled to museums abroad.

When the African slave trade ended, Chinese and East Indian workers were brought to the Americas to work on the plantations, build railroads, and join the long chain of victims in the diaspora. The kidnapping and selling of African slaves was replaced with colonialism. The transition from slavery to colonialism had many causes. The demise of outright slavery was brought on by fears of slave rebellion, heightened by sporadic revolts, worries about the growing slave population that might overwhelm the "master race," and concerns about the plight of white sailors in slaving ships. But the most important factor was that the innovations and expansion of industrial capitalism imposed new requirements in production, social relations, and markets. The slave trade that provided New England, Lancashire, and the English Midlands with much of their capital for the industrial revolution surely would not be given up until a more effective and acceptable alternative to slavery loomed on the horizon. Thus when the era of colonialism and gunboat diplomacy began, Euro-Americans readily adjusted their conscience to the new economic exigencies and the call of abolitionists, previously ignored and despised, found wide respectability.

Even the noble efforts to suppress the slave trade were mainly a prelude and justification to the colonial conquest in Africa. Britain took the lead in the suppression of the slave trade, whereas other countries, particularly the United States, resisted such efforts for years. Significantly, however, the British Navy, which was to enforce the law of 1807, had two missions: to suppress the "illegal" trade in human cargoes and to protect "legitimate" trade in nonhuman commodities. The first mission of suppressing the "illegal" trade marked the end of the era when millions of Africans were shipped abroad in bondage. The second mission of protecting "legitimate" trade, entailing the

---

[6]See, for instance, Abate (1978, p. 14); also see Paxton (1975, pp. 3–4).

opening up of new markets for manufactured goods and new source of raw materials, began the era of colonialism when the whole African continent became a huge labor camp.

The historic greed for profit, the glory of conquest abroad, the wish to ensure internal peace by conquering "enemies" in distant lands, and the collective conceit to save heathens from hellfire—all these motivated and justified colonialism. Every Western European power—mighty and small—prepared for the assault on people of color. Each nation grabbed what colony it could and forced its subjects to foot the bill. Between 1850 and 1911, Europe's scramble for subjects and raw materials brought almost the entire world under domination. By 1914, Britain boasted of an empire 140 times its size. Belgium, 80 times; Holland, 60 times; and France, 20 times. This remarkable expansion of territories and the exercise of brutal might was to have not only catastrophic repercussions in economics and politics in the world, but also profound consequences for human psychology and particularly the relationship between people of European descent and the rest of humanity.

The violence of slavery is well known, but little appreciated is the striking continuity of slavery in colonialism, particularly in its pre-World War II variety. Each colonial power perfected its own style and system of exploitation. However, the effect on Africans was the same everywhere. In the French Congo, for instance, some 9 million Africans were coerced to undertake the extremely dangerous labor of gathering and preparing India rubber. Women and children were held in unsanitary and crowded "hostage houses" to compel relatives to work. In the Congo Free State, the kidnapping of women and children for ransom in rubber was so common that "hostage houses" became familiar and common institutions. Where rubber did not grow, inhabitants were forced to furnish food for soldiers and serve as carriers. Within 20 years, a population of nearly 30 million was reduced to about 9 million. (Chinweizu, 1975; Morel, 1969).

Similarly, the long railway known as the Congo-Ocean, stretching through the difficult equatorial terrain, was built by forced labor between 1921 and 1932. It required no less than 127,250 "fit adult males," 138,125 "years of absence" from villages, and a minimum of 141,100 deaths for its completion. At about the same time, 42,000 Africans from the Ivory Coast were conscripted to build the railway linking Abidjan and Ferkessedegan, while at least 16,000 others were put to work in transport and agriculture (Davison, 1978). The Italian fascist government, which ruled a portion of Somaliland, was also known for its practice of capturing thousands of "contract workers" whom they put to hard labor or leased to private companies. The same practice was also common in Portuguese colonies, particularly in Angola. And yet if all such killing labor illustrates the greed and sadism of earlier generations, apartheid in South Africa is today but a veritable amalgam of past cruelties of slavery and colonialism. One simply has to look at current practices in that country to observe *in vivo* the harrowing experiences under slavery and colonialism, but with all the trappings of modernity and essential complicity of such countries as Britain, France, the United States, and Israel.

With the demise of colonialism in most of Africa during the early 1960s, the era of *neo-colonialism* was upon us. Today, neo-colonialism exists side by side with *auto-colonialism*—the highest stage of oppression in which the victim actively participates in his own victimization.[7] Besides Europe's insatiable greed to own and control, three components of this historical oppression of blacks by whites are worth emphasizing. The first is a class of men called "factors" during the slave trade. The second is the role of alcohol and the fostering of a self-destructive *homo consumen* among the oppressed. The third and perhaps most important is the use of gunpowder for Europe's global pillage.

FACTORS, ALCOHOL, AND GUNPOWDER

The middlemen on the African coast who bought and delivered blacks for the Atlantic voyage were called *factors*. They often represented large firms and sometimes dealt with any slaver who was willing to pay for the human merchandise. Some of them were a degraded lot of European convicts, sadists, and fortune seekers. Their contemporary representatives are the white mercenaries today serving apartheid and the subversion of Zimbabwe for money. Others were Africans who adopted European manners and greed, capturing and selling any human being for money. These African factors have since increased and found new disguises. In the plantations, they emerged as the "house niggers," attending to all the master's needs and reporting on the "field niggers." In colonial Africa, they appeared as "domestic boys," petty civil servants, and agents of colonial administrators. Conversion and Western education later became the effective tools for making and disguising a modern African factor. Today, factorship is a pervasive psychosocial phenomenon among the black intelligentsia and many black leaders.

The role of alcohol in slavery and colonialism also requires greater appreciation. The historical origin of alcohol and the use to which it was later put are significant. Although beer was made in Egypt around 3000 B.C., the first steps in the distillation of strong spirits were developed by Arab alchemists around A.D. 800. Religious prohibitions prevented them from taking the crucial step to distill alcohol. Thus they were content to distill perfumes. The increase in the range and potency of alcohol coincided with Europe's conquest of the rest of the world. The first distillation of strong spirits was for medical purposes in the twelfth century (Bernal, 1977, vol. 1). During the fourteenth-century bubonic plague, called the Black Death, the demand for whisky and brandy wine intensified. Alcohol of different varieties was soon produced in large quantities for Europe's conquest of other lands and psyches.

As mentioned earlier, the introduction of alcohol to Native Americans hastened their subjugation and now sustains their victimization. It is remark-

---

[7] A great deal has been written on colonialism and neo-colonialism, referred to by Kwame Nkrumah as "the highest stage of imperialism." During the past decade, however, *auto-colonialism* has become quite real and rampant in Africa.

able how much land and lives have been lost for a few drinks. The Dutch bought Manhatten Island for three barrels of rum in 1626. Indeed the name of the island means "the place where we got drunk" (Bernal, 1977, vol. 1, p. 325). Alcohol was also a potent and effective tool in the Atlantic slave trade. A highly profitable commodity, it contributed significant capital to finance the Industrial Revolution. African dealers in the slave trade were often induced to drink and, while drunk, better bargains were struck. The dealers themselves were sometimes kidnapped. What is more, addiction to alcohol ensured numerous dependent dealers willing to exchange anyone for a few drinks.

Using alcohol primarily, American slave traders of the middle eighteenth century perfected the triangular trade. They used three commodities: *rum, slaves,* and *molasses.* They took rum from New England and exchanged it in Africa for slaves. They sold the slaves in the West Indies and bought cheap molasses for their voyage back to New England. The molasses was distilled into more rum at home and the rum was later used to buy more slaves in Africa. Much like the triangular trade of Liverpool, this exchange of three commodities brought enormous profits for white predators and more torment for black victims. In Europe as in America, alcohol distillation brought about more industries and advances in chemistry.[8] But for Native Americans, as well as people of African descent, alcohol consumption forced them into bondage and today sustains their auto-destruction.

That alcoholism is a major and pervasive problem among Black Americans is well known. Not only is it a significant health hazard for Black Americans, but also the sale and purchase of alcohol have an amazing ripple effect. The National Institute of Alcoholism and Alcohol Abuse estimate that Black Americans spent six and one-half billion dollars on alcohol in 1974–1975 alone. The loss of sorely needed income is also concurrent with much suffering of alcoholics and their loved ones. Just as there is a chain of profiteers, starting from the owners of liquor stores to the owners of the distilling industries, there is also a chain of victims for every alcoholic. Loved ones and community members pay an immeasurable toll for every alcoholic in the community. For instance, more than 70% of murderers use alcohol regularly.[9] Alcohol consumption in the black community reaches its peak on weekends and so do such violent crimes as homicide, suicide, spouse beating, and child abuse. Indeed, the alcohol blood level of the black community is higher than when bargains were being struck long ago between slavers and dealers on the African Coast. More specifically, today's soaring alcohol blood level in the black community only hastens its auto-destruction.

Equally appalling is the rate of alcoholism and alcohol-induced black-on-black crime in South Africa. The relation between alcohol and oppression is here more blatant and more ominous. The racist government of South Africa hardly disguises how it uses alcohol for social control and for the subjugation of black people. For instance, the West Rand Administration Board, charged

[8]See Bernal (1977, Vol. 1); see also Williams (1966, pp. 78–81).
[9]See Harper (1976); also see Rose (1981).

with administrative control of Soweto, held a monopoly on all legal sales of alcohol in the huge township. In Soweto alone, it used to sell 160 million barrels of beer annually. The blood and tears shed due to this level of induced and manipulated consumption are impossible to measure. The number of lives lost, homes broken up, psyches destroyed—these retell the same story of ordained auto-destruction. The willful designs of a racist government knows well the helplessness and painful withdrawal symptoms it can inflict on so many in the black community. Thus in retaliation for the 1976 rebellion in Soweto, the government deliberately burned many beer halls and liquor stores (Harsch, 1980, p. 19).

Yet alcohol and factors would not by themselves be sufficient to force slavery and subjugation on a people without the power of deadly and superior arms. The ever-increasing sophistication of Euro-American weapons reflects an unwavering determination to perpetuate that historical rampage and the *status quo* of bondage. The development and use of gunpowder is itself revealing. Indeed no invention has created as much havoc in the world as did the development and application of gunpowder. The Chinese first invented gunpowder, but they used it for only fireworks. Medieval Europe learned of it from the Arabs. It is said that, even in Europe, the introduction of gunpowder had the greatest impact politically, economically, and scientifically. Gunpowder and its early complements—the cannon and the musket—initiated a technical revolution in warfare and drastically changed the balance of power in the world. This new technology of death undermined the independence of the land-based European aristocracy and brought to ascendancy those who had access to the necessary technical skills and sources of metal. Meanwhile, the non-European majority of the world was being decimated and subdued with gunpowder.

The African inability to develop gunpowder had a most devastating consequence. To be sure, Africans had long elaborated advance cultures and fashioned huge empires like Ghana, Mali, and Songhay. The mining of gold, copper, and iron was known centuries before Europe unleashed its historical avarice. Higher centers of learning, like the University of Sankore at Timbuktu, existed while Europe stagnated in the Dark Ages. Remarkable advances were also made in medicine, jurisprudence, and art. African craftsmen were in fact able to make muskets before and during the slave trade. But, in spite of these advances, only few African societies had developed their own gunpowder. In a world made gruesome and cynical by Europe's violent onslaught, little wonder that some historians consider gunpowder "the hallmark of an advanced culture" (Mannix, 1962, p. 14).

During the early phases of European encroachment, Africans fought the best they knew how, with whatever they could lay their hands on. This was not sufficient, however, and the continent was an easy prey to Europe's relentless rampage and violence. An effective defense against European predation was therefore impossible. In time, the noose of bondage became ever tighter and more suffocating. All defenses and human values were dislocated. Subsequently, there remained but two possibilities: *slavery* or *collaboration*.

Europe's guns and gunpowder forced some into chattel slavery, others into sinister collaboration. The ethic of skinning others before being skinned spread like a contagion. Internecine wars became endemic, guns and gunpowder ever more indispensable. Europe gained at once more slaves, more collaborators, and a market for its new technology of death. These gains reinforced each other in geometric proportion. So did the agony and bloodletting of Africa.

During the eighteenth century, for instance, Birmingham guns and gunpowder were notorious in the slave trade. Birmingham was the center of gun manufacturing and trade for more than two centuries. There was in fact a common saying that "the price of a Negro was one Birmingham gun." Not only were Birmingham guns and gunpowder cherished by slave traders, but Africans were also importing them in huge quantities. Africa was indeed the most important customer of Birmingham guns and gunpowder. It is estimated that African imports of Birmingham guns alone amounted to from 100,000 to 150,000 annually (Williams, 1966, p. 82). Thus Europe's new technology of death at once enslaved millions, forced others to degrading collaboration, and created a new market all for profit.

Birmingham guns and gunpowder were early harbingers of what was to follow on a global scale. The technology of death has now become more sophisticated and more destructive. It comes in all sizes, range, and efficiency. It is made and sold by the West, and by the East, with countries like Israel and Brazil profiteering through the manufacture and auctioning of arms. Meanwhile, many African countries squander more on foreign arms than their combined budgets for health and education. Internecine conflicts and wars still rage as the fervor for alien arms reaches reckless and maddening peaks. Sorely needed resources, human and material, are thereby wasted. Under the false and confused pretext of national security, the carnage within and without borders becomes more and more wanton. Heavily equipped African armies are today conquering none other than their own people.

The avarice and violence Europe unleashed upon the rest of the world also came to haunt Europe. The dictum that violence begets violence is nowhere better illustrated than in Europe's history. World War I was in fact more bitter and bloody than the Thirty Years' War of the seventeenth century. An unprecedented number of European youth were hurling steel and explosives at one another, while others were dying of poison gas in rat-infested trenches. John Buchan, a British diplomat commenting on World War I, wrote: "Everywhere in the world was heard the sound of things breaking" (Paxton, 1975, p. 97). Two decades later, a more total and consuming fire engulfed Europe. World War II was a veritable demonstration of a civilization gone mad. As the high priests of science presided in concentration camps and gas chambers, everywhere was heard the sound of things breaking and the agony of millions dying, maimed, or psychologically broken.

World War II was both a tragic culmination and a clear warning to those who cuddled up to Europe. This war also marked a historical watershed in the awakening of people of color in Africa and Asia. Duped into defending the "motherland," willy-nilly dragged into Europe's bloodbath, people of color were able to scrutinize Europe more closely—its people, techniques, and family quarrels—in battlefields and distant lands. Peoples previously separated by geography and history also came in contact with one another and shared their common aspirations for freedom. As veterans of World War II returned to the colonies bitter and awakened, nationalism and their people's will to freedom were rekindled. What happened in Hiroshima and why Japan was selected for that shameful experiment left little doubt that a civilization built on the toil and torment of others will readily explode its technology of genocide and do anything to ensure its supremacy.

That today the United States and the Soviet Union—specifically, the dominant *European* strain in both countries—compete for world hegemony does not change the historical rampage and self-aggrandizement of Europe. The superpower competition merely extends the historical violence to a colossal proportion: Korea, the Congo, Vietnam, and Afghanistan recall the same pattern of victimization, the same European greed to own and control at whatever cost. But when African or Asian leaders plead for more deadly arms from Washington or Moscow to reconquer only their own people, this indicates that factors come in many guises and that factorship is today more insidious and pervasive than ever before. Slaves no longer have to be chained or transported in ships. They come on their own to Europe or America, possessed and compromised long before they have reached these shores. Haitian refugees pathetically show that the Middle Passage is still as real and harrowing as ever. These refugees, victims of factors at home and of racism abroad, embark on risky sea voyages only to be herded to American prison camps and treated as criminals. The plight of African students is similar but more subtle. The master–slave dialectic to date remains intact (Bulhan, 1979).

Even the best in human achievements, such as the first heart transplant and the landing of men on the moon, betray the same pattern of exploitation and the same persistent wish for conquest. The first heart transplant was made by a *white* South African physician. Predictably, the unwilling "donor" was a *Colored*. The lucky beneficiary was an ailing *white* South African. Undocumented, but not unreasonable to suspect is that many South African blacks were experimented with before this historical, successful heart transplant. Similarly, the spirit and ambition of Columbus is now reaching outer space. That historical wish to own and control, relentless self-aggrandizement that disemboweled others and stripped them of their humanity, is today seeking to conquer other planets. The same persistent motivation also now threatens a nuclear holocaust and total annihilation. Indeed the greed that consumed other peoples and hoarded earthly resources may soon cannibalize itself before it has conquered outer space. Yet what have psychologists said and done about this historical rampage and potential self-annihilation?

THE HERITAGE OF PSYCHOLOGY

The earliest roots of Euro-American psychology can be traced to Greek tradition and philosophy. Greek civilization laid the initial foundation for certain problems that persist in Euro-American psychology. The body–mind dualism, the nature–nurture debate, the individualistic orientation, and the fascination with numbers characterizing Euro-American psychology found early expression in Greek thought. Socrates and Plato sharpened the distinction between soul and body, whereas Aristotle sought their unity. Pythagoras believed that the soul is at home with numbers. He argued that the world of beauty and of science were ordered mathematically (Murphy & Kovach, 1972, p.9) Hippocrates insisted that mental disorders were due to a diseased brain. He also emphasized the importance of heredity and predisposition.

Greek scholars often distinguished between *nous* and *psyche*. The former meant "mind"; the latter translates to "spirit." Their concept of mind emphasized the human capacity to receive impressions as does a blank wax tablet. Their notion of spirit stressed animating force, movement, and particularly emotional experience. The distinction between thought and feeling as between inherited attributes and environmental influences has since persisted in Western thought. With the demise of ancient Greek civilization, the Church and its doctrines became dominant. Promoting the view that the world is sick and sinful, it made guilt and restitution common European preoccupations. The Church also instigated and directed a bloody era of witch-hunting and burning. Estimates are that, between 1603 and 1628 alone, one-quarter of a million persons were burned as witches in Europe. During these 25 years, there were, respectively, 70,000 and 100,000 persons burned in England and Germany (Mears & Gotchel, 1979, p. 5).

The emergence and consolidation of the bourgeoisie brought forth new social reforms and innovations in various fields. But this emergence and consolidation of the bourgeoisie also brought new problems in the relation of classes in Europe and of races abroad. The cult of reason justified and supported the cult of profit. Speculations about human nature, the relation of mind and body, and debates about the differences between social classes or races were given a new impetus by the discovery of the Americas, the infamy and guilt of slavery, the sociocultural dislocations of industrialization, the mass migration to urban centers, and later, by the imposition of colonial domination on people of color. The major thinkers who profoundly influenced the emergence and content of psychology often provided ample rationalizations for the exploitation of the "lower classes" in Europe and the "inferior races" abroad. These early rationalizations and the stature of their proponents had in turn a formative impact on the future development and amnesia of Euro-American psychology.

Psychology was for a long time subsumed under philosophy. Problems of ethics, the nature of human emotions, the power of human will—these were some of the questions examined through introspection and erudition. By the late eighteenth century, psychology had developed a closer affinity to experimental physiology. Early experiments centered on physiology and biophysics. Sensation, reaction time, and the function of the cortex were carefully scrutinized. These early experiments were mainly of academic interest. On a few occasions, however, some researchers ventured out of their laboratories into the real world. Early studies like those of Canabis in France anticipated what later was to become a hallmark of establishment psychology—namely, the fetish of experimentation on narrow, technical problems even as the life and death of others is in balance. Canabis studied the process and consequence of execution by the guillotine, wondering if victims died speedily and painlessly. Following observations of that macabre practice, Canabis reasoned that the brain was not the region of direct assault. He concluded that death by guillotine was not painful, since only mechanical responses of lower reflexes followed execution (Murphy & Kovach, 1972, p. 39).

The beginning of scientific psychology is by common consent dated at 1879 when Wilhelm Wundt established his psychological laboratory in Leipzig, Germany. Wundt emphasized the need to study psychological problems through physiological and experimental methods. This meant that a psychological experiment, to be genuinely scientific, must focus on the manipulation of measurable variables, under stated conditions, and the findings evaluated on the basis of empirical criteria. As Murphy and Kovach (1972, p. 160) point out, Wundt was so successful "in turning psychology into a laboratory-based science that since his time all other aspects of psychology have suffered from feelings of second-class citizenship." By the time Watson came on the scene, experimental psychology had emerged from the shadow of experimental physiology. Watson neglected consciousness and subjective experiences. Thus the testimony of human subjects came to lose credence and experimentation on animals was seen to be more reliable and promising. As the focus shifted to behavior and its quantification, the usefulness of concepts like mind and consciousness was doubted. Yet some of the old debates in psychology persisted.

There is in psychology no debate as persistent and politically potent as that of *nature* versus *nurture*. The debate has long permeated psychological literature. The nature versus nurture controversy is certainly far from an academic debate. Fundamental to it is this implicit question: What indeed must be done with the poor, the dispossessed, and those considered somehow "deviant?" More specifically, are these wretched beings simply the veritable products of inferior heredity *or* are they redeemable victims of a deleterious environment? This is really the heart of the heated and persistent controversy. The technical jargons or the veiled terms in which discussions are often couched only obscure the sociopolitical kernel of the controversy. And when the debate is stripped of its academic and scientific trappings, one finds much that is truly scandalous.

Responses to the controversy have generally taken two classical forms. There are, on the one hand, those who argue for the primacy of inherited predispositions and, on the other, those who argue for the potency of environmental influences. Rarely does a theorist of either persuasion argue for one position to the exclusion of the other. It is rather a question of emphasis and the conclusions thereby drawn. There has recently been disillusionment with the debate and efforts made for an interactionist perspective. Through the centuries, the debate has been waxing and waning. Periods of social upheaval and agitation for reform bring the debate to prominence in the psychological literature. What is more, the position in any period often reflects the predatory or reformist mood of the ruling classes.

The list and academic stature of supporters for the "nature" position in the debate are indeed impressive—more so when the debate concerns people of color. Thomas Malthus, David Hume, Herbert Spencer, Francis Galton, Karl Pearson, G. Stanley Hall, Lewis Terman, Cyril Burt—to name only a few—had each taken a dim and disparaging view of the poor and the dispossessed. Each of them justify oppression. Attempts to refute the justifications appeared as difficult as dismantling the objective conditions of oppression. The ideas of these men of great stature also became the rallying doctrines for hateful bigots and calculating beneficiaries of an oppressive *status quo*. One of the earliest and most influential of these was Thomas Malthus who believed that any reform to improve the lot of the poor was not only unpatriotic, but also against the law of God and nature. In his view, the diseases and death of the poor were not to be prevented but actively sought. Thus in his famous *Essay on the Principles of Population*, Malthus wrote (Chase, 1977, p. 68):

> if we dread the too infrequent visitation of the horrid form of famine, we should sedulously encourage the other forms of destruction. . . . Instead of recommending cleanliness to the poor, we should encourage contrary habits. In our towns we should make the streets narrower, crowd more people into the houses, and court the return of the plague. . . .

If Malthus opposed all reforms for the dispossessed in Europe, David Hume justified slavery and the subjugation of blacks. His stature as a scholar and careful observer made him one of the most formidable spokesmen of the view that blacks are inherently inferior to whites. Hume argued that "negroes and in general all other species of men . . . to be naturally inferior to whites" (Popkin, 1977–78, p. 213). Such sweeping generalizations by a pioneering empiricist shows that, for a bigot, racism supercedes any evidence or scientific observation. Antiracists and abolitionists had first to struggle against the authority and influence of Hume, his ideas and stature. It is now hard to appreciate the difficulty this entailed and to realize the impact Hume's racism had on other thinkers. Influenced by Hume's ideas, Kant commented thus about a man of color: "this fellow was quite black from head to foot, a clear proof that what he said was stupid" (Popkin, 1977–78, p. 218).

The theory of natural selection Malthus formulated and Darwin established was soon extended to social, moral, and political debates. Spencer interpreted society and psychology in terms of a "struggle for survival" and "the survival of the fittest." His pronouncements and the Social Darwinism he espoused were quickly embraced to forestall social reform in Europe and America. Spencer himself opposed such basic reforms as universal education, minimum standards of health or occupational safety, improved sanitary conditions, and the establishment of trade unions. Not surprisingly, affluent and commercial tycoons found Spencer's ideas most congenial. Andrew Carnegie wrote that he "found the truth of evolution" in Spencer's writings. John D. Rockefeller asserted that "the growth of large business is merely a survival of the fittest . . . merely the working out of a law of nature and a law of God"

(Chase, 1977, p. 8). To oppose Spencer's Social Darwinism was not only to refute assertions of such powerful tycoons or to challenge Spencer's personal influence, it was also to contradict "evolutionary theory" itself. Here was one clear instance when capitalists and scholars combined forces to powerfully defend the *status quo*.

Equally formidable, but with more enduring consequences for psychology is the work of Francis Galton, a cousin of Darwin and an heir to a handsome fortune. A decade after the publication of *The Origin of Species,* Galton published his *Hereditary Genius,* in which he argued that individual greatness is inherited and runs in well-to-do families. Galton was the father of eugenics and of the psychometric tradition in psychology. Not only did he pioneer the study of individual differences and the quantitative method in psychology—two central features of Euro-American psychology—he also pioneered the pseudo-scientific classification of the human races into various levels of superiority and worth. Galton viewed the nature versus nurture question as a practical social problem for which his eugenics movement provided an effective solution to the elimination of the "unfit." Galton's delusion regarding the "menace of racial pollution" rapidly caught on and later formed the intellectual edifice for Nazi propaganda and genocide. It was also the impetus and justification for numerous legislations on the compulsory sterilization of the poor and oppressed in America.

The eugenics movement Galton pioneered has since developed into a highly influential force with sinister aims and programs. The power and stature of those it counts in its ranks is indeed disquieting. For instance, the First International Congress of Eugenics, held at the University of London, was chaired by the son of Charles Darwin and attended by such notables as Winston Churchill; Alexander Graham Bell; Charles E. Eliot, who was president emeritus of Harvard University; David Starr-Jordan, then president of Stanford University; and Gilford Pinchot, a future governor of Pennsylvania. The Second International Congress of Eugenics was held in New York in 1921. Herbert Hoover, then Secretary of Commerce, and the presidents of Clark University and of Smith College were listed among the sponsoring committee of this congress. The repeated call for forced sterilization of the poor and the downtrodden reached its climax during the Third International Congress of Eugenics held in New York in 1932, the third year of the Great Depression. In all seriousness, Theodore R. Robie presented the following solution for what he saw was amiss in America: the forced sterilization of at least 14 million citizens who had low IQ scores since World War I (Chase, 1977, p. 20).

The development and use of intelligence tests gradually gave psychology a new professional identity, a modicum of scientific respectability, and a lucrative social function. Most remarkable in the history of testing is the immense gains psychology derived from the twin pestilence of war and bigotry. World War I and World War II brought psychology out of its academic ivory tower. World War I enlisted the services of psychologists for the classification and screening of recruits in the armed forces. Following the war, an unprecedented and hectic pace of psychological testing exploded in schools and society. Psychological testing of European immigrants, and the deportation of thousands presumably for low IQ scores, gave psychologists new powers and the function of gatekeeper. World War II saw at least 1,500 American psychologists in the armed services. In addition to testing recruits, psychologists took on increasing psychotherapeutic roles in order to return as many men as possible to combat. The discipline of psychology—its theories, methods, and instruments—subsequently blossomed. Its students increased exponentially. The public stature of psychology also grew. New and seemingly inexhaustible sources of funding, both private and governmental, became increasingly accessible for research and training.

WASP and Jewish Trends in Psychology

The combined services of testing and psychotherapy ushered psychology into a public, lucrative arena to which the academic psychology of the past was unaccustomed. These two professional activities, two social functions, and two ways of earning a living had different origins and inspiration before they became alloyed into Euro-American psychology. The psychometric tradition had been pioneered and inspired by Galton and his eugenics movement. Permeating this tradition was WASP bigotry, delusions of Anglo-Saxon superiority, and a determined wish to keep people of color under subjugation or even eliminate other "species" of humanity. Galton and his student, Karl Pearson, introduced a method and the mathematics for their scientific racism. The development and use of intelligence tests also provided a potent tool for assessing the worth of others according to *birth* and what they *have*. Those who were not either WASP or rich were doomed to the category of the "unfit" and risked sterilization.

It was in 1890 that Cattell introduced the notion of "mental tests." In 1916, Binet and Simon published their test based on a wider sample of behavior. Henry Goddard, an ardent disciple of Galton, introduced Binet's test to America. But it was Terman's revision of the Binet Scale, now widely known as the Stanford–Binet Intelligence Scale, that was destined to have a profound influence. Lewis Terman, it should be noted, was also a firm believer in the Galtonian delusion. He was convinced that Spanish–Indians, Mexicans, and blacks have genetically inferior intelligence. "The children of this group," wrote Terman, "should be segregated in special classes and given instruction which is concrete and practical" (Chase, 1977, p. 235). This manner and content of education were to prepare them for the manual and menial jobs that they were presumably suited to by nature. As for their parents, Terman argued that "from a eugenic point of view they constitute a *grave problem* because of their unusually prolific breeding" (Chase, 1977, p. 235). His recommendation, like those of other eugenicists, was of course sterilization.

Interestingly, while insisting on such brutal pessimism about the living majority, Terman and his associates evoked the dead from their tombs and estimated the IQ of such great men as Beethoven, Darwin, Napoleon, and

Lincoln. Of all the illustrious dead whose intelligence was assessed, Galton's IQ predictably soared highest and was most impressive. According to Terman and associates, Galton's IQ approached "unquestionably in the neighborhood of 200, a figure not equalled by more than one child in 50,000" in the general population (Chase, 1977, p. 237). Such wild reveries and eugenic ranting may now be seen for what they actually are. But these conclusions were not drawn by obscure and isolated men. Terman was by then president of the American Psychological Association. Similarly, G. Stanley Hall, the teacher and mentor of both Goddard and Terman, was twice president of that association. These pioneers and countless others who followed in their footsteps left Euro-American psychology a significant heritage that only massive amnesia could repress.

Actually, it is not only the racism and influence of these men that are conveniently repressed. Hardly explored are the remarkable social network binding such racist psychologists into a powerful force and the dishonest expediency with which they furthered bigotry. For instance, Sir Cyril Burt, who died in 1971, was the most prominent psychologist in Britain for over half a century. His prolific writing and twin studies showing the primacy of heredity over environment were for years unassailable. The precision and consistency of his findings were impeccable, to the chagrin of those who disagreed with his conclusions. Jensen and Shockley, two contemporary adherents of the Galtonian delusion, rely inexorably on Burt's twin studies to bolster their racist contentions. Yet we now know that Cyril Burt simply *fabricated* much of his data.[10] Interestingly, Jensen was not only a close friend of Burt, he was also one of the last to visit Burt before his death. Burt himself grew up in the neighborhood of the illustrious Francis Galton. Burt knew Galton personally and remained enchanted with his bigotry for the rest of his life.

In short, those who argue for the primacy of genetic-biological factors in the nature–nurture debate are tightly knit and inbred. They are more ardent, more unyielding, and more organized than the so-called nurture proponents. They have the tycoons, their capital, and state violence in sympathy and complicity with their sinister aims. They oppose social reform and defend social inequity as the natural order of life. They attribute inherent, immutable deficiencies to the poor and the dispossessed. A corollary to this conviction is their implicit suggestion that the well-to-do in society deserve the wealth and power they have because of better genes and superior heredity. Their impact on psychology is formidable. They defined psychology's topical priorities, pioneered many of its methods, and formed the intellectual edifice upon which much of Euro-American psychology was founded. Leading scholars in their days, they played key roles in professional organizations and established some of the most prestigious journals of psychology. Adamant, cohesive, and expedient, they brought to bear their influential works and personal reputation to forestall new reforms and thwart hard-won legislation for the poor, the disabled and the different. In research and practice, they defended bigotry and went to any length to concoct convincing data.

[10]A detailed account of this scandal is presented by L. S. Hearnshaw (1981).

Opposing these nature proponents are the less cohesive, less uniform, and more relenting nurture proponents. The latter do not of course deny the importance of genes or heredity. What they reject is the view that these are distributed according to social or racial patterns. But beyond some general assertions, the nurture proponents hold contradictory opinions of what, if anything, must be done to change the plight of the poor and the oppressed. The majority of them, although tolerant of differences in their outlook, take a *laissez-faire* approach in practice. Others among them, although arguing for the potency of the "environment," somehow manage to blame the victim as they invoke deficit or pathological models. Even their central concept of environment is ambiguous. What they all share is the view that the environment, defined broadly to include anything external to the person, is the most crucial determinant of human psychology. But beyond this general agreement, the nurture proponents within establishment psychology are plagued with ambivalence, indecision, paternalism, and even veiled racism. They shift with the political mood of the time and they adjust their scholarship to the requirements of funding agencies. Their characteristic propensities and their *laissez-faire* approach to practice make them at best unreliable allies for "the wretched of the earth."

If the psychometric tradition in psychology is founded on Galtonian and WASP bigotry, psychotherapy as we know it today in Euro-America developed from two trends in establishment psychology. The first is the *dynamic* tradition, the second the *behavioral* perspective. The first owes much to the genius and charisma of its founder, Sigmund Freud, an assimilated Jew who personally knew the anguish of bigotry, minority status, and social exclusion. He had experienced enough to give him the impulses and pains of a *victim*. A history of anti-Semitism and his struggle with the "compact majority" gave him and his people a moral edge over others, a critical skepticism of the prevailing ethos, and the uncanny skill to transform subjective experiences in order to assimilate into the dominant social order. Thus the most important and most arduous therapy that Freud was to undertake was that of himself. He is said to have once remarked to Fliess, his doctor and friend, that "the main *patient* who keeps me busy is *myself*" (Ellenberger, 1970, p. 446).

There are ample indicators that Freud's personal anguish and self-doubts had much to do with his being a Jew in racist Europe. Not unlike Fanon, his personal suffering and victim complex provided the stimulus for creative thought. The experience of victimization in oppression produces, on the one hand, tendencies toward rebellion and a search for autonomy and, on the other, tendencies toward compliance and accommodation. Often, the two tendencies coexist among the oppressed, although a predominant orientation can be identified for any person or generation at a given time. Unlike Marx and Fanon, Freud's orientation to the *status quo* of oppression was essentially assimilationist. Moreover, the hermaneutic approach to the psyche Freud pioneered is partly Jewish in origin. But it also derives from experiences of victims in an oppressive social structure they believe immutable. From this approach, one can best understand and change the *subjective* domain so as to better adapt to and assimilate the dominant *status quo*. Thus, although the WASP trend in psychology emphasizes bigotry and active intrusion in the lives of others, preferring empiricism and control of external objects, the Jewish trend pioneered by Freud opts for an introspective approach and emphasizes the need to come to terms with one's self—a self historically tormented by a formidable and oppressive social structure.

Freud's modest beginnings and minority status in the dominant society became less significant as his pioneering efforts were crowned with success. As Freud acquired a reputation and won numerous disciples, success attenuated his victim impulse. His class identity became entrenched as his cherished goal of assimilation into the bourgeoisie was realized. His epoch-making attack on sexual repression persisted, but his ideas remained steeped in a middle-class, European outlook. This bourgeois European outlook, reinforced by the complaints and class background of his patients, had a decisive effect on the theory and practice Freud elaborated. The desire to win scientific respectability, in the Darwinian sense, also diluted his social critique. Psychoanalytic theory deflected from its radical critique as it moved into the realm of animal instincts and myth-making. What is more, the introduction and popularization of psychoanalysis in America accentuated latent problematics and added new limitations. Psychoanalysis gradually became an expensive venture, a middle-class luxury, a lucrative career, a commodity for profit. The critical edge that rendered it epoch-making was further blunted and it came to idealize mere adjustment. It blamed the victim of oppression and took the *status quo* off the hook. Today psychoanalysis serves as a rationalizing bulwark to oppression—a fact not unrelated to changes in the wealth and status of the Jewish community in the United States.

The behaviorist perspective was a latecomer in the practice of therapy. It had diverse origins and influences. Major contributors to it include a Russian, a white South African, and two Americans. Ivan P. Pavlov first demonstrated what has come to be known as "classical conditioning." John B. Watson coined the term *behaviorism* and limited himself to observable behaviors. But the two leading figures who had the most impact on behaviorist therapy are Burrhus F. Skinner, an American from a conservative Republican background, and Joseph Wolpe, a white South African reared as an Orthodox Jew. The behavioral approach to therapy became a major force in a remarkably short time. Its simplicity and efficiency appeals to the technocratically conscious. The relative ease with which its "behavioral technology" can be taught and practiced is envied by competitors for the same clientele—namely, patients who can *pay* and those who wield *power* in society. Actually, behaviorism represents a synthesis of the two major trends in psychology: It manipulates *objective* variables to effect individual *adjustment* to the *status quo*.

A fundamental problem in the behaviorist perspective is that its central concepts of behavior, control, and environment are devoid of social, political, and indeed human content. Knowledge gained from experimental rats and pigeons is extrapolated to human experience. Behavior is reduced to a specific, measurable response within a specified time. Thus it is stripped of intentionality and meaning. How such narrow definitions can explain the psychology of, say, human labor and its social character is never stated. Control is similarly reduced to simply what precedes or follows a given behavior. It is confined only to the immediate, the measurable, and the quantifiable. Systemic power and social control therefore become too complex and irrelevant for such a paradigm. Forgotten is also that the violence of racism is often more pernicious when covert than when overt. What is more, questions like who controls whom and for what end are ignored. As Mishler aptly points out, such questions are evaded with the retort that "all control is reciprocal." Thus, according to Skinner, even "the slave controls the slave owner" and, by implication, neither bears responsibility for that state of affairs (Mishler, 1976).

Similarly, the behaviorist use of "environment" has lost its human meaning and content. The experimental maze becomes its analogue. As with rats or pigeons, the experimenter attempts to manipulate people according to his or her wishes or whims. More commonly, people are portrayed as passive objects or a blank slate, a *tabula rasa*, able to receive impressions only from without. Forgotten is the fact that people are not only *objects*, but also *subjects* of history. It is they who transform the world and are in turn transformed by it. The naive materialism permeating the behaviorist perspective readily accommodates a history in which people are treated as objects. Thus Skinner and Wolpe emphasize not that a given environment or set of controls are oppressive, but that it can and should be made more effective. The net result of their arguments and practice is only this: *more effective power for the powerful and more effective control over the powerless.* If and when the question of values and ethics are posed, their answer is that such queries are irrelevant. This recalls the argument of Wernher von Braun, the German rocket engineer: "My rockets just go up. Who cares where they come down?"

Actually, the use of psychology for warfare is a thriving, but little known speciality. The abortive Project Camelot was a U.S. Army project concerned with counterinsurgency and counterrevolution in the Third World. The Army's fact sheet indicates its precise purpose as "a basic social science project on preconditions of internal conflict, and on effects of indigenous governmental actions . . . on these preconditions" (Sjoberg, 1967, p. 142). The operating budget of the project was at least 6 million. Today sea lions, porpoises, and killer whales are trained for naval warfare. Even the innocent pigeon was "drafted" for the historical rampage.

Project Pigeon was developed during World War II when guidance systems for missiles were very rudimentary. If pigeons could play table tennis, they could also be trained to guide a missile. Skinner therefore devised a system in which pigeons pecked at a symbol as long as the missile remained on course. When the missile moved off course, the symbol moved left or right and so did the pigeon's pecking to return the missile on course. "By using certain schedules of reinforcement, Skinner could guarantee these pigeons would go on pecking till they dropped dead. Various tests showed that this was a practical scheme. . . . Project Pigeon, however was abandoned in favor of the development of the atom bomb. When the Manhattan Project got going, the pigeon

missiles were grounded" (Cohen, 1977, p. 264). Skinner was openly disappointed. But his ingenuity had sparked hectic experimentation in psychological warfare. During the Vietnam War, pigeons were trained for equally lethal
assignments. What the Soviets had thus far done with Pavlovian conditioning
or Skinnerian reinforcements remains a mystery.

In short, the world is still reeling from the historical avarice and violence
Europe unleashed upon it. The global hemorrhage is by no means due to a
curse, an accident, or a death instinct. Its genesis is traceable to a specific
region of the world, to a specific era, and to definable historical circumstances.
Europe's greed to own and control has had a profound impact on human history and psyches. Because of it, the world is made grim by wars for profit and
power. Peoples of all color and hues have lost their innocence. The will to
reach out and touch the other, in good faith, has long been overcome by a
consuming desire for ownership and self-aggrandizement. Profit, gunpowder,
alcohol, slaves, factors—these have left behind a violent legacy to the world.
No people and no psyche remain untarnished. Even the pigeon and the por-
poise are enlisted in these wars for profit and power. Oppression is everywhere
and so is the technology of death.

As subsequent chapters demonstrate, the oppressed are still chained—
physically here, socially there, and psychologically everywhere. The oppressor
too remains adamant. He is in no mood for reconciliation; he has no wish for
atonement. Nor is he willing to turn over a new leaf. But he knows the gravity
of his own crimes. Restless and hypervigilant, he gropes for inner security and
peace through a more advanced technology of death. Indeed oppression has
now become so much a part of the world, so sedimented in the human psyche,
that the distinction between the oppressed and the oppressor is sometimes
blurred. The oppressed is willy-nilly forced to be an oppressor—to himself, to
his loved ones, to his neighbors. The appalling rates of alcoholism, child abuse,
homicide, and tyranny in oppressed communities are best understood in these
terms. The original and stubborn oppressor too is oppressed, but by his own
greed, violence, and fear of reprisal. How else can we make sense of today's
incredible arms race? The technology of death has so advanced that all humanity could perish with the slightest provocation or misjudgment of one superpower. Or as with madness, can we really make sense out of the irrational?

The specialists whose profession it is to make sense out of madness and
heal psychic wounds are themselves enmeshed in that historical rampage and
violence. Euro-American psychology itself is now a veritable arsenal. Those
who profess and practice it are waging wars within wars, even when the immediate victim is a child whose IQ is being tested. There is a culture of silence on
Europe's violence and a convenient amnesia among establishment psychologists. Writers on the history of psychology too remain fettered by the same
tradition of selective inattention. Europe's violent assaults within and without
its borders are sloughed off as if they never existed or mattered. Conveniently
omitted also are the bigotry and complicity of major pioneers who defined the
priorities, content, and methods of establishment psychology. History and
ideas are thereby "sanitized." Psychological theories shorn of their relation to

oppression are catalogued; technical innovation for the economics of inequity and politics of domination are brandished. In the end, the amnesia of the expert fosters more amnesia in the neophyte. Meanwhile, the oppressed and the oppressor alike court auto-destruction—each according to his style and means. Fanon broke with this culture of silence and the amnesia of establishment psychology. As we shall see in subsequent chapters, his insights in the psychology of oppression open new vistas and present exciting challenges.

II

PSYCHOLOGY, MEDICINE, AND DOMINATION

4

FANON AND EUROCENTRIC PSYCHOLOGY

Besides phylogeny and ontogeny stands sociogeny . . . *let us say this is a question of* sociodiagnostics.

—Fanon, *Black Skin, White Masks*

As part of a growing and profitable industry, books and journals on psychology inundate the market. There is now a welter and profusion of psychological studies. Multiplicity of hypotheses, findings, and dogma abound in the literature. What is more, each theoretical orientation or subspecialty in psychology has its own concepts and techniques. A line of inquiry considered important in a given perspective is condemned as trivial in another.[1] Under these conditions, it becomes difficult to isolate the kernel of psychology as a discipline. Yet behind the fragmentary findings and contradictory conclusions lie a shared world view, a specific methodology, and a common source of experiential datum for psychological research.

The previous chapter sketched the history of psychology within the history of global rampage on people of color. This chapter critically evaluates Eurocentric psychology from two vantage points. First, it examines some fundamental problematics of a psychology derived from a white, middle-class male minority, which is generalized to humanity everywhere. The first section of the chapter underscores how the self-aggrandizement and domination of that minority finds expression, confirmation, and justification in psychological theory and practice. Second, the chapter examines Fanon's encounter with Eurocentric psychology. It shows how Fanon, a committed militant, benefited from and later rejected Eurocentric psychology. Fanon's encounter with Eurocentric psychology is illustrated here by his encounter with Sigmund Freud, Carl Jung, and Alfred Adler. As pointed out earlier, Fanon's critique of this trio is best appreciated within the framework of a general critique of Euro-American psychology.

PSYCHOLOGY: SCIENCE OR SORCERY?

Interest in human experience and behavior is not of course peculiar to Euro-America. Other people elsewhere and in various eras have inquired into

[1]For a detailed discussion of conflicting findings and formulations in psychology, see David Finkelman (1978, pp. 179–199).

63

the whys of human experience and the wherefore of interpersonal behavior. Yet psychology as an organized discipline—psychology in the form today taught and practiced—is undoubtedly Euro-American in origin and substance. In concepts as in assumptions, in instruments as in outlook, this psychology is Eurocentric through and through. It is nonetheless this psychology that is now fast proliferating in education, health, industry, and social policy. Even the non-European, non-Western majority of the world is gradually adopting this Eurocentric psychology. What is more, the adoption is too often uncritical and wholesale. Yet in a world of cultural and racial heterogeneity, this Eurocentric psychology and its proliferation pose one fundamental concern: the fact of imperialism in psychology.[2]

That this Eurocentric psychology dominates contemporary studies of the human psyche is by no means an accident of history. The ascendancy and globalization of Euro-American psychology indeed correlates with the ascendancy and globalization of Euro-American military, economic, and political might. Viewed from this perspective, the organized discipline of psychology reveals itself as yet another form of alien intrusion and cultural imposition for the nonwhite majority of the world. It is strange but true that the human psyche, even in a remote African village, is today defined, studied, and mystified according to the techniques and styles of Europe and its diaspora. There is a remarkable irony here. The Europeans and their descendants who embarked on violent assaults on the rest of the world now dictate the theories and methods of comprehending the essentials of human psychology. The same Europeans and their diaspora who flourished because of slavery and colonialism have evidently set themselves up as the peacemakers and purveyors of what is human about us.

This obvious irony is itself related to a host of other ironies. For instance, in spite of numerous studies, Euro-American psychology is far from unraveling the mysteries of the human psyche. True, the difficulty depends in part upon the complexity of the human psyche itself. To solve the enigmas of the human psyche may be more complex than either splitting the atom or landing astronauts on the moon. And yet this fact alone cannot explain away the meager advances of Euro-American psychology. Even staunch supporters of this psychological tradition concede that the discipline has fallen short of its stated aims and promises. They admit that the amount of time, money, and energy devoted to a plethora of studies are hardly commensurate with the limited and uneven advances of psychology as a discipline. Explanations for the meager progress have been offered by various writers. But these explanations amount mostly to differences in schools of thought within the dominant psychology (Finkelman, 1978).

In our view, the limited and uneven advances of this psychology derive from the essentially *solipsist* character of its basic assumption, methods of

---

[2]Subsequent chapters will illustrate various manifestations of imperialism in psychology. For a discussion focused on imperialism in African psychological research, see Hussein A. Bulhan (1981a).

inquiry, and sources of experiential datum. *Solipsism* is the perspective that posits that only the "self" exists or can be proven to exist. The dominant psychology is founded and imbued with the outlook that (a) the Euro-American world view is the only or best world view; (b) positivism or neo-positivism is the only or best approach to the conduct of scientific inquiry; and (c) the experiences of white, middle-class males are the only or most valid experiences in the world. The first of these I call *assumptive solipsism;* the second, *methodological solipsism;* and the third, *experiential solipsism*. These three types of solipsism interpenetrate and influence one another. Together, they form the foundations of Eurocentric psychology.[3]

All psychological research and theorizing of course entail some basic assumptions about the world and human nature. Basic assumptions are implicit and often elusive. In their global assertions, basic assumptions are categorical and hardly permit exceptions. Basic assumptions are neither empirically derived nor open to scientific inquiry, but they nevertheless pervade our perceptions of the world and how we theorize about it. It so happens that the basic assumption of the dominant psychology is rarely examined or admitted. This avoidance in part derives from fears of undermining psychology's tenuous claims of its status as a science. To delve into the basic assumptions of a discipline that overidentifies with the natural sciences is to open Pandora's Box of untestable cultural ethos, values, and beliefs.

The assumptive solipsism of establishment psychology is manifested in its Eurocentric bias, control–prediction bias, analytic-reductionist bias, trait–comparison bias, and stability–equilibrium bias. To begin with, the dominant psychology is founded on and permeated with the implicit assumption that the only human reality is first *Euro-centric,* then *middle class,* and finally *male* in substance. What is not appreciated is that this culture-, class-, and sex-bound reality is but one instance in a universe of diverse human realities. Thus the reality of Euro-Middle-Class Males, imposed on the world through conquest, is elevated as the exemplar of human reality. The psychology of this minority is reified and generalized as the psychology of humanity everywhere. Only the "self" of this dominant and intrusive minority is recognized or considered the ideal. All other experiences are treated as chimera or caricature. What is true, typical, or beneficial for this exalted minority is assumed to be true, typical, and beneficial for all people everywhere. The (il)logic of this Eurocentric bias is peculiar indeed, but it pervades establishment psychology.

The control–prediction bias of psychology is perhaps the least difficult to discern. It is explicitly articulated in discussions of methodology when control of variables and prediction are acclaimed as the *sine qua non* of scientific inquiry. Parallel with and basic to this methodological ideal is the assumption that it is desirable to control nature and predict events long before they occur. This assumption in particular has had profound and global consequences. Although many non-European societies sought harmony with nature and with other people, Euro-America strove to *master* nature and *control* people. The

---

[3]Some variants of solipsism are discussed by Karl-Otto Apel (1972).

result was catastrophic. The wish to own and control, as we demonstrated, has forced many into the position of being the owned and the controlled. The technology that presumably was developed to meet human needs now threatens annihilation. The same technology also irreparably damages a worsening environment. Not only people and the environment, but also the future become the target of control. Anxiety about the future, which non-European cultures have resolved by other means, is mitigated by an obsession to predict events long before they occur. Indeed attempts are made to force the future to unfold according to a desired script. Psychology's uncritical embrace of a value-assumption extolling control and prediction has fostered a willing complicity in social control and oppression. Moreover, this value-assumption keeps Eurocentric psychologists from understanding the psychology of the non-white, non-middle-class majority in the world.

The analytic-reductionist bias of Eurocentric psychology entails the assumption that complex human experiences are better studied when reduced to their elemental and simple units. There is a vexing dilemma here. The dominant psychology overidentifies with the natural sciences. It aspires to adopt the methods and techniques that have proven effective in their sciences. Yet most psychological problems—and certainly all *relevant* human experiences—are inevitably complex, dynamic, and rarely amenable to neatly controlled experimentation or reducible to meaningful quantification. Establishment psychology commonly resolves this dilemma by giving precedence to positivist rigor over meaning and relevance. This overidentification with the natural sciences thus entails significant compromises in the substance and the understanding of human psychology. It also fosters two characteristic reductionisms. The first is reductionism to individual psychology or even a minor but quantifiable aspect thereof. The second is the all too familiar practice of reducing human psychology to its lowest animal denominator. People thus come to be considered as if they were rats and experimental rats as if they were human. What is more, even the experimental rats have been *white* (Guthrie, 1976). And since some humans are considered more animal-like than others, who but people of color, especially "primitive tribes," can provide simpler analogues of the complex psychology of Euro-Americans?

The trait–comparison bias of Eurocentric psychology posits that the primary task of psychology is the assessment of traits or abilities and, in addition, the comparison of individual differences of such traits or abilities. What is meant by *traits* or *abilities* and which of these are most salient to human psychology have been the subject of controversy. Typically, traits and abilities are considered to be stable, enduring characteristics of persons. Some psychologists view them as convenient constructs, whereas others insist that they indeed exist *in* persons.[4] Whether treated as constructs or entities, however, the presumed traits and abilities are often decontextualized and isolated from their socio-historical determinants. Batteries of tests and instruments to quantify them are thereby devised and debated as to their degree of reliability and

[4]For a detailed critique, see, for instance, Walter Mishel (1968).

validity. Invariably, the decontextualization of traits and abilities works to the advantage of white middle-class persons and to the disadvantage of the poor, the dispossessed, and the culturally different. This is best illustrated by the measurement of "intelligence" and the ways in which the fate of individuals are sealed long before they assume adult responsibilities. With the use of IQ tests, for instance, some students are catapulted to academic heights and promising careers, whereas others are relegated to special classes and inferior education (Kamin, 1976).

The stability–equilibrium bias has, like other biases, its function in the practice of social control and the wish to perpetuate the *status quo.* Stability, balance, and consonance are considered by Eurocentric psychologists to be more desirable than conflict, change, and upheaval (Riegel, 1976). Health is therefore defined as a state of equilibrium, and disease as a state of conflictual instincts or forces. Genuine conflicts between individuals and groups are also viewed as subjective aberrations traceable to human misunderstanding or faulty communication (Riegel, 1976). Conflicts within the person also are decontextualized and isolated from their socio-historical import. Various techniques are thereby elaborated to attain equilibrium through private utterances and insight. Such a stability–equilibrium bias is not confined to theories of psychopathology and psychotherapy. The same idealization of consistency and congruence is found in the theory of cognitive dissonance, which glorifies the maximization of internal consistency and of congruence in intrapersonal cognition. Of course, what this stability–equilibrium bias neglects is that conflict, contradictions, and change are not necessarily negative, but are indeed facts of everyday living and of human history. Not surprisingly, the stability–equilibrium bias appeals to those for whom the *status quo* is salutary and who vainly seek to stem inevitable changes. But "the wretched of the earth" finds such a stability–equilibrium bias unacceptable. Their dream, as Fanon pointed out, is only this: that "the last shall be the first."

Congruent with these basic assumptions and giving them concrete embodiment is the methodological solipsism of Eurocentric psychology, which takes two dominant and competing versions—namely, *subjectivism* and *positivism.* On the surface, the two approaches represent extremes with irreconcilable views on the source of knowledge and the conduct of inquiry. Subjectivism and its kindred approach of introspectionism found early articulation in the works of Descartes, Berkeley, and Kant. According to this approach, whatever exists and how it can be known are wholly or primarily mental. Thus Descartes found the starting point of certainty in his existence ("I think, therefore, I am"). Berkeley asserted that all reality is mental. Kant's emphasis on innate abilities gave impetus to "faculty psychology," in which such categories as memory, reason, and will gain ultimacy.

The positivist approach, in contrast, has its early roots in the works of Hume and later empiricists. Central to this approach is what has come to be called "the verificability principle of meaning." This principle maintains that (a) the truth or falsity of a statement is verifiable only by *empirical* observations; (b) the *meaning* of that statement is the mode of its verification; and (c) *values* are irrelevant to the conduct of inquiry.[5] The net consequence of this approach is that psychological reality is reduced to what can be codified, counted, and computed. In such a reduction, psychological reality is decontextualized, reified, and trivialized. The wish to attain scientific respectability forces a rigid adherence to count–measure rituals that compromise the salience of meaning and value in human experience.

The methodological solipsism of the two approaches becomes clear when both are considered from the perspective of the oppressed, the black, and the culturally different. In the first approach, the subjectivism and personal interpretations of Euro-American psychologists are imputed with utmost validity and generalized to humanity everywhere. How the Euro-American psychologist experiences his existence and what he intuits about others gain primacy first to him and later to his clients who willy-nilly accept his conclusions. Thus the factory worker resisting orders of a ruthless and exploitative supervisor may be told that his main problem is "latent, unresolved homosexuality." The female victim of rape may be urged to recognize and resolve her "unconscious wish for rape." The black patient is pronounced impervious to psychotherapy for assumed lack of "insight" or "verbal articulation." Any client who opposes such injunctions is considered neurotic or delusional. Any professional who questions such assertions comes to be known as a heretic or untutored in the mysteries of the psyche.

In the second approach, human experience is seen to exist only insofar as it permits the "operational definitions" of Euro-American psychologists. The meaning of that experience is reduced to count–measure operations and all values—except those of dominant psychologists—viewed as irrelevant or disturbing "contaminants" to the conduct of inquiry. The impression is given that operational definitions and value-free research are the royal road to scientific research. But what is rarely admitted is that concepts and instruments, and the psychologists who conceive of and use them, are inextricably fixed in a given world view, values, and interests. So long as the dominant world view, values, and interests remain unchallenged, the validity and reliability of specific operations can be disputed. Levels of statistical significance thus become potent criteria of evidence in such disputes. Questions about meaning, relevance, and values are readily resisted because they undermine the positivist foundation and cast doubt on Euro-American psychologists as the sole arbiters and validators of human experiences everywhere.

Beyond questions on assumptive domains and methodology, psychology is also plagued with experiential solipsism. The population to which most its theories pertain, the patients on whom therapeutic techniques are refined, the experimental subjects providing data for research, and the standard samples whose responses form the benchmark of psychological tests are invariably Euro-American and specifically white middle class. Conveniently ignored is the fact that a diversity of human experiences exists and that white, middle-class persons are a minority. The existential travails of a minority is thus

[5]See Kaplan (1964); see also Keat and Urry (1975).

generalized as universal human travails. The diagnostic classification and interventions elaborated for patients within this minority are considered appropriate for patients everywhere.[6] Research data generated from white middle-class samples are readily generalized to others who are neither white nor middle class. Psychological tests standardized on a sample within this minority are commonly applied to nonwhite, non-middle–class persons, often to their detriment.

The experiential solipsism of the dominant psychology is best illustrated by intelligence tests. Without exception, all intelligence tests have been developed and standardized on white and often middle-class samples. For instance, the 1937 standardization sample of the Stanford Intelligence Scale consisted of 3,184 white subjects. Later versions were little changed in this respect. Similarly, the early Wechsler-Bellevue Scale completely excluded people of color and underrepresented the rural population. Later revisions recognized this limitation, but no significant adjustments were made. Yet these scales are widely used for assessing many nonwhite, non-middle–class persons. Psychotherapeutic theories and techniques equally betray the same experiential solipsism. Although conceived and refined under different historical and sociocultural realities, these theories and techniques are readily assumed to have universal application. Benjamin Brody examined the 145 cases Sigmund Freud treated and demonstrated that the patients on which psychoanalytic theory was developed were "drawn exclusively from the upper and middle classes" (Brody, 1970, p. 11).

It would of course be foolish to deny that human psyches have some features in common across races, classes, and cultures. But it is also quite dangerous and shortsighted to ignore the solipsism and imperialism of Euro-American psychology. The fact is that the economic and political intrusion of Euro-America also entails psychological intrusion and self-aggrandizement. One of Fanon's early research projects was to delineate what aspects of the dominant psychology could be fruitfully applied to people of color. He built his initial study of racism around the psychoanalytic literature. In his first book, he invoked a wide array of recognized authorities, including Sigmund Freud, Carl Jung, Alfred Adler, Anna Freud, Otto Rank, and Jacques Lacan. But even as he invoked these authorities, Fanon maintained a critical posture toward the dominant psychology. Enriched later by the liberation struggle of Algeria, Fanon abandoned these authorities and outlined a transformative psychology unobscured by Euro-middle–class bias or solipsism.

FANON AND FREUD

In his Introduction to *Black Skin, White Masks,* Fanon (1967a, p. 10) stressed that "only a psychoanalytic interpretation of the black man can lay

---

[6]It is instructive to compare the three *Diagnostic Statistical Manuals* developed since the early 1950s, modified in 1968, and recently modified again to accommodate shifts in perspectives to psychopathology.

bare the anomalies of affect that are responsible for the structure of the [inferiority] complex." At this stage, Fanon identified himself as a psychoanalyst. Although Gendzier (1973) pointed out that Fanon had a disdain for being psychoanalyzed, he nevertheless used Freud's topographical (conscious, preconscious, unconscious) and structural (id, ego, superego) theories. At one point, Fanon seems to have even accepted Freud's pivotal notion of aggression and aim-inhibited sexuality. Thus, Fanon wrote (1967a, p. 41):

> Man is motion toward the world and toward his like. A movement of aggression, which leads to enslavement or to conquest; a movement of love, a gift of self, the ultimate stage of what by common accord is called ethical orientation. Every consciousness seems to have the capacity to demonstrate these two components, simultaneously or alternatively.

Most psychoanalysts would agree that Freud defined sexuality broadly. Some would even see a degree of equivalence in Fanon's concept of "love" with the notion of object-cathexis, which is central to the libido theory. But nowhere does Fanon clearly postulate "instincts" *per se*. Neither does he resort to explanations oriented to instinctual substrates, nor in fact is there any indication that Fanon accepted Freud's metaphysical extensions of aggression and sexuality into "Eros" and "Thanatos."

But that Fanon had an abiding interest in problems of aggression and sexuality is hardly a secret. Two chapters of *Black Skin, White Masks* focus directly on sexuality in a colonial and racist context: "The Woman of Color and the White Man" and "The Man of Color and the White Woman." In the chapter "The Negro and Psychopathology," Fanon (1967a, p. 160) elaborated the dynamic function of casting the black man as "phobogenic," a stimulus for anxiety, and then commented that

> If one wants to understand the racial situation psychoanalytically, not from a universal standpoint but as it is experienced by individual consciousness, considerable importance must be given to sexual phenomenon.

Indeed Fanon's occasional statements like "every intellectual gain requires a loss of sexual potential" (Fanon, 1967a, p. 165) are strong reminders of Freud's *Civilization and Its Discontents* as is more generally his notion of sublimated instinctual energies that must find socially acceptable means of expression.

Similarly, Fanon (1968) stressed throughout his work the significance of aggression as a central component to the human drama he studied and sought to transform. His extensive treatise concerning violence is in fact the first and most controversial chapter in *The Wretched of the Earth*. As we shall explain in Chapter 7, Fanon's treatise on violence was not, as some would have us believe, the result of an outburst of cataclysmic or anarchistic propensities. It was rather the crystallization of ideas grounded on observations of a personal and historical nature. From the very beginning, starting with *Black Skin, White Masks*, Fanon examined the clinical and political ramifications of the violence endemic to the colonial situation. He discussed covert as well as overt expressions of aggression and sexuality; their dialectical substitutions; their manifestations in language, fantasy, dreams, or psychopathology; and their relations to narcissism, masochism, and self-hate.

Yet it would be misleading to conclude from the preceding that Fanon embraced psychoanalytic theory which of course had very formative influences on his thinking. But even more misleading would be the suggestion that Freud's and Fanon's interests in aggression and sexuality derived from identical social and personal sources. Freud's theorizing emerged out of a nuclear, patriarchal, and bourgeois family context and within a sexually repressive Victorian Europe. Although he challenged the Victorian mores of his day, Freud was essentially an apologist for the *status quo* within the bourgeois family and the larger capitalist society. Reflecting his elitist mentality and class assimilation, Freud claimed that "those patients who do not possess a reasonable degree of education and a fairly reliable character should be refused" for psychoanalytic treatment. He later added with satisfaction that "precisely the most valuable and most highly developed persons are best suited for this procedure" (Jones, 1974, p. 307).

Fanon, on the other hand, was not a member of the ruling bourgeoisie or of the white race. Coming as he did out of a totally colonized island in the Caribbean, he had a firsthand knowledge of what it meant to be black and downtrodden. He observed how the search for recognition in a racist milieu was easily perverted to a consuming desire for "lactification," sometimes by means of an interracial marriage. He was a veteran of World War II who, having directly witnessed the horrors of war and torture, later gave himself uncompromisingly to a liberation struggle by the oppressed. It is therefore hardly surprising that Freud and Fanon were worlds apart in the ideological thrusts of their psychological formulations and social praxis, as they differed in their views of culture and human nature.

Fanon kept his critical outlook toward psychoanalysis even in his formative years when he wrote *Black Skin, White Masks*. Following Leconte's and Damey's critique on the classification of psychiatric syndromes, Fanon, in his Introduction to the book, distinguished between "sociodiagnostic" models and the traditional diagnosis founded on the medical model. This differentiation was preceded by a comment that both conceded Freud's contribution and exposed the weakness of his formulation (Fanon, 1967a, p. 11):

> Reacting against the constitutionalist tendency of the late nineteenth century, Freud insisted that the individual factor be taken into account through psychoanalysis. He substituted for a phylogenetic theory the ontogenetic perspective. It will be seen that the black man's alienation is not an individual question. Besides phylogeny and ontogeny stands sociogeny . . . let us say that this [Fanon analysis] is a question of sociodiagnostics.

Freud was of course the first to systematically examine personality development and to propose ordered psychosexual stages during childhood. Earlier theorists, unable to free their mind of religious or philosophical idealism, offered mystical or subjective propositions and presented commonsense views on the nature of consciousness. Others, captivated by the new discoveries of evolution, insisted on Social Darwinism with all the racist platitudes this implied. On the one hand, Freud's clinical studies ushered in an unprecedented focus on and interest in the history of the individual in contrast to earlier speculations on the history of man in the abstract. That Freud situated the individual psyche within the dynamic framework of age-specific, somatic demands in interaction with a particular environment was a revolutionary leap for psychology. With his psychological insights, Freud uncovered the content, structure, and formation of the individual psyche in a particular sociocultural context. At the same time, his clinical practice called into question the irrationalities and defenses of his society.

On the other hand, Freud revealed the narrow and reactionary kernel of his interpretations when he generalized the psychology of Europeans in a particular era to the universal human condition. He insisted that *sexuality* is the primary leitmotif of all human psychology and in addition reified the *bourgeois* family of his day as the most exemplar and most desirable human environment. One consequence of this insistence and reification was not only the analytic fragmentation and ossification of the human psyche, but also the elaboration of a metapsychology that is *a*historical if not *anti*-historical. Another consequence was the deprecatory outlook Freud consistently adopted toward the working class and particularly toward nonwhite, non-Western peoples. Time and again, Freud was to identify these peoples as having a "primitive psychology." He compared them with European neurotics or children and sometimes characterized them as infantile beings wallowing in instinctual perversity.

Fanon was bold in his critique of psychoanalytic theory even during the formative years when he wrote *Black Skin, White Masks*. Again in his introduction to his work, he took pains to dissociate his approach from Freud's ontogenetic perspective: "It will be seen that the black man's alienation is not an individual question. Beside phylogeny and ontogeny stands sociogeny." Having emphasized a sociogenetic perspective, Fanon in fact rejected Freud's ontogenetic reductionism and Jung's phylogenetic speculations. He questioned Freud's assumption of a necessary isomorphism or an unalterable antagonism between the individual and society. Equally unacceptable to Fanon were the generalizations of class- and culture-bound conflicts into inescapable human predicaments, the reduction of the human individual into a mere bundle of instincts, or the characterization of culture only in terms of a highly organized mechanism of repression under which weight people must renounce, delay, or modify tyrannical instincts of sex and aggression.

But nowhere was Fanon's critique of psychoanalysis more acute than in his outright rejection of the Oedipus complex. Forming the very edifice upon which rests Freud's interpretation of individual psychology and social organization, the Oedipus complex is crucial to psychoanalysis. Fanon (1967a, pp. 151–152) left no ambiguity about his views of this theory.

> It is too often forgotten that neurosis is not a basic element of human reality. Like it or not, the Oedipus complex is far from coming into being among Negroes. It might be argued, as Malinowski contends, that the matriarchal structure is the only reason for its absence. But, putting aside the question whether ethnologists are not so imbued with the complexes of their own civilization that they are compelled to try to find them duplicated in the peoples they study, it would be relatively easy for me to show that in the French Antilles 97 percent of the families cannot produce one Oedipal neurosis. This incapacity is one on which we heartily congratulate ourselves.

Taken too literally, one may with justification question Fanon's statistics and how he arrived at such a percentage. In fact his estimation of 97% is an example of his tendency to make a categorical affirmation even in the absence of precise data to support it. But taken figuratively and as a means of emphasis, Fanon's argument against the relevance of Oedipus complex is hardly surprising.

Many other giants besides Fanon have similarly questioned Freud's Oedipus complex, even within the Euro-American cultural context in which it was formulated. Adler, Jung, Horney, and Fromm are notable examples in a long list of psychologists for whom the dogmatic insistence on this theory and generally the libido theory was the primary reason for a serious rift with orthodox psychoanalysis. Among anthropologists, Kroeber's (1920) review of *Totem and Taboo* was the first serious challenge of Freud's hypothesis that the Oedipus complex formed the basis for culture and society. Nearly 20 years later, Kroeber's (1939) second review found "no reason to waver" in his earlier criticism of Freud's recapitulation theory.

A careful reading of the subsequent Jones–Malinowski debates and the equally heated Roheim–Kardiner sequel would lead to a greater appreciation of Fanon's contentions. Such a reading would also suggest a necessary caution against a glib and uncritical defense of what Gendzier has called the "sacred principles" of psychoanalysis. For instance, it is instructive to know that the most extreme conclusions of Freud's anti-historical reductionism found expression in Geza Roheim's ontological theory of culture. For according to Roheim (1943–44; 1943), the domestication of animals has not economic, but rather sexual motivations; agriculture represents an incestuous relation with "mother-earth"; trade is merely the ritualistic exchange of feces; even "war and international relationships are specifically based on the Oedipus situation."

On the surface, Fanon invoked the arguments of cultural relativity, ethnocentrism, and the prevailing moral collapse of Europe in his attack on the Oedipus complex. But on a more fundamental level, Fanon's rejection of the complex derives from a revolutionary perspective toward the notion of "culture"—a perspective that is implicit in *Black Skin, White Masks*, but finds greater explication in his succeeding works. Fanon's rejection of the Oedipus complex highlights his determination to explain human psychology within its essential socio-historical coordinates. He found unacceptable Freud's thesis that neurosis was an inescapable consequence of all cultures and thus inherent in the human condition. Fanon (1967a, p. 152) saw neurosis and all psychopathology as expressions of a given culture: "Every neurosis, every abnormal manifestation, every affective erethism . . . is the product of the cultural situation."

Thus the notion of culture is crucial in Fanon's thinking. He of course did not view culture according to the idealistic conception that isolates beliefs, values, and norms from their material foundation. In a 1956 speech before the First Congress of Negro Writers and Artists, Fanon defined culture as "the combination of motor and mental behavior patterns arising from the encounter of man with nature and with his fellow-men" (Fanon, 1967a, p. 32). Amilcar Cabral (1973, p. 41) later elaborated the same view of culture:

> In fact, culture is always in the life of a society (open or closed), the more or less
> conscious result of the economic and political activities of that society, the more or
> less dynamic expression of the kinds of relationships which prevail in that society, on
> the one hand between man (considered individually or collectively) and nature, and,
> on the other hand, among individuals, groups of individuals, social strata or classes.

Since the level of productive forces and the mode of production form the
material base of culture, psychological reductionism has no place in the Fanonian conception of culture and personality. Nor is culture assumed to be only
an instrument of repression, as Freud had in fact assumed. For if culture is the
dynamic synthesis of man's encounter with nature and with his fellowmen,
these encounters can turn out to be as deadly and repressive as they are life-
sustaining and liberating. Fanon had demonstrated these two possibilities of a
given culture. On the one hand, he showed how the black man's encounter
with his European fellowman entailed a profound depersonalization under the
weight of a repressive colonial culture. On the other hand, he outlined how the
struggle for liberation from an oppressive culture frees creativity and leads to a
capacity to transform that culture into an invigorating, nurturing force. The
Fanonian perspective therefore embraces man's vocation as both the *object*
and *subject* of history. The Freudian formulation, in contrast, is grounded in a
pessimistic and Schopenhauerian philosophy, negating man's ability to transform nature and himself.

FANON AND JUNG

It is primarily this radical approach to man and culture that led Fanon to
reject Jung's Lamarckian explanation of the "collective unconscious." Jung
distinguished three levels of the human psyche: *Consciousness, the personal
unconscious,* and *the collective unconscious.* He identified the personal unconscious as the repository of the individual's experiences that have been
repressed or temporarily discarded because of childhood trauma or unresolved
conflicts or of seeming irrelevance. The collective unconscious is, according to
Jung, a portion of the psyche that does not depend on personal experience. It is
instead the reservoir of "primordial images," which are inherited from the
ancestral past, extending to even prehuman (animal) ancestors. Using an er-
roneous conception of evolution, Jung explained these original images as inherited predispositions for experiencing and responding to the world.[7]

That Fanon made use of Jung's insights and concepts is without question.
In *Black Skin, White Masks,* he adopted Jung's notions of extroversion, intro-
version, complex, archetype, shadow, anima, animus, and the collective unconscious. In one study, for instance, Fanon (1967a, p. 166) used Jung's Word

[7]Jung relied on the discredited Lamarckian Theory of Evolution. The theory argued that change in
organic structure occurs in three main steps. First, the organism makes adaptive responses as it
encounters the physical environment. Second, this gradually results in a higher development of
those parts of the body that, in making adaptive responses, get more exercise and use. Third, the
developed feature of the organism is then passed on to offspring as an inherited characteristic.

Association Test. He interviewed some 500 members of the white race and on occasions inserted the word "Negro" among 20 other words. In almost 60% of his subjects, the word "Negro" brought forth associations of biology, penis, strong, athletic, potent, savage, animal, devil, sin, et cetera. From such Jungian approaches to the unconscious, Fanon (1967a, p. 190) concluded that in Europe "the Negro has one function: that of symbolizing the lower emotions, the baser inclinations, the dark side of the soul." Fanon in fact incorporated these denigrating symbolisms into the psychology of the "Manichean world," which we elaborate in Chapter 7. What is significant here is that Fanon readily made use of Jung's insights, as he had done with Freud's.

At the same time, however, Fanon did not hesitate to point out a serious limitation in Jung's contributions. In a characteristic manner that is by now familiar, he (Fanon, 1967a, p. 190) conceded the value of Jung's insights and simultaneously offered a devastating critique:

> I believe it is necessary to become a child again in order to grasp certain psychic realities. This is where Jung was an innovator: He wanted to go back to the childhood of the world, but he made a remarkable mistake: He went back only to the childhood of Europe.

Implied in this critique is of course the recognition of the same kind of ethnocentric orientation in Jung as in Freud's Oedipus complex theory. It was not so much Jung's insights into the European psyche that prompted Fanon's rejection. What Fanon resisted in particular was the effort to generalize this psychology into the universal human condition. Fanon turned to Jung in order to explain the unconscious processes by which blackness is associated with denigrating and sado-masochistic symbolism. But he was disappointed to find that Jung too had confused European man with man everywhere. Even Jung's research in non-Western cultures did not provide the necessary corrective. In addition, Jung failed to appreciate the traumatic effects of colonialism on the peoples of color he studied. These criticisms of Jung centered on his interpretation of the "collective unconscious" (Fanon, 1967a, p. 187).

> Continuing to take stock of reality, endeavoring to ascertain the instant of symbolic crystallization, I very naturally found myself on the threshold of Jungian psychology. European civilization is characterized by the presence, at the heart of what Jung calls the collective unconscious, of an archetype: an expression of the bad instinct, of the darkness inherent in every ego, of the uncivilized savage, the Negro who slumbers in every white man. And Jung claims to have found in uncivilized peoples the same psychic structure that his diagram portrays. *Personally, I think that Jung has deceived himself.* Moreover, all the peoples that he has known—whether the Pueblo Indians of Arizona or the Negroes of Kenya in British East Africa—have had more or less traumatic contacts with the white man.

Actually, Jung's (1930, pp. 83, 193–199) self-deception and racism are most blatant in an article that seems to have escaped Fanon's attention. The article, "Your Negroid and Indian Behavior," was addressed to an American audience. Jung recounts there his impression of Americans during a visit to the United States. His initial impression was that white Americans have "an amazing amount of Indian blood." But to this first impression of Indian strain in most Americans, Jung then asserted that the white American psyche and culture have a significant Indian and Negro component. But in addition to simply drawing this conclusion, Jung openly deplored the "racial infection" this nonwhite component entailed and moreover traced many American "peculiarities" to Indian and Negro influences. The American peculiarities for which people of color were held responsible include childlikeness, exhibitionism, emotional incontinence, high promiscuity, Negroid mannerism in whites, and an overall propensity toward the primitive and primordial. Thus for instance: "It would be difficult not to see that the Negro, with his primitive motility, his expressive emotionality, his childlike immediacy, his sense of music and rhythm, his funny picturesque language, has infected American behavior" (Jung, 1930).

Living in close proximity with "primitive peoples" and particularly "Negroes" was said to seriously contaminate whites, psychologically, culturally, and even physiologically. What is more, the primitivizing and "heavy downward pull" of uncivilized neighbors was viewed by Jung (1930) as nothing short of a contagion like the plague.

> Now what is more contagious than to live side by side with a rather primitive people? Go to Africa and see what happens. . . . The inferior man exercises a tremendous pull upon civilized beings who are forced to live with him. . . . To our subconscious mind contact with primitives recalls not only our childhood, but also our prehistory.

Jung's bigotry was thus neither subtle nor tentative. His racism was not simply intellectual. Jung lived out his racism in interpersonal contacts. For instance Jung recounts one incident during a visit to "a stiff and solemn New England family whose respectability was almost terrifying." At dinner, Jung attempted to crack jokes but without success. He then decided: "Well, Indian blood, wooden faces, camouflaged Mongols. Why not try some Chinese on them?" Jung in addition points out that a "Negro servant" was waiting on the table and that the great expert of collective unconscious was "cautiously scrutinizing the dishes, looking for imprints of those black fingers." Here then is one major pioneer of Euro-American psychology—a pioneer who established for himself a reputation for going beyond the superficial, the immediate, and the pedestrian. And this is what his claims of the sublime, universal, and fundamental has come to: *simply, the obscenities of a shameless racist enthralled with his own racism.*

Yet it would be incorrect to suggest that Fanon rejected Jung's notion of the collective unconscious in the categorical manner with which he debunked Freud's Oedipus complex. With marked ambivalence, Fanon endorsed Jung's concept of the collective unconscious: "Unless we make use of that frightening postulate—which so destroys our balance—offered by Jung, the *collective unconscious,* we can understand absolutely nothing" (Fanon, 1967a, pp. 144–145). What Fanon objected to was not therefore the notion of the collective unconscious *per se,* but rather Jung's interpretations based on it. For the Jungian interpretation of the collective unconscious was not only ethnocentric, but also too archeological, both approaches defying historical and rational comprehension. In particular, Fanon (1967a, p. 188) found the Lamarckian underpinnings of Jung's interpretation too strong a brew to swallow.

> Jung locates the collective unconscious in the inherited cerebral matter. But the collective unconscious, without having to fall back on the genes, is purely and simply the sum of prejudices, myths, collective attitudes of a given group.

Thus Fanon substituted a cultural-historical formulation for the evolutionary interpretations of Jung. He differentiated *instinct* and *habit* on a philosophical level. Instinct, according to Fanon, is inborn, invariable, specific; habit is acquired, learned. Making this distinction, he then charged that "Jung has confused instinct and habit" when he located the collective unconscious in cerebral matter and characterized it as "permanent engrams of the race." This evolutionary conception clashed with Fanon's radical conception of man and culture. He (Fanon, 1967a, p. 188) instead maintained that "the collective unconscious is cultural, which means acquired." By following such a cultural-historical orientation, however, Fanon did not of course deny the significance of biological substrates of the psyche. He only asserted that the sociological dimension is more *viable* and *determining*—a radical conception that increasingly dominated Fanon's world view.

This radical conception was later explicitly elaborated by Cabral (1973, pp. 64–65) in another context. According to this sociogenetic perspective, man's biological constitution defines a given set of advantages and limitations that is more or less constant among nationalities and races. Conscious, organized, and collective praxis defines man's ontological vocation as the subject of history. Through this praxis and because of it, he transforms nature, harnesses his environmental and biological resources, dominates others, or liberates himself from repressive social structures. Thus for Fanon (1967a, p. 80), even "the organic, or constitutional, is a myth only for him who can go beyond it." Jung failed to go beyond the organic and the hereditary. The mythological and mystifying thrust of his Lamarckian theories were thus incompatible with Fanon's radical conception of man and culture.

Fanon and Adler

More than Freud and Jung, Adler comes closest to Fanon's psychological perspective. Adler was an ardent socialist in his youth and continued to take a passionate interest in the social problems of his day.[8] In contrast to both Freud and Jung, Adler had grown up amidst a working class population with whom he maintained a degree of emotional attachment. His earliest work, *Health Book for the Tailor Trade*, reflects the degree of Adler's class consciousness. More particularly, it established him as a pioneer in the field of social medicine and public health. In subsequent works, Adler emphasized the social origin of

---

[8]Adler's socialist leanings are underscored by his thoughts as in *Understanding Human Nature* (1965, see, e.g., pp. 34–35).

neurosis and elaborated the importance of the familial (particularly the sibling)
constellation for personality development. Education, social praxis, and
creativity occupy a more central position in Adler's individual psychology
than either Freud's psychoanalysis or Jung's analytical psychology.

Fanon readily adopted Adler's concepts of inferiority, superiority, domi-
nance, compensation, life-style, and social interest. He was in fact using an
Adlerian formulation when he (Fanon, 1967a, p. 157) remarked that "the white
man behaves toward the Negro as an older brother reacts to the birth of a
younger." Fanon made a number of references to Adler's *Understanding
Human Nature* and *The Nervous Character.* The chapter "The Feeling of
Inferiority and the Striving for Recognition" in Adler's *Understanding Human
Nature* seems to have had a particular impact on Fanon. Summarized in this
chapter were some of Adler's central concepts: organ inferiority, subjective
inferiority, compensation, striving for superiority, life-style, social feeling, and
sibling constellation. Fanon adeptly used some of these concepts to unveil the
psychopathologies endemic in the colonial situation. In contrast to Freudian or
Jungian theories, the Adlerian influences on him were more pervasive in his
original work and less discordant with his ideological persuasion.

In *Black Skin, White Masks,* Fanon in fact devoted a whole section to the
Negro and Adler. Fanon (1967a, p. 211) stated here what he called "the first
truth": The Negro is a *comparison* who is constantly preoccupied with self-
evaluation and self-validation.

> The Antilleans have no inherent values of their own, they are always contingent on
> the presence of the other. The question is always whether he is less intelligent than I,
> less respectable than I. Every position of one's own, every effort at security, is based
> on relations of dependence, with the diminution of the other. It is the wreckage of
> what surrounds me that provide the foundation of my virility.

Underlying this preoccupation with comparison, this obsession with self-validation, is a diffuse aggression, a wish to dominate, a striving for superiority,
and more fundamentally, an inferiority complex to which the rest are only
compensatory reactions. The black man is obsessed with his manhood because
the oppressor emasculated him. But since the black man is yet unable to
liberate himself from the arsenal of internalized complexes, his compatriots or
individuals less fortunate than he become easy prey for his reactive aggression
and false sense of superiority. This "Adlerian leech" is of course historical in
origin (Fanon, 1967a, p. 213).

> If we are strict in applying the conclusions of the Adlerian school, we should say
> that the Negro is seeking to protest against the inferiority he feels historically. Since
> in all periods the Negro has been an inferior, he attempts to react with a superiority
> complex.

By self-analysis and observation Fanon discerned the overt and subtle manifestations of the Adlerian dynamics in such diverse contexts as language
acquisition, sex, marriage, family constellation, child-rearing practices, and
intellectual endeavors. It was indeed a central theme of his first book that
neither "authentic love" nor creative self-actualization is attainable until

"one has purged oneself of that feeling of inferiority or that Adlerian exalta-
tion, that overcompensation, which seems to be the indices of the black
Weltanschauung (Fanon, 1967a, p. 42). In subsequent chapters, we will demonstrate Fanon's remarkable use of the inferiority complex and his views on how
best to purge oneself of debilitating complexes.

Yet in spite of having assimilated these Adlerian influences, Fanon's critical and creative mind could never allow him to embrace any formulation
conceived under other skies and for a different population. Here again, as in
many other instances, Fanon needed to re-formulate and re-interpret. Freud's
psychoanalytic theorizing was found wanting mainly because of the unwarranted generalizations of the Oedipus complex. Jung was debunked when he
resorted to the Lamarckian theory of evolution to explain the collective unconscious. Adler too was criticized for his limited and somewhat incidental emphasis on sociopathogenic factors in the development of neurosis and character
disorder. For in his central theory of organ inferiority as in his conception of
social conflict, Adler was deeply entrenched in the tradition of the medical
model and the Social Darwinism of his day. Fanon (1967a, p. 213) was particularly critical of his teleological and ontogenetic explanations.

> In effect, Adler has created a psychology of the individual. We have just seen that
> the feeling of inferiority is an Antillean characteristic. It is not just this or that
> Antillean who embodies the neurotic formulation, but all Antilleans. Antillean soci-
> ety is a neurotic society, a society of "comparison." Hence we are driven from the
> individual back to the social structure. If there is a taint, it lies not in the "soul" of
> the individual but rather in that of the environment.

When Adler paid sufficient attention to sociogenetic factors, his theorizing did not extend fundamentally beyond the parameters of family dynamics
and sibling constellations. What he conceded *ideologically* but failed to accomplish *in fact* was a grounding of his theories in a socio-historical and
cultural foundation in which the family itself is a mediator and a microcosm.
Fanon was dissatisfied with Adler's delimitation of the "environment." It is of
course true that Adler attempted to rehabilitate the previously fragmented and
reified psyche with a unitary and holistic psychology. But the development of a
genuine sociogenetic psychology eluded him. Social reality remained for him
an encounter between separate and distinct egos, interacting with and dominating each other within the limited space–time coordinates of the family.
This narrow and personalistic overemphasis of Adler was indeed incompatible
with Fanon's repeated observations. The black man feels inferior *historically*,
not because of an organic defect or a simple familial dysfunction. Hence Fanon's personal dissociation from Adlerian psychology (Fanon, 1967a, p. 215).

> All the facts that I have noted are real, but, it should not be necessary to point out,
> they have only a superficial connection with Adlerian psychology. The Martinican
> does not compare himself with the white man *qua* father, leader, God; he compares
> himself with his fellows against the [cultural] pattern of the white man. . . . The
> Adlerian comparison embraces two terms; it is polarized by the ego. The Antillean
> comparison is surmounted by a third term: its governing fiction is not personal but
> social.

In short, Fanon sought to unravel the debilitating consequences of economic and cultural domination. For Freud, Jung, and Adler, such an analysis was both inaccessible and irrelevant from their personal, class, cultural, and racial standpoints.[9] Bourgeois psychologists of unquestionably high caliber, they studied a particular type of psyche from affluent and central heights during the heyday of colonialism. Their patients emerged from a relatively stable sociocultural framework that had not been shaken by the violent ruptures of colonialism. *Individual differences* in health and pathology seemed to them most conspicuous and explanations of them most pressing in their clinical work with bourgeois patients whose economic and cultural realities were intact. They subsequently postulated a type of human reality—namely, bourgeois psychological reality—as the condition of man everywhere. Conformity or deviation from this bourgeois reality thus became the absolute criterion for health and pathology.

Fanon's roots were in contrast in a vastly different *historical context.* In personal temperament and social origin, he had the special advantage of experiencing and grasping the meaning of oppression from the perspective of a colonial victim. For him, sociogeny took a definite precedence over both ontogeny and phylogeny. The fragmenting effect of ontogenetic perspective and the ossifying consequences of phylogenetic explanations obscured a fundamental dimension of the human psyche. Because of their conservative thrust, both ontogeny and phylogeny negate man's vocation as a subject of history and thus dash any hopes of social change. Ontogeny reveals man the *individual*—the helpless, hopeless, and isolated object of a repressive and overpowering social structure. Phylogeny points to the futility of man's resistence against a curse that is embedded in an irretrievable past. As consistently argued throughout his writings, it was Fanon's unwavering conviction that the fundamental cause of alienation is first socioeconomic and second the internalization of societal inequity as well as violence. To be effective and meaningful, according to Fanon, all efforts toward disalienation must therefore intervene both at the socioeconomic and the psychological level.

This sociogenetic perspective prompted Fanon to guard against the abstract postulation of categorical classification of "human reality and describe its psychic modalities only through deviation from it." A psychology founded in a social dialectic was for him the only reliable basis to "strive unremittingly for a concrete and new understanding of man." As we show in subsequent chapters, this shift from ontogeny to sociogeny is indeed the precondition for a Fanonian radical psychology and therapy appropriate to the wretched of the earth.

---

[9]Fanon (1967a, p. 151) emphasized that "Freud and Adler and even the cosmic Jung did not think of the Negro in all their investigations."

5

COLONIAL RESEARCH AND MEDICINE

Science depoliticized, science in the service of man, is often non-existent in the colonies.

—Fanon, *A Dying Colonialism*

Colonialism and racism are two integral and coordinated assaults on people of color. The violence that gives them birth and sustains them inevitably reverberates in all spheres of social existence. In the colonial as in the racist society, no human activity remains untarnished. The ambience of violence is everywhere. Even the search for knowledge and the honored practice of healing become easily perverted into instruments of greed, social control, and dehumanization. A review of Euro-American research and medical practice demonstrates that colonialism is not merely a product of petty officials and that racism is not simply an emotional quirk of ignorant laymen.

Contrary to common claims, racism finds its origin and support among the "best representatives" of Euro-America. Even the tools used by Western scholars and physicians serve as a veritable arsenal for human subjugation and exploitation.

This chapter examines two crucial human endeavors—namely, the conduct of research and the practice of healing—in the context of oppression. First, it examines the kind of questions about people of color that for decades preoccupied Euro-American researchers and physicians. Second, the chapter highlights the role of medicine in conquest. We will see that not only did physicians work closely with colonial administrators, but that they also provided a new impetus to oppression where men of arms and of religion had failed. Finally, the chapter explains Fanon's seminal contributions in his critiques of such research and medical practices. It should become clear from this that Fanon's insights suggest that Western scholarship and the Western practice of medicine be critically reevaluated.

RACISM IN RESEARCH

As early as the 1700s a debate was raging among Victorian scientists regarding the educability of the African. In 1799 the Briton Charles White agreed with the conclusions of von Soemmering of Germany that the African was lacking in intelligence, and this affected the outcome of the debate just preceding the 1807 Anti-Slavery Trade Act. In spite of evidence to the contrary, White's conclusions struck a responsive chord since this provided a "scientific" rationalization of slavery. Samuel Morton, an American physician and a professor of anatomy, had also established a trans-Atlantic reputation for his conclusion that the black man was intellectually inferior to the Caucasian.[1]

What is more, with the publication of Darwin's *The Origin of Species* and the economic motives for regarding the African as subhuman, it required little originality from President Hunt of the Anthropological Society of London to assert that the black man "descended from the ape only a few generations ago."[2] Such denigration of blacks in the name of science was by no means confined to British and American intellectual circles. In 1860, for instance, the Frenchman Paul Broca reported that the brain of the African weighed 78.5 grams less than that of the European. At about the same time, the more influential de Gobineau propounded a doctrine that the "different races of humankind are innately unequal in talent, worth, and ability to absorb and create culture." He argued further that it was absurd to maintain an equality of races in any sphere of social existence. In his *Essai sur l'inegalité des races humaine*, de Gobineau laid the foundation for the supremacist Nordic School. He argued there that "the various branches of human family are distinguished by permanent and irradicable differences, both mentally and physically . . . [and] the dark races are the lowest on the scale."[3] Thus according to de Gobineau, people of color are not only unintelligent, they are also innately incapable of creating the rudiments of culture.

These early claims of inequality among the races indeed found their absurd extremes in the work of men like Caroll who set out to compile "evidence that the negro is not of the human family" (Burns, 1948, p. 22). In a work published in 1902, Caroll went so far as to assert that "all the evidence indicates that the beast of the field which tempted Eve was a *negress* who served Eve in the capacity of a maid servant" (Burns, 1948, p. 22). Innate inferiority, inherited criminality, and domestic servitude were thus suggested to be the primordal nature of the black race. The master–slave relationship between whites and blacks was not viewed as a phenomenon of a given historical epoch, but rather as a fact of nature. These early rationalizations of slavery have had lasting effects on later psychological research in Africa. The pseudo-science that justified slavery later was used to rationalize colonialism in Africa.[4]

In the 1920s, Lucien Levy-Bruhl took upon himself the task of "enlightening" his readers on the thought processes of the African. Levy-Bruhl propounded a *concreteness thesis* and the classification of a "prelogical mentality" to describe the African's mode of thought. It was accordingly surmised

[1]See, for instance, S. G. Morton (1839).
[2]Quoted in V. M. Brattle and C. H. Lyons (1970, p. 8).
[3]Quoted in Alan Burns (1948, p. 77).
[4]For a detailed discussion, see Bulhan (1981b).

that the African, unlike the European, had yet to develop the capacity for logical and abstract thinking. The African was said to rely merely on memory and lacked the capacity for individuation. A belief in mystical causation and the failure to learn from experience were also seen to be distinguishing characteristics. Assuming that the development of thought processes was genetically determined, Levy-Bruhl concluded that the African mode of thought had to belong to an earlier phylogenetic stage.

Despite some definite but indecisive opposition, Levy-Bruhl's view significantly influenced Euro-American psychologists for decades. These views of Euro-American psychologists, fostered by a particular social and material relationship, were readily used in the service of colonialism. It therefore comes as no surprise that Dougall (1932, p. 251), for one, wrote:

> The theory [of Levy-Bruhl] is supported by a mass of data and reasoned with great *persuasion*. . . . As such, it deserves the closest study, not only because it accounts for many facts in African thought and behavior but also because it would . . . have far-reaching consequences in the framing of *practical* policies and modes of dealing with the African.

In most instances, however, colonial rulers did not wait until their academicians derived from theory "practical policies and modes of dealing with the African." Colonial armies and administrators had long ensured the ruthless exploitation and forced subjugation of the African. What was needed instead was an institutionalized rationalization to stifle the consciousness and conscience of its own agents, real or potential. A scientific basis for rationalization could only further fortify colonialism.

Now it is not sufficient to attribute to the African a "prelogical mentality." The African had to be characterized in subhuman terms as a freak of nature, or at least as a subnormal human being whose infantile proclivities and dependency needs call for the exercise of external authority or the presence of a parent–surrogate. Thus Ritchie (1943, p. 61) argued for the existence of two forces in African psychology. He suggested the presence of a benevolent force giving him everything for nothing and a malevolent force depriving him of life itself. The subsequent ambivalence and conflict are said to make the African dependent on a mother or a mother surrogate. Furthermore, it is argued that the individual personality of the African "is never liberated and brought under conscious rational control." The implication here, as in Mannoni's analysis (discussed later), is that the African looks upon the European colonizer as a parent surrogate who protects him and meets his innate dependency needs.

Similar contentions of low intelligence, dependency needs, and lack of individuation recur in later psychological research on the African. For instance, Haward and Roland (1954, 1955) compared the scores of Nigerian and European subjects on the Goodenough Draw-a-Man Test. Their interpretation of the scores included suggestions of a low-level personal individuation, an inability to abstract or synthesize, a failure to develop a self-image or body-boundary, and thus "the existence of certain psychological mechanisms or frames of thought which he [the African] appears to share with the white

84 CHAPTER 5

mental patient." (Haward and Roland, 1954, p. 87). They concluded also that the African finds pleasure in routine activities and that "this love of repetition is doubtless but another manifestation of the rigid and concrete attitude of the native" (Howard S. Roland, 1955, p. 28). What is more, they argued that "his concreteness of mentation does not admit of compromise, only imitation, for it has long been established that the Negro races are natural mimics." One implication of this alleged concreteness is of course this: "When introducing him to Western work routine, one finds it convenient to adopt an approach suited to a European child of ten" (Howard S. Roland, 1954, p. 87).

More recently, Parin and Morgenthaler (1970, p. 194) used psychoanalytic concepts in a study of character formation among Africans. They concluded that the African lacks a superego, operates solely on the pleasure principle, has no work ethic and is incapable of guilt, and responds only to "command from an external authority; imitation of, and identification with, a prestige-bearer; reward and punishment." In an effort to support these contentions, Parin and Morgenthaler cited what in their view represented typical cases. One of these concerns a European missionary and an ordinary African. "The White Father" is said to have implored the African to work on a particular task as a favor. When the African refused, the missionary immediately resorted to firm command. The African is said to quickly resume the task with this retort: "You should not have asked me whether I minded it; you should have told me straight-away that I have to do it" (Parin & Morgenthaler, 1970, p. 194).

Another illustration is said to be that of African road builders who explained to their European foreman why they failed to execute a given task: "Neither you nor your deputy were watching us! As long as one of you is there, we will work quite willingly." Thus here again, as in so many other works, external authority and ruthless control were being justified in the name of science. When by 1960 many African countries gained their independence, Euro-American research in Africa changed in tone and language. This shift was in form, not in function. Reports came to be couched less blatantly, with fewer racist terms. Yet one function of research remained that of social control and rationalization of the oppressive *status quo.* As I have shown elsewhere (Bulhan, 1981), neo-colonialism and apartheid advance numerous pseudo-scientific psychological theories for the social control and exploitation of African labor.

RACISM IN MEDICINE

That racism in the era of slavery continued into the epoch of colonialism is borne out not only by the assertions of psychologists, but also by the pronouncements of Euro-American physicians. As psychologists and anthropologists persisted in the contention that the African is innately unintelligent and genetically inferior, their counterparts in medicine were busy compiling all sorts of "scientific evidence" to support these and even more pessimistic conclusions. These affirmations and conclusions had particular weight because physicians had by the nineteenth century emerged as the sole arbiters of debates on the anatomical and physiological differences among racial groups. And what obsessed Euro-American physicians about blacks, and the instruments they elaborated, illustrate the substance and method of a truly shameful aspect of medical science.[5]

There is hardly an aspect of black anatomy or physiology that has not been scrutinized by Euro-American physicians. They observed and measured the sexual organs of blacks. They determine skull size and shape. They compared brain weights and even brain convolutions with those of other races. They sought to infer human destiny from hair texture and hair color. They recorded differences in skin color and examined melanocytes. They predicted the longevity of black people and concluded that black survival is untenable. And having asserted that blacks were a menace to the Caucasian race, they set out to map the schedule and pattern of black extinction. In short, the assault on black people has been total, as physicians coordinated their activities with Euro-American men of arms, political administrators, and scholars in the human sciences. Physicians have long endeavored to provide scientific justification for slavery, colonial rule, and racial segregation.

One widely held belief of nineteenth-century physicians was that the emancipation of blacks in America would bring about their total extinction. Joseph Camp Kennedy, a noted statistician and superintendent of the Eighth Census, remarked in 1862 that the actual extinction of the black race was an "unerring certainty" (Haller, 1970a, p. 154). He argued that freedom for and gradual assimilation of blacks would only hasten the process of extinction. Physicians subsequently compiled various types of data to confirm this. The Ninth and Tenth Census of 1870 and 1880, research by the United States Army, statistical data from insurance companies, numerous reports from physicians—all these were used to corroborate the inevitable end of the black race. Having embraced Kennedy's prediction, physicians then set out to determine the causes of this impending extinction. These causes are indeed as interesting as the prediction itself.

E. T. Easley, an important Texan physician, argued in 1875, that emancipation was the major cause of the manifest deterioration of the black race. He considered the emancipation of blacks as "the most deplorable event in the history of that race" and further suggested that freedom brought to blacks social status for which they were innately ill-equipped (Holler, 1970b, p. 256). According to Easley, the white slaveowner who best knew how to be a nurturing caretaker of black slaves was now saddled with the responsibility of being the undertaker of free blacks. Eugene R. Corson, writing in the prestigious *New York Medical Times* in 1887, agreed with Easley's conclusions. He added that blacks were more prolific, but died off much faster than whites. This pattern, Corson argued, follows the biological principle that simple organisms have greater "potential prolificness," but they lack the ability of more complex

[5]For a detailed discussion of racism in psychology, psychiatry, and medicine, see Alexander Thomas and Samuel Sillen (1974). Also see Allan Chase's (1977) monumental work.

organisms for individual survival (Haller, 1970a, p. 156). That physicians like Easley and Corson were inspired by the works of Malthus, Darwin, and Spencer is not surprising.

Edward A. Ballock of Howard University meanwhile proposed several anthropometric generalities about black people. He suggested that blacks have a "lessened sensibility" at their nervous system, which made them more able to endure surgery. Physicians of the U.S. Army performed extensive postmortem examination of black soldiers during the Civil War in order to find suspected anomalies in black anatomy and brain weight. On the basis of army investigations, W. J. Burt concluded that blacks have "little elasticity of temperament" and lack "nervous endurance and moral courage." He also added that, contrary to Ballock, blacks show a "fearful mortality" in all surgical operations and thus the ordinary practice of medicine is inappropriate for black people (Haller, 1970a, p. 160).

If the prediction of inevitable extinction was intended to decry freedom for blacks, the view that ordinary medical practice was inappropriate for blacks effectively prevented the chance of blacks benefiting from advances in medicine. More fundamentally, the prediction of extinction and the contention of medical irrelevance had in effect relegated blacks to a subhuman status and tantalized the genocidal wishful thinking of the racist. Both the prediction and contention also assuaged the conscience of those who otherwise would have been alarmed by the high disease and mortality rates among oppressed blacks. As Chase (1977) clearly shows, the prediction of imminent extinction is today replaced by the fear of a high black birth rate in America: Hence the crude and subtle programs of today to sterilize the black underclass.

Yet the current effort at sterilization is but a feature of an old, morbid obsession with the sexual organs of blacks. Since the nineteenth century, Euro-American physicians have made scurrilous remarks about black sexuality. Claims were frequently made that the sexual organs of blacks were of "massive proportions." Black males were all too often depicted to have an uncontrollable "stallion-like passion" and were viewed as "a menace to the Caucasian race." Much was also made of a presumed relationship between sexual precocity of and mental arrest in blacks. Blacks were said to exhibit sexual passion at an earlier age. It was also argued that mental atrophy at a later age made them slaves to sexual impulses. The concern that black males were a menace to the Caucasian race was heightened by rape of white women by black men. The more frequent rape of black women by white men was never a cause of similar alarm or serious research.

The association often made between emancipation and "sexual bestiality" of blacks is indeed interesting. But more remarkable are the kind of solutions physicians proposed to counter the black menace. Many physicians argued against the education, assimilation, and migration of black people. William Lee Howard, a Baltimore physician, maintained, in 1903, that education will neither "reduce the large size of the negro's penis" nor "prevent the African's birthright to sexual madness and excess" (Haller, 1970a, p. 163). Dr. Charles S. Bacon of Chicago argued that education for blacks is as "out of place as a piano in a Hottentot's tent" and that blacks are "just as devoid of ethical sentiment or consciousness as the fly or the maggot" (Haller, 1970a, p. 166). What is more, miscegenation as a solution to the "negro problem" was seen as more abhorrent by Euro-American physicians than were efforts to educate and culturally assimilate blacks.

If interracial marriages and the education of blacks were unacceptable to these physicians, one would suppose that these scholars would welcome suggestions of forced repatriation of a people they consider a menace to the Caucasian race. The truth was indeed the contrary. Physicians were well aware of the place of blacks in the economy and they strongly opposed such forced migration. Dr. Charles S. Bacon indeed argued that black workers form "too valuable an economic factor to be eliminated." What he suggested instead were tactics to prevent the political and social organization of blacks. The solution he and others suggested to combat the "negro menace" was selective castration. For instance Professor Lydston at the Chicago College of Physicians once proposed that castration would make blacks "docile, quiet, and inoffensive." He added that the castration of some black men "would be a constant warning and ever-present admonition to others in their race" (Haller, 1970a, pp. 163–164). Of course, such blatant propositions were consistent with the prevailing wisdom in those days when lynching of black males was a common American ritual.

Yet none of these racist assertions are as shocking and scandalous as the recently halted Tuskegee experiment on syphilis among blacks in Macon County, Alabama (Jones, 1981). The study was conducted by the U.S. Public Health Service in collaboration with various state and federal health agencies. Syphilis is of course a serious and contagious disease, which, if untreated, in time, attacks many vital organs including the central nervous and the cardiovascular systems. The project involved a follow-up study of 400 black males and their families. For 40 years, these victims of syphilis and their families have been duped into cooperating in this research. In order to study the effects of untreated syphilis, they were never informed that they had syphilis and were not treated. The study started in 1932 and ended as recently as 1972. The ostensible aim of the study was to study the effects of untreated syphilis. More fundamentally, however, the assumption and thrust of this study derived from the racist obsession of American physicians with black sexuality.

Reading about such projects, one is reminded of Aime Césaire's assertion that we have been lied to: *"Hitler is not dead!"* What is actually most frightening is that the syphilis study could have been undertaken so recently and that physicians under the Hippocratic Oath could engage in such ruthless practices. The fact remains, however, that Euro-American physicians have all along been among the staunchest supporters of racism and colonialism. Certain of them have of course been vocal on the plight of blacks and active in social reform. But the elitist character of their training and practice has tended to insulate most Euro-American physicians from the miseries of blacks and the oppressed. Those who came into contact with the poor and the dispossessed tended to blame the victim.

It would take us far beyond the objectives of this chapter to detail the racism of Euro-American scholars and physicians. The preceding illustrations, taken from various eras, underscore the fact that Euro-American research and medicine have served as instruments of domination. A more detailed exposition would show that the charge of genetic inferiority regarding the poor generally, and people of color particularly, has reappeared in temporal clusters associated with periods of heightened social crisis and change.

An early cluster followed the discovery and effective settlement of the Americas. Exemplified by the debate between Bartolome de la Casas and Gines de Sepulveda, this charge was based on the debate of whether Native Americans should be enslaved. A second cluster emerged during the French Revolution. Gobineau and his cohorts asserted the superiority of the aristocracy and the Aryan race. A third cluster occurred during the Industrial Revolution. Malthus, Galton, and Spencer argued for the biological elimination of the poor and people of color.

Just prior to the American Civil War, we discern a fourth cluster of racism in scholarship. This racism was heralded by proslavery forces. Fifth, sixth, and seventh clusters emerged consecutively during the colonial scramble in Africa, the rising wave of immigration during the early 1900s, and the Supreme Court decision of 1954 that made segregation illegal. The seventh cluster coincided with the struggle for independence in Africa. The latest resurgence of academic racism followed President Johnson's "Great Society" program. This was heralded by Jensen's well-publicized diatribe on the IQ of blacks. Recent reactions to Affirmative Action and busing for purposes of school desegregation have obviously given impetus to scientific racism under the rubric of "sociobiology" (Wilson, 1978).

Medicine and Conquest

Disease of course occurs in all societies. Communities all over the world summon healers in times of personal distress and physical affliction. The universal desire for physical and mental well-being permits healers to wield unusual power and influence in every society. Such power and influence emanate not only from the unique function of healers, but also such power and influence are to some extent necessary for the process of healing itself. But to limit the misuse of a healer's power and influence, ethical codes govern the practice of healing in all societies. The Hippocratic Oath is the best known. The judicious use of the healers' power and influence are therefore considered sacrosanct. It can happen, however, that healers employ their power and skills in the service of social oppression and greed. The introduction of Western medicine in Africa illustrates this.

Historically, colonial subjugation has followed a well-known pattern. First to come are colonial soldiers or missionaries. The soldier "pacificied" the population by dint of superior arms. The missionary, armed with the Bible, infiltrated remote villages to self-righteously save "heathens" from hellfire.

The soldier and missionary—whoever came first—destabilized the native society. The other simply mopped-up following the devastation. The brawn and resolve of the colonized "pacified," the rear-guard personnel of colonialism were then promptly deployed. Physicians and teachers soon arrived to complete the process of subjugation. The colonized were in the end broken physically and spiritually.

The physician was often a missionary or an army doctor. It would be tedious to recount the legends, like those of Dr. Livingston, that dewy-eyed apologists of colonialism have widely propagated. But what is little appreciated is the historical role that European physicians played in colonial conquest, covert diplomacy, espionage, and social exploitation. When Europe unleashed its violence on defenseless Africans, malaria initially impeded colonial conquest (Carlson, 1977, pp. 386–390). From the fifteenth to the middle of the nineteenth century, attempts to establish colonies in Africa were effectively thwarted by the Europeans' lower immunity to malaria and yellow fever. In the fifteenth century, the Portuguese consistently failed, with enormous loss of life, to establish colonies in West Africa. The English, French, Dutch, and Danish were later to suffer similar setbacks due to the "African fever."

For instance, febrile and diarrheal diseases decimated the British colonies established at Freetown in 1789 and later in 1692. Major British expeditions to West Africa in 1832–1934 and again 1841–1942 were effectively halted by African fever. Missionary societies also lost more than one-half their personnel in their first years in Africa. If Africans could not match the superior arms of Europe, the endemic diseases to which they were generally more resistant frustrated the European. When men of arms failed to achieve imperialistic goals, European physicians rose to the occasion. Their contributions to colonial conquest thus won them a special place in the history of oppression. Their work on tropical diseases also gave a new impetus to the development of Western medicine. This is best illustrated by the history of the treatment and prevention of malaria.

The causative organism was microscopically identified in 1880 and the mode of transmission of the disease was demonstrated in 1898. Yet a treatment for and a regimen to prevent malaria were developed in Britian by 1850. The practical exigencies of the colonial scramble in Africa led to advances in treatment and prevention before the disease was understood scientifically. Prior to this, European physicians believed that malaria was caused by bright sunlight, light dew, exertion, excitation, and damp environments. Bloodletting and mercurials were common treatments. Later as contact with other continents increased, cinchona bark, arsenic, and wine were used.

British naval physicians working on the African coast first demonstrated that quinine was more effective than either bloodletting or mercurials. T. R. H. Thompson in particular, himself a physician in the 1841 expedition, established the appropriate dose of quinine for the prevention of malaria. Meanwhile, an analysis of the treatment and mortality of British naval officers in Africa and Asia allowed a naval surgeon, Alexander Bryson, to develop an effective program of quinine prophylaxis. A major test of his quinine regimen came when the British government learned that the Niger and Benue rivers were navigable and thus could serve as commercial inland waterways. To ensure that the crew took their medication, Bryson recommended that quinine be mixed with the regular supply of wine provided to participants in the expedition. Not a single person died of malaria during the entire expedition; there were only a few cases of illness and these were mild. European physicians thus removed the last barrier to colonial conquest and opened up a new era in which Western medicine, the most developed science of healing, contributed to human oppression and dehumanization.

During and after the colonial scramble, some European physicians served as spies and propagandists for their governments. For instance, the French conquest of Morocco could not have been realized without the infiltration and skillful machinations of French physicians. When other attempts at conquest failed, French physicians were dispatched to use their medical skills to win the favors of sultans, to pass along intelligence, and to sow social discord. Most notable in this regard was Dr. Rernard Linares, an agent in the French Foreign Service. From the 1870s to 1900, he was the key French diplomat at the Moroccan court. A French high official once described him as a "precious liaison capable of neutralizing rival influences . . . and preparing the way for . . . 'peaceful penetration' of Morocco" (Paul, 1978). Following the conquest, the colonial physician played a significant role in the dislocation of the indigenous culture, the disruption of traditional healing, and the erosion of social cohesion.

FANON AND COLONIAL RESEARCH

Fanon's critique of the literature on scientific racism was not extensive. It was nonetheless incisive and illustrates the limitations of research in the colonial situation. Fanon argued that previous critiques of scientific racism were scanty and half-hearted. He felt, for instance, that Sir Allen Burt's (1948) book, *Colour Prejudice*, at that time considered to espouse a highly liberal outlook, was only a partial and timid rejection of the racist formulations of such men as Gobineau, Gordon, and Carothers. Fanon paid particular attention to the works of H. L. Gordon and J. C. Carothers. Psychiatrists, Gordon and Carothers, established themselves as authorities on African psychology. Gordon was a British physician at the Mathari Mental Hospital in Kenya. In 1943, he reported that a highly "skilled examination of a series of 100 *normal* brains of *normal* Natives has found naked eye and microscopic facts indicative of inherent *new* brain inferiority" (Burns, 1948, p. 101). This statement shows the satisfaction Gordon felt in his technique, research design, and conclusion. A new research technology was used to simply confirm an old myth. Gordon went so far as to quantify the *degree* of inferiority. More specifically, the "naked eye" and "microscopic" evidence for the presumed inferiority was this: "Quantitatively, the inferiority amounts to 14.8%; qualitatively, the cells of the brain compared with those of the average normal European show defect and deficiency" (Burns, 1948, p. 101).

The conclusions of Carothers were equally outrageous. Carothers, born and brought up in South Africa, served nine years as a Medical Officer for the British Colonial government in Kenya and was the psychiatrist in charge of Mathari Mental Hospital the following 12 years. His long term of service in Africa, his position in the colonial establishment, and his South African origin combined to make him a foremost authority on the "African mind in health and disease." In his monograph bearing precisely that presumptious title and sponsored by the World Health Organization, Carothers characterized the adult African as a child with a high emotional lability and a marked inability to grow into adulthood. He described the African as incapable of learning from experience and rigidly stereotypical in his behavior. Two years later, Carothers (1951, p. 41) was even more specific. He claimed that the African is not only unable to integrate his experiences, but he is also "remarkably like the lobotomized Western European and in some ways like the traditional psychopath."[6]

It was such crude racism, presented as science, that shook Fanon's confidence that reason can triumph against the daily abuses of colonial administrators. He found that all sorts of "scientific" evidence was collected to embolden and vindicate the colonial predator. Fanon's (1967a, p. 120) disgust was profound:

> In the first chapter of the history that the others have compiled for me, the foundation of cannibalism has been made eminently plain in order that I may not lose sight of it. My chromosomes were supposed to have a few thicker or thinner genes representing cannibalism. In addition to the *sex-linked*, the scholars had now discovered the *racial-linked*. What a shameful science!

Fanon later analyzed the various tactics scientific racism adopted in different eras. He found that the blatant negation of the black man's humanity gradually took on more subtle and refined expressions. First, there was the assertion that culture is totally nonexistent among certain groups of people. Then, as conditions changed, a heirarchy of cultures was propounded and African cultures were placed at the bottom of the scale. Later, the notion of cultural relativity gained currency to meet new historical requirements. Each claim, according to Fanon, corresponds to a socio-historical moment of oppression.

The conceptual obliteration of African cultures had meaning only when the socioeconomic domination of Africa was total and ruthless. Gordon's and Carother's contentions regarding the absence of cortical integration in the African was hence nothing but the anatomical-physiological counterpart of the same indictments by the colonial administration. Gut racism maintained by dint of arms and missionary preachings equally found further props in scientific racism. As the notion of cultural relativity emerged, one observed a more subtle re-assertion of old convictions. This is so because European civilization is totally permeated with racism. Thus, according to Fanon (1967b, p. 32):

[6]See Carothers (1951, 1953).

> The vulgar, primitive, over-simple racism purported to find in biology—the Scripture having proved insufficient—the material basis of the doctrine. It would be tedious to recall the efforts then undertaken: the comparative form of the skulls, the quantity and configuration of the folds of the brain, the characteristics of the cell layers of the cortex. . . . Such affirmations, crude and massive, give way to a more refined argument. Here and there, however, an occasional relapse is to be noted. . . . This racism that aspires to be rational, individual, genotypically and phenotypically determined, become transformed into cultural racism.

Yet nowhere was Fanon's critique of colonial psychological research as strong as in his detailed rebuttal of Mannoni's thesis of "dependency complexes." A whole chapter in *Black Skin, White Masks*, "The So-Called Dependency Complex of Colonized Peoples," dealt with this. The chapter is significant for at least three reasons. Mannoni was a prominent French psychoanalyst whose views could hardly be taken lightly. His analysis of African psychology was also more sophisticated than previous interpretations of the colonial situation. More significantly, Mannoni's work had come to public attention at a critical point in the burgeoning anticolonial struggle in Africa. In 1964, after Fanon's death, Mannoni (1968, pp. 7–8) himself stated that his book had willy-nilly served colonial designs: "The administrators, military officers, and even missionaries who dealt with practical problems of colonial life adopted the book in order to exploit it, and extract from it methods and gimmicks to use in pursuit of their own ends." Thus Fanon's careful and reasoned critique of Mannoni's "dependency complex" theory was indeed timely.

Mannoni called his book *Prospero and Caliban: The Psychology of Colonization*. The author stated that the book was inspired by a desire to comprehend certain elusive features of the colonial situation. Traditional ethnographers and economists had hitherto one-sidedly focused on the traits of colonized peoples or used abstract concepts devoid of human content. Mannoni set out to unravel the psychological coordinates of colonialism. This necessitated the study of the psychodynamics of both the colonizer and the colonized. He used cultural myths, folklore, personal conflicts, dreams, and observed behaviors in his analysis. The colonial experience in Madagascar was used in an effort to isolate the psychology of both the colonizer and the colonized. The subsequent analysis, undoubtedly original in approach, had also given scientific trappings to the common vagaries of colonial racism.

Colonial racism, Mannoni argued, is only the work of petty officials, not the work of the best representatives of European civilization. In his view, France was the least racist country in the world. The colonial situation, Mannoni further asserted, was a condition of mutual misunderstanding and incomprehension. It is the meeting of two distinct personalities and of different cultural adaptations. But behind this apparent and shared misunderstanding, Mannoni found a complementarity that, in his view, was unconscious and most fundamental. The European "inferiority complex" leads to a need to dominate and paternalize. The African in turn suffers from a "dependency complex," which leads to a need for a nurturant authority to rule and protect him. This dependency complex was assumed to predate the arrival of the European—an arrival that, in Mannoni's view, was long awaited by Africans.

The African's dependency complex, he argued, thus found a happy gratification in colonial domination, whereas failure to meet this dependency complex was said to leave the Malagasy with consuming anxieties of "abandonment."

Moreover, the Malagasy were seen as perennial children. Mannoni (1968, p. 56) argued that the Malagasy in particular and the African in general are "obviously totally unfit for the orphaned state, and . . . absolutely never, clumsily or in any other way, [try] to 'grow up' as we do." Even his attempt at liberation from French colonialism (in particular, one abortive rebellion during the late forties) was explained as an ineffectual effort to resolve infantile conflicts. Indeed, using psychoanalytic language, the conclusion was drawn that the Malagasy lack the "honor" of living out their Oedipus complex (Mannoni, 1968, pp. 59–60):

> The psychological sequence in the Malagasy rebels was probably this. The father image was projected into the Vazaha [the European] they were attacking. The rifles symbolized the male sex organs. . . . In order to be able to attack the father, in the person of the Vazaha, the Malagasy rebel had persuaded himself that the father, too, was only a harmless child. . . . Thus, instead of protesting, like the European, that he is man like his father, the Malagasy appears to claim that all men are children. He projects his own dependency on everyone else.

Calmly, and with incredible politeness, Fanon exposed Mannoni's psychological reductionism and racism. Colonial racism, Fanon argued, is not merely the work of petty officials. Nor is France the least racist country in the world, as Mannoni had claimed. Racism has an economic, structural, and cultural foundation in European societies. A given society is either racist or it is not. But once racist, none of its members—most of all, its best representatives—remain unaffected. Indeed, whether racist or not, every citizen of a racist society is responsible for the crimes committed in the name of his nation. Fanon (1967a, p. 86) thus argued that scapegoating petty officials is an evasion of the responsibility of the European bourgeoise for colonial racism. What is more, to claim that one form of racism is better than another is simply to deny the essential character of racism: "Is there in truth any difference between one racism and another? Do not all of them show the same collapse, the same bankruptcy of man?"

Most disturbing to Fanon was Mannoni's proposal of a "dependency complex" and the psychological reductionism underlying his analysis. Like colonialists before him, Mannoni had simply misconstrued the traditional hospitality of the African. For instance, shipwrecked Europeans were welcomed with open arms. Early visitors were called "honorable strangers." But this was not appreciated as a gesture of goodwill and a courtesy. Colonialists took unfair advantage of this hospitality. Mannoni also used it to elaborate a theory blaming the victim of colonialism. Mannoni thus misunderstood the true nature of the colonial situation he had set out to explain. Contrary to his claims, colonialism was by no means the coalescing of preexisting complexes into a complementary whole.

First and foremost, colonialism entails economic and cultural subjugation motivated by greed and brought about by dint of superior arms. Colonialism also abhors reciprocal influence and cultural authenticity. Its hallmark is the disruption of the basic structure of the life of the oppressed. Because of it, the indigenous culture and economy are dislocated. The psychological patterns of the oppressed are thus disrupted. Colonialism is therefore neither a harmonizing force nor a phenomenon allowing the simple grafting of its elements into what already existed. Once the native submits, he ceases to exist as an independent, self-defining entity. He becomes defined and then defines himself only in relation to his oppressor. Thus the dependency complex Mannoni categorically attributed to traditional Malagasies and the inferiority complex he detected among the Malagasies are only the products and not antecedents of colonialism. Mannoni had simply confused the *cause* for what actually has been the *effect.*

Fanon was also critical of Mannoni's analysis of seven Malagasy dreams. Without empirical grounds, Mannoni (1968, p. 89) assumed these seven dreams to be "typical of the dreams for thousands of Malagasies." He interpreted all seven dreams in psychoanalytic and intrapsychic terms, all the while invoking his theories of abandonment and a dependency complex. Moreover, Mannoni assumed the universality of European symbolism and unconscious meaning. The tree was said to stand for the mother; the bull, for the father; rifles and bull horns, for the father's penis. The seven dreams were then interpreted to indicate oedipal conflicts pointing to a fundamental insecurity in Malagasy psychology. Fanon objected to this global, ahistorical interpretation of symbols. He argued that one must place dreams into their proper sociohistorical *time* and *place* in order to reveal their true meaning.

Fanon was convinced that psychoanalytic theory itself was inadequate to explain the colonial situation. For to grasp the actual import of the Malagasy encounter with colonialism, Fanon argued, "the discoveries of Freud are of no use to us here" (Mannoni, 1968, p. 104). In particular, Mannoni's application of the Oedipus complex and primal scene hypotheses to the colonial situation is most inappropriate. The nightmares Mannoni analyzed were but dream eruptions of lived experiences under the tortuous realities of colonialism. The black bull does not represent the phallus, as Mannoni claimed, but the Senegalese colonial soldier. Nor does the rifle of this colonial soldier represent a penis. The rifle has a more deadly reality: it is nothing but a "genuine rifle, model Lebel 1916" (Fanon, 1967, p. 106). In short, Mannoni used psychological reductionism to denigrate the Malagasy. In the end, he justified colonial subjugation and abstracted into mere symbols the deadly effects of actual guns.

FANON AND COLONIAL MEDICINE

The transition from metropolitan France to the harsh realities of the colonies led Fanon to new preoccupations. An interest in academic dispute, like that with Mannoni, gave way to a confrontation with the stubborn facts of the life, sanity, and death of the colonized. Fanon was soon struck with how Western medicine itself was readily used as an instrument of oppression. He subsequently presented a brilliant critique of Western medicine in his book, *A Dying Colonialism* (1967c). The book is a sociological and psychological masterpiece. Its analysis of the Algerian Revolution contains rare insights into domination and human transformation.

There are several interrelated themes to Fanon's analysis of Western medicine in the colonial situation. Fanon explained how two contrasting world views and conceptions of disease confront each other within the Manichean, colonial arena. Even the doctor–patient relationship reveals the struggle between the two irreconcilable protagonists in the colonies. Implicit in Fanon's view is also a rejection of glib explanations for the frequent failure of European health programs for the colonized. Most scholars traced the causes of such failures to problems in the indigenous society. Some argued that health programs fail because the colonized maintain a rigid attachment to the indigenous culture. Others, baffled by the outright rejection of health programs, gave up the search for explanations or solutions. Fanon sought the answer in the colonizer–colonized dialectic itself and insisted on an interesting principle: "Every time we do not understand a given problem in oppression, we must tell ourselves that we are at the heart of the drama" (Fanon, 1967c, p. 125).

In European societies, Fanon argued, medicine is a highly respected profession. The community accords doctors due regard and remuneration. Hospitals too are considered to be places of concern and compassion—institutions to care for the sick members of the community. They are a sanctioned refuge for those in distress. Moreover, the doctor–patient relationship is considered sacrosanct. It is characterized by trust, confidence, and goodwill. The patient yields the privacy and integrity of his body to the hands and even the scalpel of his doctor. If inconvenience and pain increase in the course of treatment, the patient accepts this as a necessary step for a cure. The doctor's diagnosis, prognosis, and prescriptions are readily accepted and in good faith.

This trust and confidence of the patient also finds a happy complement in the doctor's ethical disposition and professional practice. The doctor listens, probes, and touches. The measured and empathetic tone of his words reassures and encourages the patient. He acts as a trusted ally of this patient and of potential patients in the community. What is more, explicit legal and professional edicts govern his social behavior and medical practice. They define the doctor's responsibilities and the patient's rights. He cannot breach these legal and professional edicts with impunity.

Western medicine in a colonial society is, in contrast, quite integral to the prevailing system of economic, legal, and cultural exploitation. Though avowedly committed to ease pain, Western medicine partakes in the most tragic feature of the colonial situation. It intensifies rather than alleviates pain. Indeed, as we have shown earlier, the introduction of Western medicine in a colony coincided with and facilitated the imposition of colonialism and racism. The doctor claiming to heal helpless natives was as much a colonial pioneer as the missionary claiming to save heathens from hellfire. Often the two roles coincided in the same person. The doctor, always white, was also sometimes an army doctor.

It is not surprising therefore that the colonized view the doctor's treatment, home visits, and sanitary improvements as extensions of the colonizer's intrusion that violates the integrity of the body, family, and community. His questions, statistics, and surveys are seen only as covert forays to gain further spoils. His hospitals are not considered places of care and compassion. They are dreaded institutions to be visited when all else fails and then only briefly and guardedly. The colonized is keenly aware that the doctor, the policeman, and the teacher are inextricably connected. The hospital, the prison, and the school are viewed as veritable institutions of colonial humiliation. The colonized quickly forget the differences in the ostensible intent and function of these institutions. Their view of the oppressor is invariably undifferentiated and categorical.

It so happens that a degree of assimilation, or a serious and persistent illness, brings a patient to the hospital. Even then, a striking ambivalence prevails. Cure itself only heightens the ambivalence. One is willy-nilly forced to choose between appreciating the curative innovations of Western civilization or retaining one's sociocultural nexus. Indeed open acceptance of the colonizer's health innovations is easily misconstrued as wholesale endorsement of colonial oppression. Long ago, the colonizer convinced himself that the native could not exist without him. To admit the superiority of Western medicine is therefore to confirm the colonizer and his conviction. Either one accepts the medical innovation and hence implicitly acquiesces to colonial humiliation *or* one rejects the innovation and retains one's familial, cultural, and spiritual moorings. In short "the truth objectively expressed is constantly vitiated by the lie of the colonial situation" (Fanon, 1967c, p. 128).

Fanon's analysis was particularly original in unveiling and articulating the doctor–patient relationship in the colonial situation. He elaborated how the perverse drama of the Manichean world is played out even in the privacy of that relationship. The doctor and the patient, belonging to two irreconcilable species, simply reenact the colonizer–colonized dynamic in its crudest forms. The encounter between the doctor and the patient, which takes place at a moment of human distress, crystallizes the veritable clash of two cultures and two group interests. Culturally, the encounter underscores a contrasting conception of disease, treatment, and even death itself. A mutual incomprehension is thus unavoidable.

The doctor–patient relationship is also a dramatic microcosm of dynamics in the larger society. The doctor is white; the patient is a person of color. The doctor has power; the patient has none. The doctor acts; the patient is acted upon. The doctor is highly privileged; the patient is downtrodden. The doctor is a fighter, in this case ostensibly against disease. The patient is only a victim, now to disease and always to the colonial system. The doctor is paternalistic and expects gratitude. The patient resents this and his condition of forced dependence. The doctor is convinced that life without him is impossible. The patient is amused by this and resorts to covert tactics of sabotage, even if this makes his illness worse.

The visit to the doctor is always an ordeal to the colonized. Face to face with the doctor, the patient is often diffident. He is at once facing a technician and a colonizer. If he speaks at all, he does so in monosyllables. His responses to inquiries regarding his ailment are too few and uninformative to suggest a diagnosis. The doctor grows impatient. He searches for other clues. He turns to clinical examination, hoping to find the body more eloquent. But the patient's body is tense and rigid. His muscles are contracted and the doctor's efforts are to no avail. Hence starts the vicious cycle of mutual suspicion, incomprehension, and disparagement so pervasive in the colonial situation. Fanon (1967c, p. 127) illustrated the point with the following remarks:

> The doctor . . . : "The pain in their case is protopathic, poorly differentiated, diffuse as in an animal; it is a general malaise rather than a localized pain."
> The patient . . . : "They ask me what is wrong with me, as if I were the doctor; they think they are smart and they aren't even able to tell where I feel the pain, and the minute you come in they ask you what is wrong with you. . . ."
> The doctor . . . : " Those people are rough and unmannerly."
> The patient . . . : "I don't trust them."
> The doctor . . .: "They don't know whether to stay sick or be cured. . . . With these people you couldn't practice medicine, you had to be a veterinarian."
> The patient . . .: "I know how to get into their hospital, but I don't know how I'll get out—if I get out."

It so happens that such mutual incomprehension or distrust between doctor and patient does persist under conditions of oppression. Serious doubts about the essential humanity of the other lingers throughout the encounter. Further contacts only exacerbate the doubt into a categorical conviction. The doctor, baffled and pressed, conjures up a hurried guess. He diagnoses the ailment and starts a course of action. If he recommends hospitalization, the patient feels doomed. His instincts prompt him toward fight or flight. A sudden death in the hospital signals to relatives a deliberate murder.

If the doctor offers only a prescription and an appointment, the patient considers this a momentous victory. He leaves the hospital in a rush and congratulates himself on a narrow escape. It often happens that the patient never returns on the appointed date, although the importance of keeping the appointment has been explained and reexplained. Now if the patient shows up, he does so months later in the gravest, least reversible stage of the illness. Moreover, an interview reveals that he did not take the prescribed medicine. Or he may not have taken it according to instructions. For instance, he may swallow a month's supply in a single gulp in order, literally, to get even with it. More often, the patient takes the medicine and simultaneously visits an indigenous healer.

Fanon explained the psychology of such a baffling subversion of Western medicine. If, for instance, the patient realizes that penicillin is more effective, endorsement of its efficacy entails political, psychological, and social dilemmas. The patient becomes the battleground for opposing cultural and political forces. Accepting Western medicine somehow validates the colonizer's techniques. Yet the press of his ailment forces the patient to try anything that may work. Thus every pill or injection accepted must be complemented with a visit to the traditional healer. This simultaneous action is hoped to bring what

Fanon called the "double power" of the two therapies and at the same time subvert the validity of Western medicine. Fanon in addition makes the important point that this predicament of being a battleground for opposing forces gives rise to stresses that affect the original ailment adversely.

The problem is not only that ambivalence forces the colonized to view Western medicine through "the haze of organic confusion." The European doctor himself gives proof, in word and action, that he has an inordinate stake in colonial oppression. His privileged position requires that he callously defend and serve the system of oppression. Soon after his arrival, he vies for control and is seized by a get-rich-quick mentality. He quickly becomes a landowner and attaches himself to the land. Moreover, colonial society imposes neither professional nor ethical codes on his practice. No governmental agency, professional association, or community organization safeguard the rights of patients. Medical practice in situations of oppression therefore becomes literally a "system of piracy."

In colonial Algeria, as Fanon explained, the colonized were used as guinea pigs for the most hideous experiments. French doctors produced epileptic fits in Algerian patients and African soldiers. These experimental studies were designed to estimate the specific threshold of the different races. The results of such experiments only served to bolster racism and oppression. What is more, these experiments were combined with rampant fraud in clinical practice. For instance, twice-distilled water was sold as penicillin. Vitamin B_{12} was sold to treat cancer. A doctor with no radiological equipment offered radiotherapy by simply placing patients behind a sheet for 15 or 20 minutes, and subsequently collected exorbitant fees.

Indeed French doctors boasted about their knack for fraud when treating the colonized. Some claimed to take X-rays with a vacuum cleaner. One doctor filled three different-sized syringes with saline solution and sold them for 500, 1,000, and 1,500 francs. The patient, equating quantity with high cost, always chose the more expensive injection. This doctor was said to earn a handsome profit of 30,000 francs in a single morning. The colonial machine that subjugated and plundered a defenseless people was clearly operative in the privacy of doctor–patient relationship. The Hippocratic Oath aside, it takes a poverty of the heart and utter greed to mercilessly exploit humanity in distress and affliction. In reality, European physicians rarely acted otherwise in the colonies.

The abuses of European doctors were not of course confined to harmful experiments and fraudulent practices. The physician himself was often a colonial agent. During the Algerian struggle for liberation, Fanon explained, physicians constantly violated the principle of confidentiality. They reported the name and ailment of a suspected nationalist, his address and the names of his companions, and any other information deemed useful to colonial authorities. Physicians also readily complied with the ban on medicine or treatment for wounded nationalists. If an inquiry as to the death of a tortured person was ever made, the doctor always vindicated the police and torturer with a certificate of "natural death."

Indeed some doctors, themselves colonial agents, deliberately inflicted pain in defense of the colonial system. For just as they were property owners who in addition were doctors, so too did they readily become torturers who happened to be doctors, bringing their technical expertise to the practice of torturing nationalists. Fanon explained how French physicians used truth serum and electroshock for interrogation. The former technique involved the injection of a drug to produce loss of control and blunting of consciousness. Suspects given electroshock were questioned when they were confused and offguard. Such doctors also collaborated with torturers to break a nationalist. Commonly, the doctor intervened during each session of torture to prepare the prisoner for yet another session. "Everything—fear stimulant, massive doses of vitamins—is used before, during, and after the sessions to keep the nationalist hovering between life and death. Ten times the doctor intervenes, ten times he gives the prisoner back to the pack of torturers" (Fanon, 1967c, p. 138). The result was often a dead prisoner or else a "personality in shreds." The surviving prisoner, now a patient, finds suspect all communication and human contact. "Months after the torture, the former prisoner hesitates to say his name, the town where he was born. Every question is first experienced as a repetition of the torturer–tortured relationship" (Fanon, 1967c, p. 138).

Scientific advances are of course responses to given needs and challenges. Europe's historical need has been to have more and more. The self-imposed challenge was to control others and make them less. To satisfy that historical greed, to fulfill that shameful mission, Europe employed all in its power—war, religion, deception, and of course science. The personal experience and collective unconscious of the oppressed thus prompt a fight–flight reaction whenever Europeans, including European scientists and physicians, are confronted. Some form of resistance, passive or active, becomes unavoidable and indeed necessary. As we will show in Chapter 13, Fanon was convinced that science depoliticized is nonexistent, but science in the service of people is indeed possible.

6

MASTER AND SLAVE PARADIGMS

> *The colonial world is a world cut into two. The dividing line, the frontiers are shown by barracks and police stations . . . this world cut into two is inhabited by two different species.*
>
> —Fanon, *The Wretched of the Earth*

Social oppression may indeed be a perennial scourge in human history. However, as we argued earlier, Europe's global conquest had fundamentally changed the character, scope, and intensity of oppression. We have already discussed how Europe's greed for land and labor entailed the occupation of continents, the enslavement of millions, and the unleashing of violence, leaving victims in every corner of the globe. We also sketched how a remarkable arsenal—gunpowder, alcohol, the Bible, and Eurocentric psychology—has readily been used in the historic mission for property acquisition and self-aggrandizement. This rampage has given rise to, in Fanon's words, a Manichean world inhabited by different "species"—namely, masters and slaves, colonizers and colonized, bourgeoisie and workers. In time, the occupation of land culminated in the occupation of psyches.

This chapter examines three major paradigms of the master–slave dialectic. First, it presents Hegel's influential ideas on the dynamics of bondage. These Hegelian ideas on the master–slave dialectic are both seminal and historic. Their impact on later formulations on oppression has been profound. Karl Marx, Jean-Paul Sartre, and Frantz Fanon—to mention only three giants—greatly benefited from Hegel's thoughts on bondage. Second, we present the ideas of Mannoni, a French psychoanalyst, who offered a psychological, controversial analysis of "the colonial situation." We will see here not only Mannoni's remarkable originality, but also the pitfalls of a perspective founded on both Eurocentrism and psychological reductionism. Third, we summarize Fanon's implicit paradigm regarding dialectics of white masters and black slaves. Though details of this paradigm are dispersed throughout the book, it is necessary to outline here how Fanon's contributions benefited and diverged from earlier formulations. Finally, the chapter concludes with a synthesis of paradigms and presents our own reformulation on the oppressor–oppressed dialectic.

Hegel's Master and Slave

Hegel presented the details of his master–slave paradigm in *The Phenomenology of the Mind.* Full of insights and highly seminal, the work has had a profound, far-reaching influence. Many thinkers—including Karl Marx and Jean-Paul Sartre—found in it ideas with which to understand, critique, and attempt to transform Europe. In particular, Hegel's discussion on master and slave has since shaped intellectual discourse on oppression. The chapter dealing with master and slave is condensed, abstract, and elliptical. But it is rich with ideas and suggests intriguing hypotheses on the origin and dynamics of oppression (Hegel, 1966, pp. 229–240).

In a nutshell, Hegel argued that man becomes conscious of himself only through recognition by the other. But when the desire for recognition is frustrated, there is a struggle, a conflict. He who attains recognition without reciprocating becomes the master. The other who recognizes but is not recognized becomes the slave. Not only does the master gain recognition, he also reduces the slave to a mere instrument of his will, a convenient means of fulfilling his needs. Yet these advantages only serve to limit and compromise the master. Alienated from human labor, the master loses the critical means of transforming his world and himself. The slave, however, works on objects and transforms them with his labor. The objects he transforms in turn crystallize and reflect his humanity. By transforming nature, he also transforms himself. Thus the slave—not the master—is in the end the real victor and the one who is self-actualized.

The philosophical and intellectual language in which the Hegelian dialectic is couched obscures its rich psychological import. An interpretation of Hegel by Alexander Kojève clarifies the original formulation and presents it in ways more amenable to psychological conceptualization. The interpretation of Hegel by Kojève was itself a momentous achievement and highly influential. It was at the *Écoles des Hautes Études* between 1933 and 1939 that Kojève presented a series of lectures on Hegel. Present in his audience were Sartre, Merleau-Ponty, Hippolite, Lacan, and others within a significant intellectual elite of Europe. This intellectual elite and its subsequent contributions owes a considerable debt to Kojève and his lectures on Hegel. Fanon too was indirectly influenced by the Kojèvean interpretation of Hegel by way of his discussions with Sartre. Because of its historical significance and psychological relevance, Kojève's interpretation requires closer examination. The following is therefore a review of Hegel's master–slave dialectic as articulated, elaborated, and clarified by Kojève.

Self-consciousness differentiates man from animals. One is self-conscious inasmuch as he is conscious of his identity, dignity, and human reality. Man alone attains self-consciousness; animals can have only a sentiment of self. Yet both self-consciousness and sentiment of self have a common origin in "desire." This is so because biological reality always presupposes desire, such as the desire to eat. Action itself is prompted by desire, not by contemplation or reflection. Indeed cognition fosters "passive quietude"; desire "dis-quiets" and precipitates action. Action born of desire has a dual effect. On the one hand, it objectively destroys or at least transforms the desired object. On the other hand, it creates a "subjective reality" when the content of the alien, desired object is assimilated and internalized. Indeed self-consciousness and sentiment of self are born of desire, but which of the two will emerge is determined by the type of desire and by the quality of the assimilated content.

Animal desire, like the desire to eat, is bound to the immediate given reality and to preservation of life. It is desire directed toward a natural object. Assimilating the desired natural content (e.g., meat) produces only an animal I, a sentiment of self. Self-consciousness is born of human desire directed toward another human—namely, the desire for "recognition." This human desire goes beyond the immediate given reality and beyond the instinct of preservation of life. This desire entails risking life for "pure prestige" and recognition. When human desire is directed toward another human desire, the content of the internalized is neither a static nor a natural object. Self-consciousness is therefore a dynamic, intentional becoming.

Of course the desire for recognition, the desire to have others affirm your values as theirs, presupposes that people are fundamentally social. Recognition is possible only in the presence and confrontation of the other. Thus recognition by the other confirms one's self-worth, identity, and even humanity: "It is only by being recognized by another, by many others, or—in the extreme—by all others, that a human being is really human, for himself as well as for others" (Kojève, 1969, p. 9). Without recognition from others, what one believes and attributes to himself could simply be a delusion. The highest ideal and most authentic self-validation derives from mutual and reciprocal recognition. But such a reciprocity is too often unattainable without a struggle. For it so happens that some gain their humanity because they are recognized, whereas others lose theirs for lack of reciprocal recognition. This state of non-reciprocal recognition is what gives rise to the master–slave dialectic.

The search of recognition necessarily entails a perilous struggle between two adversaries who want to force recognition from another, without reciprocating. The struggle that gives rise to the master–slave dialectic involves a fight to the death. But if both adversaries risk their lives and die, neither is recognized. If one alone dies, the other is deprived of recognition. Thus for recognition to be possible, both adversaries must live. This can be so only if the adversaries adopt two different behaviors in the fight: one risking life till recognized, the other submitting for fear of death. The one who is recognized but does not recognize becomes the *master*. The other who recognizes but is not recognized becomes the *slave*. The first adopted this principle: Conquer *or* die. The second decided: Become a slave *and* remain alive.

Because the master is recognized, he is intersubjectively confirmed. His idea of himself and his self-worth are reflected back to him by recognition from the slave. He thus attains "objective truth" for what was to him "subjective certainty." In contrast, the slave is not recognized and thus lacks both objective confirmation and subjective certainty of his human worth. The master elevates himself and is elevated to human life; the slave is reduced and reduces himself to animal life. The first reveals himself as an autonomous, determing consciousness; the second becomes a dependent, determined consciousness. The master not only attains recognition from the slave, but he also consumes and enjoys what the latter produces. The slave thus becomes only an extension of the master's will and body. Herein lies the foundation of human oppression.

Yet this master–slave relationship also entails a hidden tragedy for the master and a promising future for the slave. For sooner or later, the master finds himself in an "existential impasse." The recognition for which he risked his life proves to have no authentic value. This becomes clear upon considering why, in the first place, the master engaged in the fight and the disappointing way in which the victory concluded. Before the fight, the master was an autonomous person seeking validation through the other's recognition. After the fight, the master attained recognition from one whom he made less human, merely an animal or a thing. What initially precipitated the fight was a human desire directed to another human desire. Now it has become a desire directed to a slave—a thing or an animal. The master is therefore recognized by a mere thing or an animal. The recognition he attains is inauthentic because he is recognized by someone not worthy. Finding he is on the "wrong track," he is never satisfied. Thus the master is a prisoner in a situation of his own making.

Yet in spite of his "tragic" predicament, the master lacks the will and wish to change himself or to get out of his existential rut. Nor can he be educated, convinced, or rehabilitated. He is too accustomed to being master. He is fixed in the status of master and views mastery as the supreme value, the cherished goal. Idle and unproductive, comfortable in mere consumption, he finds little motivation to change himself or his ways. He clings to his principle of conquer or die, being either a master or a slave. Now if he cannot change on his own, if he can neither be educated nor rehabilitated, there remains only one way to overcome the master–slave relationship: *The master can be killed.*

For the master to be killed, for the master–slave relationship to end, the slave too must cease to be a slave. He must somehow rediscover his lost humanity and fashion it in his image. His experience in slavery was full of torment and sacrifice. But these torments and sacrifices actually give him a decisive edge and a substantial advantage. He alone is destined for authentic recognition and satisfaction. Unlike the master, who is fixed and imprisoned in a situation of his making, the slave is the embodiment of change and is ready to transcend the oppressive situation he finds himself in. Slavery eroded every stable anchor for him; nothing is fixed. Before the fight, he did not risk his life for freedom. Now as a slave, he knows what it is to be free. Knowing that he is not free, he wants to become free. Change, which the master dreads, the slave desires by any means. Indeed "if idle Master is an impasse, laborious Slavery, in contrast, is the source of all human, social, historical progress. History is the history of the working slave" (Kojève, 1969, p. 20).

The slave has thus every reason to overcome slavery. To overcome his bondage, he first overcomes his fear of death and embraces liberating work. Originally, he became a slave because he did not risk his life for recognition and freedom. Having become a slave, his fear of death persisted and was incarnated in the person of the master. This constantly lived fear shook him to his foundation. "By this fear, the slavish consciousness melted internally; it shuddered deeply and everything fixed-or-stable trembled in it" (Kojève, 1969, p. 21). Later, however, this fear of death and fear of the master is demystified. It can no longer overwhelm him or enslave him. Indeed this fear educates the slave and gives him new ideals for which he can now risk life, which is now a wretched life. He who knows he cannot escape death and overcomes the fear of death is potentially a revolutionary. But before the slave imposes himself on the master, he reconstitutes and transforms himself through work.

The work the slave performs was imposed on him by the master. This imposed work nevertheless creates for him new possibilities. It frees him from being a slave—first of nature and later of his master. In the first fight, he refused to risk his life. He submitted to the imperatives of a natural instinct— the instinct of preservation. He thus chose to remain a slave of nature. A slave of nature, he also became a slave of the master. But through work, the slave frees himself from nature and his master. Work for the slave requires that he "repress" the desire to consume. He accepts a delay in gratification. Thus he sublimates and transcends the immediate through work. Work also educates him and permits him to transform things as well as himself. His work creates a nonnatural world—a cultural, historical, human world. Through work and the product of his labor, the slave objectifies himself, his personality, his humanity. "The product of work is . . . the realization of his project, of his ideas; hence it is he that is realized in and by the product . . . it is by work, and only by work alone, that man realizes himself objectively as man . . . and only in this real and objective product does he become truly conscious of his subjective human reality" (Kojève, 1969, p. 25).

Whereas the slave is thus an objectified history, the master is only the catalyst of this historical process. Without the master who imposed bondage and work on the slave, this historical process, this objectification of personality and history, would not have taken place. The master imposed work through terror. He consumed the product of work while requiring the slave to delay gratification of his needs. The master's consuming behavior required more work, more discipline, more production from the slave. It is this imposition of work, discipline, and production that nonetheless creates the conditions in which the slave transforms his world and himself. By transforming his world and himself, the slave puts his objective world in harmony with his subjective experiences—a harmony the master cannot obtain. When the slave overcomes terror and engages in liberating work, he once again takes up the fight for recognition. In the end, the slave succeeds where the master failed. The slave alone attains authentic self-consciousness and objectifies history. In short, the slave embodies the future and human history. The warlike master is simply a catalyst who must perish. The master–slave dialectic is thus the dialectic of history.

This interpretation of the master–slave dialectic at once clarifies and extends Hegel's original formulation. How much is Hegel's and how much Kojève's is a matter for debate. But there is no doubt that the Kojèvean interpretation of the master–slave dialectic has been influential and is rich in psychosocial import. Kojève's integration of Hegel and Heidegger influenced both Sartre and Merleau-Ponty. His views on the role of desire and speech have also been pivotal in the psychoanalytic contribution of Jacques Lacan. Indeed Sartre's perspective on desire and action has the same origin—namely, Kojève and Hegel. A human being for Sartre is a being in need. This world of scarcity conditions an incessant struggle to meet needs, to fill a void. The need for food, sex, shelter, and recognition from the other stirs man to material production and action toward the other. These central notions of Sartre bear clear Kojèvean influences.

It is significant that Kojève has been criticized for an overly "social interpretation" of Hegel's master–slave dialectic. George A. Kelly (1972, pp. 191–192), for instance, argues that Kojève's exegesis ignores "the subjectivity of the scenario" and unduly injects "anachronistic overtones of the Marxian class struggle." Kelly purports that Hegel's master–slave dialectic is primarily a metaphor for inherent traits of domination and servitude within individual psyches. He concedes that Hegel broached the social and interpersonal dimensions more explicitly. Nevertheless, Kelly understands Hegel to mean that the social and interpersonal expressions of the dialectic are derivatives of more basic psychological traits of mastery and slavery. Kelly argues that the master–slave dialectic originates in "natural inequities" and "internal imbalance." How else, Kelly asks, can we explain why, of two protagonists locked in combat, one becomes master and the other slave?

Unfortunately Kelly does not explain what he really means by "natural inequities" and "internal imbalance." But one thing is clear in his argument: The oppressed is held responsible for his oppression. He who enslaves, conquers, and colonizes is implicitly vindicated. Kelly (1972, p. 25) finds support for his contention in the following quote from Hegel:

> if a man is a slave, his own will is responsible for his slavery, just as it is its will which is responsible if a people is subjugated. Hence the wrong of slavery lies at the door not simply of enslavers or conquerors but of the slaves and the conquered themselves.

Our intent here is not to join the debate on what Hegel really said or meant. Rather, we wish to emphasize that maneuvers to blame victims of oppression are time-worn efforts to both rationalize an unjust social order and to assuage a guilty conscience. As we have seen in earlier chapters, such maneuvers abound in the psychological literature. What is remarkable is that victim-blamers never put the onus on the initiators, maintainers, and initial beneficiaries of oppression—namely, the oppressors themselves.

The psychological preconditons for oppression no doubt need further study. But resorting to immutable group characteristics or racial differences leads only to the solipsism and racism we discussed earlier. Contrary to Kelly's claims, the Kojèvean interpretation is pregnant with many psychological insights, as shown by its formative influence on Lacan's psychological thought. Fanon's version of the master–slave dialectic, in particular, avoids the pitfalls of genetic or psychological reductionism. Moreover, Fanon situated the mythical master and slave of Hegel in a lived, historical drama in which the disaster and inhumanity of one led to the disaster and inhumanity of the other.

MANNONI'S MASTER AND SLAVE

It can be recalled that Mannoni proposed two psychological complexes to explain the origin and dynamics of colonialism. His proposition of inferiority complex, on the one hand, and dependency complex, on the other inform the conceptual edifice of his analysis. In his efforts to understand and analyze the colonial situation, Mannoni attributed a basic inferiority complex to the European and a basic dependency complex to the colonized. Though Mannoni's analysis focused particularly on the Malagasy he studied, he argued that these two complexes underlie colonial domination in general. Moreover, he assumed that the two complexes predated colonialism and have long existed in the collective psyches of the two groups. Fanon's critique of Mannoni regarding the attribution of a dependency complex to the colonized has been discussed in Chapter 5. Yet in spite of its serious limitations, Mannoni's work has some heuristic value in the exploration of the psychology of oppression.

Of particular interest here is how Mannoni arrived at the two basic complexes and how he used them to analyze the colonial situation. Even though Mannoni may have erred in his analysis of the colonized, one thing is certain: He approached the psychology of oppression with a courage and commitment rare in psychological literature. What Kelly and others of his persuasion had obliquely suggested or groped for with such ambiguous terms as "internal imbalance," Mannoni presented with unusual boldness and detail. He offered his own theory on the psychological preconditions of colonialism. Though his assumptions and conclusions illustrate the pitfalls of psychological reductionism and Euro-centrism, his method of analyzing the collective unconscious is indeed valuable. Mannoni's ideas on the colonial situation therefore deserve more consideration than either Fanon or our previous discussion gave it.[1]

The title of Mannoni's book, *Prosper and Caliban*, is itself revealing. Prospero and Caliban are two central characters in Shakespeare's popular play, *The Tempest*. This is the story and human drama of shipwrecked travelers who find their way to an enchanted, remote island inhabited by alien and less developed people whose humanity is in question. Prospero, the Duke of Milan, comes to preside over life on the island. Though an incompetent Duke of Milan and with little promise of accession to power on his return, Prospero attains power, authority, and a measure of respectability on the island. He dominates the action of the play, commands people as well as spirits, and is depicted as a benevolent ruler. Significantly, he uses *white* and not *black* magic. He has the power of creating and subduing storms. He asserts his will

---

[1]Fanon's critique of Mannoni was based on a few essays written before the book *Prospero and Caliban* appeared.

on others and, with varying degrees of success, foresees and controls their actions. He is a symbol of reason, knowledge, and authority. He educates, protects, and commands. In short, his characterization resembles the self-perception and practices of the European colonizer who ventures to distant lands and usurps power.

Caliban is the islander the shipwrecked party meet, enslave, and domesticate. He is said to be the son of the devil and a witch. He resembles a monster—a hybrid of man and beast. He possesses little mental capacity beyond an ability to acquire practical education. Prospero taught him language, at least European language, and expects of him devoted service and complete obedience. His name is an anagram for "cannibal," even though there is in fact no indication of his being one. He is the servant who must attend to the needs and wishes of alien intruders. Shapespeare calls him "this thing of darkness," which Prospero detests, and describes his function thus: "He does make our fire, fetch in our wood, and serves in offices that profit us." Caliban is despised, castigated, and ordered around by the intruders who now claim his island. Caliban, of course, resents his mistreatment and yearns for freedom. Yet he is portrayed as one who neither comprehends the meaning of freedom nor possesses noble qualities. He is poetic and affected by music, but he also embodies urges that are primitive and hedonistic. His consuming ambition is to kill Prospero and rape his daughter, Miranda, who symbolizes beauty, innocence, and chastity. In effect, Caliban represents the enslaved, exploited, and dehumanized on whom are projected all the unacceptable impulses of the oppressor.

Mannoni was long preoccupied with efforts to comprehend the origin and dynamics of the colonial situation. He was particularly intrigued with *why* Europeans ventured afar so perilously. The search for answers prompted him first to undertake his own psychoanalysis and then to observe behavior in the colonial situation. He also analyzed the projective content of dreams and folklore of the colonized with the intent of delineating the psychological determinants of colonialism. His analysis combined psychoanlytic perspective, Adlerian notions of complex and compensation, and Jungian concepts of archetype and the collective unconscious. Though he concedes the importance of economic and political considerations, Mannoni gave primacy to the psychological determinants of colonialism. In his view, economic dominance and political rule become reality only for those who in the first place are "psychologically prepared" for such eventualities. According to him, the Europeans and the colonized were psychologically conditioned for colonial relations long before colonization occurred.

The colonial situation, in Mannoni's view, is above all the encounter of two different personality types. By personality he meant the sum total of beliefs, habits, and propensities that make the individual a *member* of his group. Underlying his contention was the assumption that each culture or civilization fosters a typical personality structure that is passed on from one generation to the next. This typical personality structure was said to constitute a "psychological heredity" that represents the crystallization of individual, family, and group experiences within a history and an environment. The complexes of inferiority and dependency, considered two fundamental and mutually exclusive alternatives, form the axes upon which personality and culture develop. Each is believed to be nodal but repressed. Where one prevails, the other is thought to be nonexistent or at most potential. Each is conceived to underlie a particular form of mentality and civilization. One is considered to engender higher development of personality and culture; the other socioeconomic and technological stagnation. One is seen to foster dominance and a need to rule; the other to condition submission and a need to be ruled.

To support his thesis of the dependence complex, Mannoni relied on his analysis of Malagasy behavior, folklore, and dreams. Among the Malagasy he encountered, he found a marked prevalence of "dependent behavior." A favor done once is said to be taken for granted, without gratitude by the Malagasy. What is more, this favor is viewed as a license for expecting more favors from the European. In such behavior Mannoni (1968, p. 43) finds clear evidence for a deep-seated dependence: "In fact, gifts which the Malagasy first accepts, then asks for, and finally . . . even demands, are simply the outward and visible signs of this reassuring relationship of dependence." The absence of gratitude is also seen as a further manifestation of the dependence Mannoni viewed as an enduring and essential component to the personality of the "native." Feelings of gratitude presuppose a weakening in the bond of dependence—a weakening the native allegedly avoids. And since gratitude can exist only among persons who are equal and autonomous, it is considered simply futile to expect gratitude from a dependent Malagasy.

According to Mannoni, the dependency complex of the Malagasy is not confined to individual behavior. It is also deeply entrenched in the collective unconscious. Mannoni found evidence for this in what he called the "cult of the dead" and also in his analysis of Malagasy dreams. He viewed ancestor worship as the key to the collective unconscious of the Malagasy. The belief in the power of dead ancestors permeated everyday life and was clung to with remarkable tenacity. Life, peace, and fertility were all explained in terms of their omnipresent wishes and influences. For the Malagasy, the dead ancestors are the sole and inexhaustible fount of all good things. They are the originators of custom, the pillars of life in the family as well as in the community, and God of the Universe. The living are nothing but their deputies. What power and authority the living fathers claim derive from the dead ancestors whose will and wishes are inferred from dreams, portents, and prophesies. Indeed the cult of the dead is said to be so firmly lodged in the personality and collective unconscious of the Malagasy as to be impervious to logic, rationality, or science. Even conversion to Christianity has not, according to Mannoni, shaken the foundation on which ancestor worship and the dependent personality structure are founded. Conversion to Christianity only becomes a *social mask* and, as Mannoni (1968, p. 51) would have it:

> The mask is adopted readily enough, but beneath it there subsists an archaic type of personality founded, not upon the belief in a remote eternal Father, but upon the nearer and much more powerful image of earthly fathers who have died.

Mannoni views the dependency complex of the Malagasy to be an archaic, childhood fixation that "only the West has the courage" to outgrow. More bluntly, the Malagasy are seen to be children who lack the courage, desire, or temperament to grow to mature adulthood, not even a ripening adolescence. Child-rearing practices, particularly the Malagasy practice of indulgent breast-feeding and delayed weaning, are seen as perpetuating the dependency complex. This pattern of dependence in which the individual Malagasy is believed to be entrenched is also seen to characterize the Malagasy culture, behavior, and collective unconscious. Moreover, Mannoni considers the *threat of abandonment* the greatest threat the Malagasy individual and community could conceive of. Having reasoned that growth to adulthood entails an "orphaned state" in which parental nurturance and authority are outgrown, Mannoni asserts that "the non-civilized man" is without doubt "totally unfit" for a pattern of life without absolute authority and hence needs colonial domination to satisfy his naturally infantile needs.

Once the trickling dam of ethnocentrism bursts, Mannoni's analysis takes a predictable course. Rebellion and national liberation struggles are interpreted in terms of the dependency complex and of the threat of abandonment. The Malagasy personality and collective unconscious are said to be incompatible with national independence. Thus what appears as a genuine struggle for freedom is said to be only a reaction to frustrated dependence needs or the threat of abandonment. What is more, the Malagasy are said to have been psychologically prepared for colonial rule long before European colonizers arrived on the shores of Madagascar. Indeed from the analysis of several dreams and a limited forage in ethnographic literature—all on the Malagasy—the conclusion is that *all* colonized peoples have anticipated, desired, and readily submitted to colonial rule: "Wherever Europeans have founded colonies of the type we are considering, it can safely be said that their coming was unconsciously expected—even desired—by the future subject peoples" (Mannoni, 1968, p. 86).

In contrast to the dependency complex of the colonized, the inferiority complex is said to characterize the European personality and collective unconscious. In fact, the struggle with a feeling of inferiority is assumed to be the primary stimulus for the more advanced psychocultural and technological development of Europeans. The inferiority complex constitutes, in Mannoni's words (1968, p. 128), "the main driving force of Western man, and provides him with the energy which sets him apart from all other peoples in the world." The struggle with this complex is considered to underlie European initiative, independence, creativity, and dominance. Mannoni attempted to distinguish this inferiority complex of the European from the inferiority complex that arises as the result of a devalued skin color or a minority status. The former he suggested to be a fundamental trait to the European, something rooted in the history and collective unconscious; the latter he viewed to be superficial, transient, and a mere reaction to social disadvantages. In Mannoni's view, social inequity is not necessarily the cause of an inferiority complex.

An inferiority complex in itself could not have led to colonization of distant peoples. According to Mannoni, there had to be another trait equally

fundamental to the European personality structure and collective unconscious. Thus Mannoni proposed that behind the European need to rule people
in distant lands there exists both an inferiority complex and a trait he called
"misanthropy." The first refers to a basic feeling of inadequacy; the second a
basic mistrust and hatred of mankind. Mannoni argued that these two traits—
an inferiority complex and misanthropy—constitute the driving force of European colonialism. Both traits are repressed, but they nonetheless find expression in the behavior of the European. The inferiority complex is defended
against through compensatory efforts to dominate others, paternalize them,
and be superior to them. The misanthropy is expressed in flights from people
and impels thousands of Europeans to travel to distant lands. Mannoni (1968,
p. 32) argues that the inferiority complex and "the lure of a world without
men" are more potent motivations than the wish to earn profits:

> The "colonial" is not looking for profit only; he is also greedy for certain other—
> psychological—satisfactions, and that is much more dangerous. Accurate observa-
> tion of the facts would no doubt show us that he very often sacrifices profit for the
> sake of these satisfactions.

To corroborate his thesis of inferiority complex and misanthropy in the
European, Mannoni found proof in certain recurrent themes in popular European literature. He argued that the same basic traits underlie major characters
in such works as *The Tempest, Robinson Crusoe,* and *Gulliver's Travels.*
These works often recount the stories of shipwrecked, lost, or exiled Europeans who become heroes, display exceptional virility or technical ingenuity,
and flaunt the superior quality of their nature or culture. The natives they
encounter in distant lands are depicted as subhuman, semihuman, or at least
immature people who are easily outwitted, used for advantage, and paternalized. Mannoni contends that the traits of inferiority and misanthropy have
characterized the European psyche as early as 1572 and certainly before colonialism. He further argued that Shakespeare and Defoe, for instance, had no
models for Prospero and Crusoe other than their own personalities, which
exemplify European character structure. He also indicated that such literary
works have lasted and have wide appeal to Europeans because they strike a
chord in readers and vicariously gratify shared needs. These works offer imaginary characters on whom are projected feelings, thoughts, and fantasies salient
in European psychology.

Mannoni traces the origin of such an inferiority complex and misanthropy
to childhood and cultural conflicts of the European. Both traits are said to
derive from deep-seated sexual guilt, parental prohibitions, and an intense
need to project unacceptable impulses on others. If the inferiority complex is
the impetus for development, it is also what sets the European psyche in a
state of war with itself and with others. Misanthropy entails a wish for a world
emptied of human beings as they really are. The flight to distant land fulfills
the need that requires massive dehumanization and projection. The inhabitants of these lands are thus treated as if they were Calibans or Lilliputians.
Either they are seen as "monstrous and terrifying creatures" to be brutally
subdued or considered as "gracious beings bereft of will and purposes" and

hence readily paternalized. In either case, an unconscious misanthropy drives Europeans to distant lands and dictates a familiar course of action (Mannoni, 1968, p. 104):

> The same unconscious tendency has impelled thousands of Europeans to seek out oceanic islands inhabited only by Fridays or alternatively, to go and entrench themselves in isolated outposts in hostile countries where they could repulse by force of arms those terrifying creatures whose image was formed in their unconscious.

Once in the colonies and having usurped power, the European uses these "inferior beings" as convenient scapegoats on whom are projected the evil intentions of the European. Prospero is thus readily resuscitated and the colonized, treated as Caliban, are imputed with a beastly urge to rape one's daughter or sister or the neighbor's wife. But what is imputed to the colonized are the very impulses and fantasies inherent to the colonizer. The indictment of the colonized *en masse* is simply a defensive maneuver against fundamental conflicts in the European. The more intense these conflicts, the more often racism rears its ugly head. Europeans in the colonies confided their views to Mannoni. Most not only assumed the racial inferiority of blacks, but some also explained this to be a consequence of excessive masturbation. The assumption and explanation only demonstrate the perversity underlying colonialism and racism.

The colonized are of course resented whenever they assert personhood—most of all when they claim the right to freedom. In both instances, the colonizer feels outraged. He knows more is at stake than economic or political domination. Also threatened is a psychological *status quo* of projection and exploitation, which he defends relentlessly and viciously (Mannoni, 1968, p. 117).

> In other words, we are perfectly happy if we can project fantasies of our own unconscious on the outside world, but if we suddenly find these creatures are not pure projections but real beings with claims of liberty, we consider it outrageous, however modest their claims. Further, it is not their claims themselves which makes us indignant, but the very desire for freedom. Racialism, properly speaking, is simply a rather poor rationalization of feelings of indignation.

And yet Mannoni, with all his bold insights, flounders most and reverts to the dilemmas of the colonizer when he confronts the question of national independence for the Malagasy. His thesis of a basic dependency complex and the threat of abandonment, both assumed to predate colonialism, override all other considerations. It is claimed that the Malagasy transfer their basic feelings of dependence to the colonizer who himself has a need to dominate, infantalize, and paternalize. Mannoni himself actually infantalized and paternalized the Malagasy. He assumed an eternal dependence of the Malagasy on their colonizers, the French. Recommended is "the painful apprenticeship to freedom" to a people whose psyche is thought to be undeveloped. Granting complete independence is said to be out of the question and contrary to psychological imperatives: "We might as well ask Caliban and Prospero to meet on equal footing, expect Prospero to behave as Caliban's guest or Caliban to treat him like one"—an impossibility "perfectly obvious" to Mannoni. What is more, any Malagasy hopes for freedom and "complete personality" require the kind deliverance and magnanimity of the colonizer: "In trying to deliver the Malagasy from his dependence . . . we should be leading him along the rocky road of inferiority" (Mannoni, 1968, p. 65). Then and only then, could the colonized be *human* and *adult* like us. In the end, Mannoni rationalized and defended colonialism. This is what Fanon attacked, as we have seen in Chapter 5.

FANON'S MASTER AND SLAVE

Fanon has a section, "The Negro and Hegel," in his *Black Skin, White Masks*. He summarized there Hegel's master–slave dialectic and used this paradigm to analyze the relationship between contemporary whites and blacks. That Fanon took up the discussion of Hegel so directly is not at all surprising. Hegel's paradigm had theoretical relevance to a topic that for a long time had engrossed Fanon—namely, the relationship between *white* masters and *black* slaves. Moreover, as we noted earlier, Kojève's interpretation of Hegel had considerable impact on French intellectual thought, particularly that occurring during Fanon's formative years. Jean-Paul Sartre, whom Fanon admired and read with much interest, had already used Hegel's paradigm in *Anti-Semite and Jew*. This book in particular had greatly impressed and stimulated the young Fanon.

Yet, although Fanon benefited from Hegel's master–slave dialectic, he also needed to reformulate and extend the abstract paradigm so that he could apply it to concrete, lived experiences under slavery and colonialism. As we have seen, Fanon needed to reformulate, extend, and create paradigms in his critical thinking. The same need asserted itself in regard to his treatment of Freud's psychoanalysis, Jung's analytic psychology, and Adler's individual psychology. That Fanon benefited from and then reformulated a paradigm on the important topic of oppression was quite understandable. European philosophers, including Hegel and Kojève, had characteristically ignored the wretched servitude and torment of blacks under slavery and colonialism. Even when they studied the problem of oppression in Europe, they tended to approach it from academic ivory towers. Their thoughts on oppression ineluctably had the quality of philosophical fascination and subjective distance.

To Fanon, in contrast, the experiences of slavery and colonialism had a personal immediacy and urgency. He was himself a descendent of slaves, at least on his maternal side. His country and people were still languishing under colonialism. Moreover, his daily encounters with racism in France continually brought home to him the tormenting residues of slavery. His clinical observation of tortured and shattered personalities, as in colonial Algeria and elsewhere, again underscored for him the global dimensions of Europe's assault on people of color. His identification with the victim was unambiguous since, as he admitted, the oppressed were his brother, his sister, his parents. Fanon

could not therefore approach the master–slave dialectic with the cold detachment of the academician. His emotional engagement and clinical insights
combined to unravel hitherto neglected but crucial aspects—namely, the
human anguish and psychopathology of the master–slave dialectic.

In recapitulating Hegel's master–slave dialectic, Fanon underscored the
necessity of recognition to transform "subjective certainty" into "objective
truth." He also concurred that recognition is unattainable without struggle
and that this struggle entails the risk of life. In particular Fanon emphasized
the essentiality of *reciprocal recognition* for human life and relatedness. Without reciprocal recognition, there can be no identity, no self-worth, no dignity.
One is human to the extent he surpasses the immediate, projects himself into
the future, and above all, reaches out for the other in order to confirm and be
confirmed. Denied this possibility, one becomes steeped in wretched servitude
and objecthood. Psychic and social development is undermined, suppressed,
and arrested. Under such circumstances, there is only one human and liberating response: a "savage struggle" and possibly a "convulsions of death" (Fanon, 1967a, p. 218).

> I am not merely here-and-now sealed into thingness. I am for somewhere else and
> for something else. I demand that notice be taken of my negating activity insofar as I
> pursue something other than life; insofar as I do battle for creation of a human
> world—that is, a world of reciprocal recognition.
>
> He who is reluctant to recognize me opposes me. In a savage struggle, I am willing
> to accept convulsions of death, invincible dissolution, but also the possibility of the
> impossible.

This is Fanon when he wrote *Black Skin, White Masks*. These remarks
stay close to Hegel's formulation, but they also reflect Fanon's initial emphasis
on reciprocal recognition. Despite many efforts as an individual, Fanon's desire
for reciprocal recognition was frustrated in the racist France he knew. The
frustration precipitated a psycho-existential crisis. The other, white and narcissistic, insisted that he not only be recognized but also worshipped. At the
same time, he was reluctant to even concede the humanity of the black man.

Yet in this early stage, despite the stubbornness of the other, Fanon hoped
that an all-out, violent showdown could be averted. His frustration and anguish were tempered by his belief in the potency of reason. The comment
about "savage struggle" and possibly "convulsions of death" was at this period
only a statement of conviction, not a program of action. Fanon was still convinced that reason would prevail over unreason. All one had to do was explain
and make the other understand. Unfortunately, the white master proved stubborn and impervious to reason. The other remained adamant. He continued to
hurl his accustomed racial obscenities. His subtle but corrosive glances persisted. He patronized, oppressed, and exploited. Thus, inevitably, his concern
over the master–slave dialectic remained with Fanon till death. Its formulation changed in time and with experience, but the theme and concern
persisted.

In the Introduction to his first book, Fanon pointed out that there are two
camps: one white, the other black. The two camps represent a Manichean

opposition in perpetual conflict. Each camp suffers its own disaster. The disaster of the white man, Fanon asserted, derives from the fact that he killed man. The disaster of the black man rests on the fact that he was once a slave. Because of this dual disaster, human history and psyche have taken a peculiar turn. The white man is sealed in his superiority complex; the black man is insulated in his inferiority complex. The former wants to elevate himself to the status of a demigod and seeks to keep blacks in "their place." The black man wants to become white or, this wish frustrated, reacts with envious resentment.

The superiority complex of the white master and the inferiority complex of the black slave pervade all race relations and the psychology of the two camps. The white master imposed his language and culture on the black slave. The latter subsequently strove to adopt the master's diction, outlook, and behavior. The white master used black women as sexual objects. He raped with impunity, and his sexual escapades brought forth a new breed, the so-called mulatto, who made the two camps ever more fluid. The mulatto wanted to avoid slipping back; the black wanted to turn white, a notch higher in his being. But the white master frustrated this wish for assimilation. He warily guards the boundary dividing the two camps, even though his sexual adventures blur it significantly. Whenever blacks strove to achieve racial lactification and cultural assimilation, the master redefined the boundary, dividing the two camps to suit his whims and tenaciously defending it. If and when he was not swinging rifle butts and kicking with leather boots, he simply patronized, condescended to, and infantalized the black slave.

Applying the master–slave paradigm to conditions in the diaspora, Fanon emphasized that risk of life is a precondition for freedom. He thus made a distinction between the black slave in the French Antilles who, argued Fanon, was set free without a fight and the black American who constantly "battles and is battled." The former, granted freedom without a fight, is said to know nothing of the value of freedom. He misconstrues freedom to mean simply the granting of permission to eat at the master's table, assume his attitudes, and adopt his behavior. Worse still, he feels grateful for hollow proclamations and camouflaged slavery. The change he has undergone is superficial and deceptive. It is simply a shift from one style of life to another, not a fundamental transformation from one life to another.

Fanon was more optimistic about the future of the black American who battles and is battled than that of the French Antillean who is granted freedom by his master. He believed that a magnificent monument of reconciliation was about to be erected on the battle fields where black American freedom fighters had fallen: "And on top of this monument, I can already see a white man and a black man *hand in hand*" (Fanon, 1967a, p. 222). Fanon's characterization of the French Antillean as the slave granted false freedom without a fight may be a matter for debate. The debate would most likely be on the presumed absence of a fight, not on how superficial this freedom is, which recent developments confirm. Present conditions in the United States hardly justify Fanon's obvious optimism for blacks.

Fanon's master–slave paradigm was particularly enriched by a committed praxis and clinical observation in colonial Algeria. His conception of freedom subsequently changed; his thoughts about the best means of attaining it shifted; and the target audience for his writings became less diffuse. His previous hopes for reciprocal recognition gave way to an emphasis on reclaiming freedom and self-determination for the oppressed. Appeals to rationality and sensibility of the oppressor, having proven futile, were supplanted with a determination to precipitate a violent showdown. Underscored were the significance of violence, the primacy of land and national consciousness, the importance of political organization, the ethics of responsible leadership, the need for creative thought, and the betrayal of "native intellectuals" long pampered by the European oppressor.

In *The Wretched of the Earth*, Fanon's (1968) masterpiece of decoloniza-tion, the violence in the master–slave dialectic takes on a paramount, cata-strophic significance. Colonialism also reveals itself simply as another stage of slavery; the colonizer–colonized relationship is thus a derivative of the mas-ter–slave relationship. Analysis of one reveals the essential of the other. Con-cern with general master–slave relations in Fanon's first book give way to an analysis of colonizer–colonized relations in his later works without a shift in substance. Indeed praxis and experience in colonial Algeria illuminated the coordinates of the oppressor–oppressed dialectic. Fanon again emphasized that the colonial world is divided in two. It is a Manichean world—two camps inhabited by two different "species" in perpetual conflict. The two pro-tagonists live in reciprocally exclusive zones. Their neighborhoods, their nutri-tion, their health, their manner of life and death—all these are in stark con-trast (Fanon, 1968, p. 39):

> The settler's town is a strongly built town, all made of stone and steel. It is a brightly lit town; the streets are covered with asphalt, and the garbage cans swallow all the leavings. . . . The settler's town is a well-fed town, an easygoing town; its belly is always full of good things. The settler's town is a town of white people, of foreigners.
>
> The town belonging to the colonized people, or at least the native town, the Negro village, the medina, the reservation, is a place of ill fame, peopled by men of evil repute. They are born there, it matters little where or how; they die there, it matters not where, nor how. It is a world without spaciousness; men live there on top of each other, and their huts are built one on top of the other. The native town is a hungry town, starved of bread, of meat, of shoes, of coal, of light. . . . It is a town of niggers and dirty Arabs.

The contrast is as much in environment and health as it is in values, thought, and destiny. For in every respect, the colonizer and the colonized are locked in a deadly combat that affects all aspects of life. The colonizer consid-ers himself the embodiment of supreme good, but portrays the colonized as the incarnation of evil. The colonized in turn is amused with this self-delusion of the oppressor as he covertly entertains his moral superiority or prepares for the final assault on his oppressor. The colonizer, ruthless and exhibitionistic, ap-plies maximum violence—bayonets, cannons, and napalm. Sooner or later, however, the colonized learns that his salvation lies only in greater violence.

The colonizer is convinced that he alone is the forger of history and others are simply its fodder. His history books are replete with self-adulations. One reads about the exceptional valor of conquering generals, the remarkable justice of colonial administrators ruling savages, the inspiring dedication of European educators literally illuminating a "Dark Continent," and the selfless devotion of missionaries saving "heathens" from hellfire. With the exception of misguided converts and assimilated intellectuals, however, the colonized know deep down that these claims of the oppressor are but self-delusions elaborated into a culture of lies. More fundamentally, they realize that this educational propaganda and religious proselytization are but different expressions of the same violence the colonizer imposes on society, culture, and psyche.

Yet so long as the colonized accepts servitude for fear of death, so long as he is unwilling to die for freedom, the colonizer is tyrannical and violent without limit. Meanwhile, the colonized patiently marks time and ekes out his existence in an ever-narrowing margin of survival. His accumulated rage deflects from its deserving target—namely, the oppressor. He turns it on himself and his own people. He seeks magical means to exorcise and explain away this rage. But when such maneuvers fail to achieve the freedom and dignity of which he dreams twenty-four hours a day, the more his oppression intensifies. And when he discovers that the oppressor can be killed, this discovery shakes his social and psychological world to its foundation. Acting on that discovery demystifies the omnipotence of the oppressor and restores his self-confidence and self-respect. This discovery ushers in the long-awaited revolutionary struggle to ensure that "the last shall be first and first last."

Thus according to Fanon, oppression is above all else the practice and institutionalization of violence—both crude and subtle. This pervasive violence imposes a Manichean world, corrodes basic human values, and dehumanizes all involved. The exploitation that motivates and perpetuates this violence is not only economic, but also psychological and cultural. Fanon's experiences in the Algerian war for independence forced him to reformulate his earlier view. Hopes of reciprocal recognition through reason have long proven futile. The oppressor was still adamant and impermeable to reason. There remained one and only one recourse: *To practice and organize counterviolence against the oppressor.* Freedom is not given; it must be taken and defended. The oppressor, having become the oppressor through the practice of violence, only understands and yields to counterviolence. The practice of counterviolence in addition fosters cohesion among the oppressed, purges them of their complexes, and rehabilitates the alienated. In short, the revolutionary counterviolence of the oppressed brings forth a new language, a new people, and a new humanity.

MASTER AND SLAVE RECONSIDERED

When Hegel wrote his classic *The Phenomenology of the Mind* in 1807, Europe's conquest of the rest of the world was in its heyday. Hegel was, foremost, a historian and philosopher. Europe's violent past and unfolding present he knew too well, with the acuity of a brilliant insider. His master–slave paradigm no doubt contains significant insights into one of the most tragic aspects of human relations. Hegel focused attention on the pervasive problem of oppression that many other European giants, including Freud, had either completely ignored or at best indirectly intimated. Hegel thus stimulated needed discourse on an important human problem that seemed esoteric and irrelevant to many of Europe's intellectual elite who knew or cared little about the downtrodden and oppressed.

What is more, Hegel's clarification of self-consciousness, recognition, conflict, and the necessity of risking life for freedom remains pivotal in understanding and transforming situations of oppression. That Euro-American psychologists have ignored Hegel's paradigm and the subsequent discourse on oppression has had the effect of insulating them into a mode of thinking in which the concept and reality of oppression lack meaning and urgency. Familiarity with that paradigm and participation in the subsequent discourse would underscore for them the fact that oppression is a crucial feature of social existence and, moreover, that the question of oppression is primarily a problem of psyches confronting each other in society.

Kojève's interpretation and extension of Hegel is also highly instructive and stimulating. It is replete with psychological hypotheses, which, if taken seriously, could significantly shift how psychologists study human problems and what human problems they study. The centrality of "desire" for human action, the meaning and consequences of "action" itself, the difference of self-consciousness and sentiment of self, the primacy given to man as a *social* being, the role of conflict and intersubjectivity in history—these and others suggest a different perspective than the psychology currently taught, practiced, and used for profit. The current emphasis on sexual and aggressive instincts, the reduction of human action to simple, discrete, and quantifiable behaviors, the application of "social psychology" to a narrow subspecialty of tangential relevance to clinical, personality, and developmental concerns—this tradition of selective inattention and reductionism must change if psychology is to have relevance to the global and urgent problems of oppression. For however brilliant and helpful in certain conditions, the insights gained from Victorian Europe or the principles distilled from studies of rats cannot, without significant modification, be responsive to the priorities and concerns of the oppressed. Hegel's and Kojève's formulations thus add important considerations that psychologists often ignore or address superficially.

Yet in spite of Hegel's momentous contributions, his paradigm is sorely limited for us inasmuch as it is purely academic and European in outlook. In particular, the paradigm narrows the complex problem of slavery into a contestation only for abstract ends (i.e., recognition) when in fact socioeconomic motivations are at least as significant. The paradigm also reduces to individual combat what indeed has been a deadly confrontation of peoples, cultures, and psyches. Moreover, Hegel ignored the unprecedented devastation of that colossal slavery in which the master was *white* and the slave was *black*. Experiences under actual slavery—not to mention the agony of enslaved blacks—

were too remote and speculative for Hegel. Indeed one wonders if his paradigm reveals more about the psychology of enslaving Europe than universal travails of the human condition. His views on the redeeming effect of work is, for instance, an interesting version of the Protestant Ethic. Hegel romanticized the effects of forced labor because he lacked the intimate awareness of the crushing weight of real slavery and colonialism.

Mannoni's analysis of the colonial situation is no doubt bold and original. Particularly instructive is his method of self-analysis and examination of the projective content of literary works to study the collective unconscious. It was crucial to inquire into, as Mannoni did, what actually impelled Europeans to distant lands in order to conquer, dominate, and dehumanize others. Why, for instance, have Europeans and their descendants historically been so obsessed with the delusion of racial superiority and the wish to dominate. Equally important is the speculation whether there existed psychological precondi-tions like a dependency complex among the colonized long before their would-be oppressors arrived. Mannoni posed these neglected questions and provided some tantalizing answers.

In our view, Mannoni is at his best when he analyzes the psychology of colonizers and the core conflicts spawned by European civilization. In con-trast, his analysis of the colonized psyche falters because it is Eurocentric, ahistorical, and misleading. Not only did Mannoni relegate the colonized psyche into a perpetually infantile stage of development, but he also er-roneously assumed that colonized peoples willingly submitted to European domination without the bloody wars of resistance which I discuss elsewhere.[2] His pseudoliberal and paternalistic outlook confounds his analysis of the colo-nized psyche. The dependence complex is, as we argued earlier, not a cause but rather a consequence of colonialism. In thus confusing an effect for a cause and thereby blaming the victim, Mannoni remained true to the psychological tradi-tion analyzed in Chapter 5.

It is very significant that both Hegel and Mannoni emphasized that domi-nation originates in the quest for self-realization achieved only through con-quest of the other. For Hegel, self-consciousness is unattainable without recog-nition from, and conflict with, the other. Man is human only to the degree he imposes his will on the other, forces this other into bondage, and thereby transforms subjective reality into objective truth. Whatever else may follow in the Hegelian dialectic, at least this much is assumed as given in human histo-ry. For Mannoni, the European psyche is afflicted with an inferiority complex and a misanthropy that, on the one hand, fostered elaboration of a higher civilization and, on the other, prompted a superiority complex as a defense and desire to dominate others, and provided a lure to live in a world of half-witted, subhuman Calibans. Hegel's formulation is certainly more complex and richer than Mannoni's. Yet the analyses of both reveal more the dilemmas and pro-pensities of Europe's collective psyche than what is necessarily universal or

---

[2]In a work currently in progress, entitled *Capitalism & Cannibalism—A Psychological Inquiry into Racism and Violence*, I explore in more detail various aspects of domination, exploitation, and resistance.

inevitable in the human condition. Intended or not, admitted or denied, both analyses shed light on that very collective psyche of Europe that required massive dehumanization of others in order to validate its own humanity.

If both Hegel and Mannoni illuminated the core conflicts and violent propensities of the European psyche, if they shed light on what impelled Europeans toward domination of others, neither however was able to clarify the actual travails and dilemmas of the oppressed psyche. Their analyses of the enslaved and colonized were less penetrating and illuminating. Hegel's analysis of the oppressed was romantic and speculative, whereas Mannoni's was marred by ethnocentrism and paternalism. Their accounts of the oppressor are richer precisely because the predatory history of Europe permeated their personal experience and background. Little wonder then that what they revealed through self-analysis, examination of the projective content of European literature, and philosophical inquiry form a coherent exposition of Europe's psyche enmeshed with violence, misanthropy, and domination.

But their analysis of the enslaved and colonized faltered because the experiential domain of the oppressed and downtrodden was for them remote from the perspective of personal circumstances and values. For in the Manichean world Europe had created, the gulf separating the existential imperatives of two irreconcilable "species" pitted against each other—oppressor and oppressed, whites and blacks—could not simply be bridged by a leap of imagination, however brilliant or well intended. To comprehend life in the camp of the oppressed, to penetrate into the experiences of those in the inferno below, more was required than analytic acuity or an academic view from the shores of the oppressor.

When Fanon focused his discussion on oppressed blacks, he directed attention not so much to the *whys* of oppression (as Hegel and Mannoni did) but to *how* the violence of oppression dehumanizes all involved. This shift from the why to the how of oppression reflected Fanon's sense of urgency and search for the practical solution neither Hegel nor Mannoni sought. Moreover, Fanon analyzed the dynamics of oppression with the passion of a man deeply scarred by the harsh realities of the enslaved and the colonized. He too was at once enriched and limited by his existential grounding in one of the two Manichean camps. And because he was rooted in the world of the oppressed with which he completely identified, Fanon was at his best in clarifying the dilemmas and dynamics of the downtrodden. Thus his major contribution was in unraveling the psychology of the oppressed. He used self-analysis, clinical data, and social analysis to reveal the travails and conflicts of the oppressed. Unfortunately, his untimely death at the age of thirty-six did not permit him to further develop his seminal ideas or implement his proposal for psychosocial rehabilitation. Nevertheless, when his contributions are considered along with the history of slavery and apartheid, crucial features in the master–slave dialectic and the psychology of oppression can be delineated.

First and foremost, as Fanon pointed out, the problem of oppression is a problem of violence. The violence may be crude or subtle; often it is both. Yet it is this aspect of oppression that is most prone to confusion and mystification. This is so precisely because those who monopolize and benefit from violence find it convenient to obfuscate and mystify the meaning and reality of violence. They enlist the services of religion, the law, science, and the media to confound and bewilder even the oppressed who otherwise would recognize that the social order is founded on and permeated by violence. But this pervasive and structural violence is often masked and rationalized as the natural order of life. Thus there is "legitimate" and "illegitimate" violence—the former deriving legitimacy by use of superior force and convenient legal edicts, not by the actual consent of the oppressed.

Those who monopolize and benefit from violence typically judge their violence as necessary, justified, and for the good of all. Any exercise of self-defense to ward off the violence of the social order is viewed with alarm and considered illegitimate. The oppressed are permitted no right of self-defense, no due process of law. Any remark by one of their leaders concerning self-defense, as when Malcolm X stated self-protection "by any means necessary," is quickly denounced as scandalous, a threat to society, or even the delirious rantings of a man gone mad. But the policeman who, unprovoked, shoots one of the oppressed or breaks heads with batons is likely to be hailed as the protector of justice, the defender of "law and order." Simply put, in the oppressor's system of justice, might is right, and weakness eternal guilt.

The dynamics of oppression and the violence it entails are best exemplified in the master–slave relation. Hegel's paradigm no doubt overstates the primacy of *individual* traits like courage and risk of life in the genesis of oppression. He did not consider the potency of superior arms, better organization for war, and European guile in the enslavement and colonization of Africans, as we pointed out in Chapter 3. Yet Hegel stated a fundamental of oppression when he assumed that the two protagonists are necessarily locked in a deadly combat and that, once oppression is imposed, freedom cannot be regained without risking life. In this sense, then, the Hegelian paradigm acknowledges the centrality of violence in the imposition, maintenance, and eventual negation of oppression.

If freedom requires the *risk of life*, oppression too requires the *fear of physical death*. It is axiomatic that oppression can never be imposed or maintained without the exercise and threat of violence. Historically, most of those on whom oppression was imposed had first put up a violent resistance. Many among them fought heroically and gave their lives for freedom. Oppression took root only when the fear of physical death exceeded the will to freedom. Defeat often heralds fear of physical death among survivors. Thus more than to superior arms, the oppressor owes his power to fear of physical death. This is one of the reasons why the psychological dimension of oppression is so significant. For if and when the oppressed overcome this fear, superior arms, violence, and the oppressor lose their potency.

The fear of physical death without which oppression cannot be imposed is first of all a characteristic of individuals. At its most elemental level, this fear is experienced individually and existentially. This fear inevitably crystallizes as a conflict between an individual wish for physical survival and the community's socio-historic survival. This fear pits immediate and animal instincts against long-range, higher ideals. One cannot succumb to fear of physical death and at the same time work to preserve the cultural values and collective goals that are challenged. Whenever fear of physical death gains prominence, tyranny and exploitation flourish. The individual who places a premium on biological survival becomes uprooted from his community's ideals, history, and destiny. And the more the oppressed seek physical survival, the more their oppression deepens and the more frequent betrayal becomes.

The fear of physical death not only hinders the possibility of freedom, but also limits productive and meaningful living. Those who submit to oppression may continue to breathe, eat, and sleep. They may congratulate themselves for having preserved biological life. Unfortunately, however, they only exchange one form of death for another. This is so because as they submit to oppression and preserve biological life, they invariably suffer a degree of *psychological* and *social* death. Even their physical survival remains tenuous. They enjoy a stay of execution so long as they serve the interest of the oppressor. But their psychological and social death continues without interruption so long as their fear of physical death persists.

Orlando Patterson (1982) came to a similar conclusion in his brilliant and comprehensive study of slavery. He identified three constituent elements of slavery that are worthy of note. First, the master–slave relation was founded on interpersonal and institutional violence. The master's absolute power and the slave's total powerlessness rested on the use and threat of violence. Forced to a state of powerlessness and helplessness, the slave became a human surrogate and instrument of the master's self and will. Second, the slave was subjected to a state of "natal alienation," whereby his genealogical and cultural moorings were obliterated. To be without a legitimate or recognized bond with others—be they dead, living, or unborn—amounted to being a "socially dead person." Third, a distinctive feature of the slave was his generalized condition of dishonor. For in his eyes and those of others, his person and status lacked integrity, worth, and autonomy.

From this it follows that slavery was the ultimate of human domination and exploitation. Those on whom slavery was imposed were spared physical death as long as they remained living tools of their masters. In exchange they submitted to death in three domains—personality, social bonding, and culture. They suffered depersonalization, desocialization, and deracination. Their outward behaviors were incongruent with their wishes, needs, and psychic life. Their relations to others, even to their loved ones, were rendered illegitimate and meaningless. Their culture and history were also uprooted, derailed, and made appendages to those of their masters. To a varying degree and intensity, these three forms of "death" exist in most situations of oppression.

It is important to appreciate, in situations of oppression, the various mechanisms of social control that complement, refine, and deepen the violence of the oppressor. Brutal and blatant violence is insufficient to produce an obedient slave. For a situation of oppression to be effective, various methods of social control must pervade the life of the oppressed. Among the first freedoms to be curtailed are basic freedoms like those of movement, expression of opinion, and assembly. The oppressed is made a prisoner within a narrow circle of tamed ideas, a wrecked ecology, and a social network strewn with prohibitions. His family and community life is infiltrated in order to limit his capacity for bonding and trust. His past is obliterated and his history falsified to render him without an origin or a future. A system of reward and punishment based on loyalty to the oppressor is instituted to foster competition and conflict among the oppressed. Such methods of social control, best exemplified in slavery and apartheid, make the psyche and social relation of the oppressed the locus of control and domination.

When the oppressor's harsh prohibitions and threats are enacted in family and interpersonal relations, problems of oppression and hence of violence become infused with a confounding ambivalence and guilt. This intensity of oppression, when even loved ones have adopted the oppressor's values and norms, is most difficult to change. Any attempt toward change thus entails the confrontation of those one has come to love or respect or consider significant others. What is more, the institutionalization of oppression in daily living also entails an internalization of the oppressor's values, norms, and prohibitions. Internalized oppression is most resistant to change, since this would require a battle on two fronts: the oppressor within and the oppressor without.

Prolonged oppression reduces the oppressed into mere individuals without a community or a history, fostering a tendency to privatize a shared victimization. Thus one observes contrasting attitudes and behaviors between the two protagonists in situations of oppression. When a member of the oppressing group meets a member of the oppressed, the first always acts as a majority; while the latter behaves simply as a minority of one. The former demands more space and privilege; the latter tends to settle for less. The former exudes confidence and a sense of entitlement; the latter betrays self-doubt and a readiness to compromise. Consciously and unconsciously, each know that their personal encounter is also an encounter of two collectives with unequal power. The prevailing ideas, values, and rules of conduct serve the former; they entrap and frustrate the latter. The one who is a member of the oppressing group exploits all this; the other compensates with his personality and individual resources.

The oppressed find everyday living a challenge. The narrow and rigid confines in which the oppressed are entrapped by laws and rules of conduct require a marked degree of repression and personal versatility. Stripped of a collective aura, the oppressed tend to think, dream, and act as a helpless minority of one. The oppressed learn to wear many masks for different occasions; they develop skills to detect the moods and wishes of those in authority, learn to present acceptable public behaviors while repressing many incongruent private feelings, and refine strategies for passive-aggressive behavior. This pattern of adaptation no doubt entails a personal toll, an excessive use of energy, and a higher vulnerability for psychopathology. Though the human capacity for adaptation is remarkable, there is also a threshold for what is tolerable. It should therefore not be surprising if the oppressed often complain of many somatic afflictions and "wandering organ syndromes" or suddenly erupt in rage, persecute scapegoats, abuse substances, and take murderous actions against relatives or friends.

Oppression pervades more aspects of life the longer it prevails. Its various forms of violence also become harder to discern the more one is oppressed. Yet as suggested by Professor Chester Pierce, it is possible to identify several key indicators for objectively assessing degree of oppression. All situations of oppression violate one's space, time, energy, mobility, bonding, and identity.[3] The oppressed finds his or her physical and psychological space unacknowledged, intruded into, and curtailed. The oppressed is not allowed any claim to territoriality nor is his or her privacy respected. Of the twenty-four hours of each day, there is less time the oppressed can call his or her own, to be used at will for self-development and/or leisure. The energy of the oppressed is often depleted, expropriated, and harnassed to advance the oppressor's interests. The movements of the oppressed is controlled and curbed. Equally crucial, his or her bonding with others is subverted, weakened, and rendered conflictual. His or her personal, as well as collective, identity is also challenged, undermined, and confused.

The slave best exemplifies the relevance of these six indicators of oppression. The male slave was allowed no physical space which he could call his own. The female slave had even less claim to space than the male slave. Even her body was someone else's property. Commonly ignored is how this expropriation of one's body entailed even more dire consequences for female slaves. The waking hours of the slave were also expropriated for life without his or her consent. The slave labored in the field and in the kitchen for the gain and comfort of the master. The slave's mobility was curbed and he or she was never permitted to venture beyond a designated perimeter without a "pass." The slave's bonding with others, even the natural relation between mother and child, was violated and eroded. The same violation of space, time, energy, mobility, bonding, and identity prevails under apartheid, which, in effect, is a modern-day slavery.

Life is actually inconceivable without space, time, energy, mobility, bonding, and identity. How a community allocates and uses space, or in the most materialist perspective, how it distributes ownership and control of land reflects its values, economics, health, and quality of life. Equally, the rhythm of life and all developmental processes presuppose the category of time. As man strives for immortality, a fleeting present recedes into a forgotten but potent past. Developmental milestones are passed in time; plans are made for an unfolding and uncertain future. Moreover, the capacity to act and particularly to work—in a word, energy—is a measure of how and by what means an individual lives and objectifies his or her potential. Mobility permits fulfillment of needs and flight from danger in an environment of action and reaction. Bonding with others is so basic that, without it, neither development of self nor life is possible. And identity provides the anchor for individuality and continuity with others.

These six dimensions thus define, determine, and sustantiate the human psyche. The space and time we inhabit, the energy and mobility available to

---

[3]Personal communication; I added "bonding" and "identity" to Pierce's original four—space, time, energy, and mobility.

us, and the social bonding that forms, fulfills, and nurtures us, the sense of self and awareness of its possibilities—these are the foundations for human psychology. Any attempt that seeks to elucidate the psychology of oppression, but ignores the importance of these dimensions is misleading and evasive. This is so because, when all is said and done, the question of oppression is also a question of control and/or violation of at least these basic dimensions of life. Oppression is motivated by economic, social, and psychological gains that, in the end, entail the manipulation and usurpation of these life domains. To focus only on inferred needs or debates on innate racial qualities serves to distract attention from these nodal dimensions that could empirically be studied and changed. Thus by emphasizing the distribution and control of these nodal dimensions, we can objectively answer whose needs are fulfilled or frustrated, how this is achieved, and what psychology of the self is subsequently elaborated.

Every psyche of course indulges in a degree of narcissism while defending against attributes it finds disturbing. Having distinguished between self and other, it seeks a convenient line of demarcation, a tangible anchor for an ever-shifting boundary. A collective consciousness too has a need to establish visible markers that distinguish it from others while it must also negotiate internal contradictions that threaten disintegration. The individual psyche may deny, relegate to a ghetto, and project that which it finds unacceptable or threatening. As much as it needs affirmation from others, it also develops through confrontation with others. The collective consciousness too finds it easier to identify external scapegoats to reaffirm its boundaries and to regulate internal conflicts. The more the internal conflicts threaten disintegration, the more the collective consciousness resorts to disparagement and persecution of others in the hope of obtaining a semblance of cohesion. Even in times of peace and relative tranquility, it performs rituals in which old warriors are remembered and earlier victories recounted.

This dual process of differentiation and integration, negation and synthesis, is basic to the development of individual and collective psyches. It so happens that people are oppressed not only to satisfy economic needs, but also to resolve marked ambiguities, deep insecurity, or conflict in identity. Oppression affords a partial solution for the oppressor inasmuch as it redefines an illusive boundary, provides scapegoats on which to unload unacceptable attributes, and fosters a sense of superiority. Thus what Hegel discussed in terms of a struggle for recognition is essentially a struggle for identity. By introducing violence into the natural process of differentiation and integration, oppression transforms normal conflicts into veritable crises. And if the development of identity requires both affirmation from others and negation of at least some attributes, oppression renders all affirmations inauthentic and turns negations into violent confrontations.

The processes of internalization and objectification that Kojève explained so well also are relevant to the psychology of oppression. For in prolonged oppression, the oppressed group willy-nilly internalize the oppressor without. They adopt his guidelines and prohibitions, they assimilate his image and his social behaviors, and they become agents of their own oppression. The oppressor without becomes an *introppressor*—an oppressor within. The well-known inferiority complex of the oppressed originates in this process of internalization. Because of this internalization and its attendant but repressed rage, the oppressed may act out, on each other, the very violence imposed on them. They become *autopressors* as they engage in self-destructive behavior injurious to themselves, their loved ones, and their neighbors. Introppression refers to something more specific than Freud's supergo. It is an ensemble of internalized aspects of oppression that prompts a betrayal of self and loved ones and plots of resistance. Often, the oppressed acquire a *victim complex* and hence view almost all actions and communications as further assaults or simply other indications of their victim status. This is one expression of the "adaptive paranoia" seen among the oppressed.

The oppressors too are profoundly affected by the violence and dehumanization they impose on others. Their violent and dehumanizing actions in time turn against them and reverberate in their psyches and social lives. Violent and niggardly to so many, yet wanting to love and be authentic to kin, the line of demarcation between *we* and *they* gradually blurs. Their violent and niggardly proclivity to others comes to dominate their intimate social existence. The oppressors assimilate the cruel and harsh image they provoke in the oppressed. This fact of *retroppression*, whereby violent and dehumanizing actions boomerang on their perpetrator, further harden the oppressors, and their oppressive practices become further entrenched. The harsh actions on the oppressed, the unjust exercise of authority, and the subsequent lack of compassion—these gradually invade their family life and their dealings with loved ones. This state of affairs takes its toll and leaves its own psychological scars. Repressed guilt and fear of reprisal also come to dominate the psyche and social relations of the oppressor.

One common way in which oppressors attenuate the guilt and discomfort that arises from their violence and dehumanization is to impose further violence and further dehumanization. This is the *Nero complex*.[4] Like Emperor Nero of Rome, the oppressor's injustice prompts only further injustice. To repent and to make amends are not possible. Oppressors only concede to a relentless demand, rarely to reason or compassion. Skillful in creating self-fulfilling prophesies, they conjure up and actualize victims who "deserve" to be victimized. Oppressors find justification and legitimacy only through greater violence and injustice. If Rome had to be burned to save it, the oppressed too are dehumanized to make them more human. The logic here is no doubt peculiar, but it is quite prevalent in oppression. Considered children and in need of guidance, the oppressed are thought to benefit from rigid discipline and raw injustice. And if the victims cannot be physically annihilated, they can at least be psychologically mutilated. The oppressors meanwhile extol themselves

---

[4]This term was introduced by Albert Memmi (1965).

and boast of their glory while devaluing and debasing the oppressed. All these reinforce their feelings of omnipotence and superiority.[5]

The decision to die for freedom is a decision to eject or kill introppressors as well as real oppressors. To attain freedom, to change one life for another, the oppressed must risk not only a deadly combat with the real oppressor, but also a perilous dislocation of the oppressor within. This dual struggle may thus result in death, madness, or freedom. It so happens that victims of prolonged oppression are more familiar with death and madness, which pervade their social existence, than with how to obtain their freedom and take control of their destiny. Indeed as we pointed out earlier, prolonged oppression blurs the great divide between life and death as well as that between sanity and madness. Mortality, incarceration, psychiatric hospitalization—in effect different forms and stages of death—are appallingly pervasive among the oppressed. Yet the freedom for which they yearn requires that they first overcome their fear of physical death and their illusion of individual redemption.

All individuals are mortal, and physical death can at best be postponed but never avoided. Communities and cultures outlive individuals. Those who fear physical death and submit to oppression invariably condemn themselves to psychological, social, and historical death. Depersonalized, desocialized, and deracinated, they become surrogates of the will and self of others. Their psychological and social death only hasten their physical death, as is well shown by the excess rates of morbidity and mortality among the oppressed. This is indeed one of the ironies of oppression. The oppressed submit for fear of physical death, but because they submit, they become ill more frequently and die at an earlier age.

The search for security in conditions of oppression, the quest for personal harmony in circumstances of social violence, or the wish for private success at the cost of betraying collective aspirations require little originality and risks because such efforts accept the *status quo* of oppression as immutable. Freedom requires new courage, new vision, and new commitments. The dehumanizing master without must be killed—at least psychologically—just as the slumbering slave within must be ejected. Neither can occur without willed, organized action. Both entail risking a psychological crisis and even physical death. For then, and only then, can a given generation of the oppressed effect change and reclaim their history.

[5]The relation and dynamics of concepts introduced here—for instance, the relation of *introppression, autoppression, victim complex, retroppression,* and *Nero Complex*—are detailed in the work cited earlier and now in preparation (see footnote 2).

III

TYPES OF VIOLENCE
AND FORMS OF DEATH

7

Violence and Manichean Psychology

Colonialism . . . is violence in its natural state, and it will only yield when confronted with greater violence.
—Fanon, *The Wretched of the Earth*

A situation of oppression is essentially a caldron of violence. It is brought into existence and is maintained by dint of violence. This violence gradually permeates the social order to affect everyday living. In time, the violence takes on different guises and becomes less blatant and more integral to institutional as well as to interpersonal reality. It even invades the deeper recesses of the individual psyche, permeating fantasies and dreams. Thus to study oppression is, in the final analysis, to delve into the problems of violence in both its subtle and crude manifestations.

This chapter examines the problem of violence from a Fanonian perspective. We begin with a discussion of current definitions of violence, point out their limitations, and redefine violence from the perspective of the victim. We then review Fanon's theory of violence in situations of oppression. It should be clear from this that Fanon traversed the ordinary, sanctioned, mystifying zone of discourse on violence. Finally, we summarize and evaluate the critiques of Fanon and his theory of violence. We hope to show that those who vilify Fanon for his perspective on violence distort the militant humanism on which his ideas are founded.

Violence Defined and Redefined

As suggested, many internalized prohibitions and prevailing social controls condition us to view violence too narrowly and selectively. We tend to recognize violence mostly in those instances when it is blatantly destructive and contrary to the established norms of society. A cold-blooded murder in a dark alley, a shocking case of child abuse in a neighborhood of ill-repute, a devastating and senseless war in distant lands—we commonly associate violence with such events. The media, with its selective and sensational "news," also reinforces our limited and controlled conception of violence. Moreover, as we are informed each day of these shocking occurrences, we come to reassess our less than ideal predicament and feel lucky that we have been spared such cruel assaults. And since we often are socialized into the prevailing ideology of law and order, we may even breathe a sigh of relief in the belief that the machinery of the state—the police, the courts, and the prisons—exist to protect *all* of us from such wanton acts of violence.

This narrow and selective conception of violence no doubt has an adaptive function both in the psychodynamics of the individual and in the maintenance of the social *status quo*. The fact remains, however, that violence is more pervasive in life than we commonly believe and that it undergirds more of our cherished ideals and institutions than we care to admit. All societies rely on the use and threat of violence; the family itself is as much an arena of violence as of love; and the final arbiter of justice is indeed violence. Law and order depend on violence and so do lawlessness and disorder. Without the use and threat of violence, fundamental changes rarely occur in a social order. All this seems paradoxical and violence is paradoxical indeed.

First, what do we mean by *violence*? This is actually a difficult concept to define. What constitutes violence has been debated over the centuries and the debate continues. One central problem is that *violence* refers to many actions, processes, and conditions. Each definition invariably emphasizes some aspects more than others and includes some to the exclusion of others. The concept of violence has both literal and figurative meanings. It may refer to actions causing physical injury or it may figuratively emphasize intensity of feelings and of words. *Violence* may be confined only to those harmful actions lacking social sanction. It may refer to a phenomenon between individuals or groups. A definition may include intent to cause harm, even if the violence led to no actual harm, or the occurrence of any harmful actions, however unintended and unpremeditated. Violence may be considered to be a result of such intense emotions as rage and hate or of impersonal circumstances as racism and war. The consequences of violence may be immediate or long term. Violence may be taken to depend upon the personal traits of an individual or it may be seen as embedded in social conditions. In short, violence is an omnibus concept that can be defined in various ways and viewed from different perspectives.

Which of these aspects is included or excluded in a given definition has significant import to the range of human experience examined and the kind of conclusions drawn. Behavioral scientists who study the problem of violence tend to offer definitions that are individual oriented and fit the canons of (neo-)positivist tradition. This approach narrows violence to what is measurable and quantifiable. It assumes an identifiable perpetrator and an equally identifiable victim. It searches for the immediate observable antecedents and consequences of violence. Less immediate causes and long-term effects introduce unwanted complexities and overload established methods of verifiability. This approach to the study of violence has contributed significantly to criminology and clinical work. But it presents serious limitations when one is considering the problem of violence under conditions of oppression. A few examples underscore the point.

Newman (1979, p. 2) defined violence as "that which leads to physical injury or damage, since historically and statistically it is the only aspect of violence that we are able to observe or record." Wolfgang (1976, p. 316) defined violence as "the intentional use of physical force on another person or noxious stimuli invoked by one person on another." Straus and Steinmetz (1974, p. 4) similarly defined violence as "the intentional use of physical force on another person." Gelles and Straus (1979, p. 554) later modified their definition of violence as "an act carried out with the intention of, or perceived as having the intention of, physically hurting another person."

A distinction often made in the literature is between "instrumental" and "expressive" violence. *Instrumental violence* refers to the infliction of pain and/or injury, or the use of physical constraint in order to induce another person to carry out some action against his wishes. *Expressive violence* is the use of pain or injury as an end in itself. Another distinction also made is that between "legitimate" and "illegitimate" violence. *Legitimate violence* refers to the socially sanctioned use or threat of harm as in police action and war. *Illegitimate violence* is that which goes against laws and the accepted norms of society. Criminal homicide and forcible rape are clear examples of illegitimate violence.

These definitions and their taxonomy illustrate how behavioral scientists usually approach the problem of violence. In general, behavioral scientists use some or all the following criteria to define violence. First, one must demonstrate the use of physical force against another person. Second, there must be an intensity of feelings, like rage and hate, which prompts the "violent action." Third, one must have some ground to infer an intent to inflict harm. Fourth, the action or intent must lack social or legal sanction. Fifth, one must demonstrate the effects in terms of physical damage. These five criteria are useful in ordinary areas of research on violence, but they become serious problems in the study of social oppression.

Obviously, not all acts of violence require face-to-face contact or the exertion of physical force. Shooting with a gun, spraying a territory with poison gas, and pushing a button that fires a missile are examples of deadly violence. The feelings associated with interpersonal violence are not necessarily identical to those associated with collective violence. Reliance on intent may be useful in defining individual violence but less useful in defining systemic violence. Many actions and conditions that cause harm may not necessarily be intentional, but their consequences are no less devastating. Indeed it is one thing to emphasize *intent*—hence the perspective of the actor and perpetrator—and quite another to emphasize *consequences*—hence the perspective of the acted-upon and victim. In a world of powerful perpetrators of violence, it is hardly surprising that in law, as in the behavioral sciences, intent gains primacy over consequence.

Even more of the ideological and value biases of the preceding definitions are revealed when a definition of violence is limited to that which is "illegitimate." Thus slavery and apartheid, both given legal and social sanction, would not be considered "violent." The plunder of people's land and labor too comes to be viewed as having little or no significance to the study of violence, whereas a minor robbery involving a member of the propertied class would readily qualify as "violent." What is more, the narrow view of physical injury or damage often neglects the long-term somatic, psychological, and social consequences of systemic violence.

Newman (1979, p. 4) best illustrates the limitations of the current definitions. She uses the five criteria stated previously and concludes that the notion of a "violent system" is untenable and meaningless because "there is no intensity of feeling, no purpose or direct infliction of physical injury or damage." For her, inequities in a social order, even if they cause physical injury or damage, cannot be considered violent because such "suffering is more by default than intent." This emphasis on emotional intensity, intent, and direct infliction of injury obviously limits the range of human behavior one can consider violent. Ironically, Newman's narrow definition of violence is argued in a book ambitiously titled *Understanding Violence.*

The criteria of emotional intensity, intent, and direct infliction of injury may be useful in making sense of certain types of violence. But insisting on these criteria to define violence leads to obvious absurdities. Thus for instance, those who order a pilot to bomb an enemy territory may have the stated intent of killing armed adversaries. But would killing innocent children more "by default than intent" make the bombing less "violent?" Would a Nazi war criminal who coldly and dispassionately sent victims to gas chambers be considered nonviolent because of claims that he personally did not inflict direct physical force or that he simply followed orders and had no personal "intent" to harm anyone? Is the action of a parent who committed infanticide less violent because one can prove this murder occurred in a moment of psychotic rage?

In fact, only a small fraction of human violence can be explained in terms of intent. Even in that fraction, there is room for dispute as to what constitutes actual "intent" and the accuracy of such attributions. Much human violence occurs with little rational content or individual deliberation. Violence is integral to relations and social conditions. We would comprehend less of its essence if we reduce it only to a moral question just as we would be remiss if we limit it to what a social order designates illegitimate. For in any given social order, violence often occurs vertically—from top to bottom—in the struggle for power, property, security, and "justice." This form of violence is often sanctioned as legitimate, whereas violence from bottom to top is considered illegitimate. Even if we cannot always identify the perpetrators of vertical violence, we find countless victims and their survivors who bear indelible scars. The victims and survivors of vertical violence may in turn vent their anger and frustration through horizontal violence, victimizing themselves, their relatives, and their peers.

The definition of violence we offer here is closer to that offered by Gil (1981) who defines violence as "human-originated relations, processes, and conditions which obstruct free and spontaneous unfolding of innate human potential, the human drive toward growth, development and self-actualization, by interfering with the fulfillment of inherent biological, psychological, and social needs." This definition may seem awkward or abstract, but it is certainly more useful than most traditional definitions. It permits the study of violence in its various manifestations—without of course excluding legitimate violence or unintended violence from consideration. We propose a more succinct but related definition: *Violence is any relation, process, or condition by which an individual or a group violates the physical, social, and/or psychological integrity of another person or group.* From this perspective, violence inhibits human growth, negates inherent potential, limits productive living, and causes death.

The proposed definition rests on several assumptions. First, violence is not simply an isolated physical act or a discrete random event. It is a relation, process, and condition undermining exploiting, and curtailing the well-being of the victim. Second, these violations are not simply moral or ethical, but also physical, social, and/or psychological. They involve demonstrable assault on or injury of and damage to the victim. Third, violence in any of the three domains—physical, social, or psychological—has significant repercussions in the other two domains. Fourth, violence occurs not only between individuals, but also between groups and societies. Fifth, intention is less critical than consequence in most forms of violence. Any relation, process, or condition imposed by someone that injures the health and well-being of others is by definition violent.

This dynamic definition enables us to examine aspects of violence the prevailing and limited definitions cannot accommodate. Moreover, the taxonomy of violence into legitimate and illegitimate or instrumental and expressive presents problems in considering situations of oppression. The question of legitimacy is a relative one depending on where one happens to be situated in the social order and depending on who has the authority—indeed ability to effect violence—to impose it on others. Might is so often right and, in the final analysis, violence is the foundation of legitimacy. Equally, the distinction between instrumental and expressive violence proves untenable when one's perspective changes from intent to consequence and from perpetrator to victim. To call a violent action expressive because the intent or aim of the actor appears to us senseless and incomprehensible is to sanction and celebrate our ignorance at that moment. In our view, *all* acts of violence are both instrumental *and* expressive. Which aspect we choose to emphasize depends on our goals, values, and state of knowledge at the moment.

If one seeks to delve into the motives behind individual behaviors or to unravel the psychopathology of given acts of violence, then the question of instrumentality and expressiveness of violence becomes dominant. If one aims to study the incidence and dynamics of "crime" while believing that the social order is sacrosanct, then it makes sense to focus on illegitimate violence. This approach thus precludes the serious consideration of a vast array of legitimized violence carried out by, say, policemen, soldiers, prison guards, and executioners. Our goal here is different because we want to explore human violence in situations of oppression. This requires that we look at various forms of violence—legitimate or not—that create and maintain a condition of oppression. That is why we suggest a different taxonomy of violence.

Human violence occurs at personal, institutional, and structural levels. Personal violence is the easiest to discern and control and its effects are easiest to assess. Typically, personal violence is a phenomenon of a dyad. It often involves direct actions and means (like a fist or a bullet) and is restricted to place as well as time. Moreover, one can identify a specific *perpetrator* whose aims can be verified and a *victim* whose injuries can be assessed. There usually exists a perpetrator–victim relation preceding and subsequent to the "violent incident." In some cases, violence indeed permeates the relationship as a whole. Nonetheless, personal violence permits the ordinary procedure of imputing intent, rendering judgment, and exacting retribution. We will see later how personal violence manifests itself in one of two related forms—namely, *interpersonal* and *intrapersonal* violence.[1]

Institutional and structural violence are higher order phenomena that subsume and supercede personal violence. Examples of microsocial systems in which institutional violence occurs are prisons, mental institutions, and the family. Even though we tend to think that mental institutions are places only for healing and the family is only an arena of love, closer observations of both institutions reveal more violence than we usually assume. Structural violence is a feature of social structures. This form of violence is inherent in the established modes of social relations, distribution of goods and services, and legal practices of dispensing justice. Structural violence involves more than the violation of fairness and justice. As the next chapter illustrates, structural violence leads to hidden but lethal inequities, which can lead to the death of those who lack power or influence in the society.

Thus institutional violence and structural violence involve more complex relations, processes, and conditions than personal violence. Personality and temperament are more likely to gain primacy in personal violence than in institutional and structural violence. Ordinarily, institutional and structural violence spans individuals and generations. The historical forces that give rise to them and maintain them override personality traits and temperament. Structural violence in particular imposes a pattern of relations and practices that are deeply ingrained in and dominate everyday living. Individuals are born and socialized into it as victims or perpetrators and, in the absence of a fundamental social change, they play out their ascribed roles. This fact in particular makes structural violence hard to discern because it is very much part of the structure of social reality, prevailing values, and everyday practices. Personal violence confronts us as acts of *individuals*. Structural violence enjoys sanctions of ruling authorities and appears diffuse and very much linked with *social reality*. Directed at individuals, it swamps them and renders them help-

---

[1]Actually, a more complete taxonomy would distinguish and relate four forms of violence: intrapersonal, interpersonal, institutional, and social-structural violence. The first is exemplified by suicide and the second by homicide, both examples constituting the most extreme instances of personal violence.

less. Collective action alone can question, harness, and redirect structural violence.

Clearly, structural violence and personal violence are at different levels of complexity and of different durations. Institutional violence is at an intermediate level of complexity and duration. It mediates personal and structural violence. All three are of course related and none of them can be understood apart from the other two. All three also reinforce and depend on one another. Structural violence cannot occur without institutions and persons to give it expression. Personal violence is doomed to scorn as "crime," incurring harsh punishment when it occurs without institutional and social sanction. Thus in a patriarchal society in which men monopolize violence, a man who beats his wife is less of an anomaly than a woman who beats her husband. Similarly, in the racist society of yesteryear, white men raped black women with impunity but black men suspected of raping white women risked lynching.

All three forms of violence occur in every society. Yet how much of each is expressed and modified varies from one society to another. There are societies with a relatively high degree of integration and synchrony among the three forms of violence. In such societies, one finds a shared axis around which revolve the prevailing laws, the rules governing family life, and the conventions guiding conduct in everyday living. The integration and synchrony of the three levels of violence are of course never total or perfect. There are also societies in which personal, institutional, and structural violence are not coordinated and do not have a common purpose. These usually are societies in marked transition and conflict. It so happens that in both types of societies only certain groups tend to bear the brunt of the violence. They die more frequently and at younger ages than others in the *same* society. The more oppressive and rigid the social order, the higher their death rate—physically, socially, and psychologically.

A situation of oppression involves structural, institutional, and personal violence. Oppression and one of its expressions, racism, legitimize structural violence, rationalize institutional violence, and impersonalize personal violence. In a situation in which oppression spans generations the violence to which it owes its origin and sustenance is masked and obfuscated. The law, the media, education, religion, work relations, the environment—the whole ensemble of cultural and material arrangements of society remain infused with violence, which becomes harder to discern the longer one lives under this condition of oppression. A search for personal or conscious intentions is futile under these circumstances. Structural and institutional violence have their own logic and momentum. This is what Fanon set out to boldly and critically unravel.

FANON'S THEORY OF VIOLENCE

In the first chapter of his classic *The Wretched of the Earth* (1968), Fanon elaborated the dynamics of violence and the human drama that unfolds in situations of oppression. He boldly analyzed violence in its structural, institutional, and personal dimensions. He brought fresh insights to a central topic of human history, albeit a topic that is difficult to unravel or study. Fanon not only demonstrated the ugly manifestations of violence, he also explained its liberative role in situations in which all other means have failed. His treatise on violence is no doubt the most controversial of his contributions.

It is important to appreciate the evolution of his thought on violence from the time he wrote his first book, *Black Skin, White Masks,* to when he completed *The Wretched of the Earth.* In his first work, Fanon analyzed the psycho-existential aspects of life in a racist society. He emphasized the experiential features and hidden psychoaffective injuries of blacks and the various defensive maneuvers they adopted. Another unstated objective was quite personal: He himself had experienced these injuries and writing about them was a way of coming to terms with himself. These objectives were more or less achieved, but no program of action to change the oppressive social order was proposed.

That the early Fanon resorted to self-analysis and a psychological approach should not be surprising. His newly acquired profession of psychiatry had conditioned him to this manner of looking at human problems. Even at this stage, Fanon no doubt realized the necessity of fundamental changes in the social order. But the outlook that dominates Fanon's early writing was a belief in the potency of reason in dealing even with matters so irrational as racism and psychopathology. Reading his early work, one cannot but be impressed with Fanon's abiding belief that, however intolerable conditions were, reason would at last prevail. Hence the task was one of explaining, marshaling evidence, and persuading: "I seriously hope to persuade my brother, whether black or white, to tear off with all his strength the shameful livery put together by centuries of incomprehension" (Fanon, 1967a, p. 12).

The optimism that underlies this approach of rational persuasion is no doubt inspiring. Unfortunately, stubborn realities rendered it untenable and perhaps too naive. It was indeed one thing to experience racism with a touch of civility in a metropole like Paris or to debate the plight of the oppressed with intellectuals. But it was quite another thing to submerge oneself in the jarring realities of a colony, such as Algeria, and witness the "natives" hounded, persecuted, and tormented in their own land. And the Europeans who presided at such a colonial inferno relied upon and understood only brute violence. Thus the question of violence had to be squarely faced and so too the question of oppression from a new perspective. The result was at once an illuminating and incendiary thunderbolt.

Fanon elaborated the crude and subtle processes by which the colonizer usurps power and property all the while reducing the colonized into objects to be used, misused, and destroyed at will. The means to usurpation and dehumanization were not reasoning, persuading, or cajoling. They were rather by a series of brutally violent acts. Guns, cannons, and a technology of death were used along with deception, and the fanning of every local conflict, and of course the deployment of an army of specialists—anthropologists, doctors, teachers, and religious zealots. What is more, the oppressor was not content to occupy the land of others or expropriate their labor. He wanted to advance ever deeper and place himself in the very center of the dominated (Fanon, 1967c, p. 65):

> There is no occupation of territory, on the one hand, and independence of persons on the other. It is the country as a whole, its history, its daily pulsation that are contested, disfigured, in the hope of final destruction. Under this condition, the individual's breathing is an observed, and occupied breathing. It is a combat breathing.

If the occupation of land thus entailed the occupation of psyches, then the war for liberation had to be waged on two fronts. The colonizer residing not only *without*, but also *within* had to be confronted on both fronts. Otherwise, the vicious cycle of domination would continue. To battle the colonizer *without* first assumes a degree of self-respect and self-validation, a conviction that one is at least as good and as human as he is. It also assumes the existence of a bond with others, a sharing of similar experiences and determination. But neither assumption is usually tenable under conditions of prolonged oppression. The confidence and self-worth of the oppressed have long been undermined. Their connection with one another, save that which is innocuous or regressive, has also been weakened. The colonized had been reduced to individuals without an anchor in history, alienated from themselves and others. So long as this alienation prevailed, the colonizer *without* could not be challenged. His abuses, humiliations, and suffocating repression permeated everyday living, further undermining the colonized's self-respect and collective bonds.

How does a community of oppressed and alienated regain its self-respect and confidence in order to challenge the colonizer *without*? Psychotherapy is out of the question for at least five reasons. First, in its most developed and traditional form, psychotherapy is a tool for the treatment of individual psychopathology. In its most extended form, it can be effective only with small groups and families. Psychologists are not of course in the business of "mass psychotherapy," which, if such a practice existed, could have offered one option for the community of the oppressed and alienated. Second, the problem is not really one of psychopathology, but rather of oppression, not of instinctual or only subjective conflicts but rather of genuine conflicts between oppressors and oppressed. Any attempt that reduces the problems of oppression to instinctual or subjective problems or of psychopathology runs the risk of blaming the victim. Third, the elitist and class foundation of traditional psychotherapy orients it toward social control and adjustment to the *status quo*. Thus psychotherapeutic endeavors with the oppressed can easily become a subtle but effective tool of oppression. Fourth, its ethnocentric orientation has tended to incorporate racist and solipsist views in its theory and practice. And fifth, psychotherapy has become a commodity to be sold and bought. It therefore follows that as a commodity, those who can afford get it whereas those who are poor and powerless seldom become the focus of genuine interest among psychologists. The question then, is this: What options are available for rehabilitation of the oppressed?

Fanon may have mused over such issues long before he became a clinical director at the Blida-Joinville Hospital in colonial Algeria. But as we shall see, his work in this hospital confirmed his fears that mental institutions in oppressive societies are places of violence, not of healing. The institution in which he worked was not only intolerably crowded and medieval, it was also used by the colonial authorities as a dumping ground for tortured and broken Algerians. Fanon was later convinced that the colonizer *without* and the colonizer *within* are best confronted simultaneously and by the same means—namely, violence. The Algerian war of independence burgeoned and Fanon committed himself to it. His earlier conviction that reason would prevail or that persuasion would change the oppressor–oppressed dialectic had lost ground. Fanon (1968, p. 147) now saw that only violence could transform the oppressive order and occupied psyches. The colonizer depended on and understood only violence and he had to be met with greater violence: "Violence alone, violence committed by the people, violence organized and educated by its leaders, makes it possible for the masses to understand social truths and gives the key to them."

By the time the chapter on violence was written, Fanon had years of direct experience on battlefields and in the circle of Algerian freedom fighters. He observed not only the ravages of war, but also the cultural and psychic revitalization that emerge as the oppressed begin to take control of their destiny. The chapter on violence is appropriately on decolonization, not on colonization. The audience for which it was intended is not everyone, but only the colonized. The style and tone of writing also changed. Fanon here did not quote European scholars nor did he confine himself to psychological concepts. He developed his own formulation and discussed violence in its various manifestations. How the oppressor uses it to maintain his unjust rule, what defensive maneuver the oppressed adopt, how the oppressor's vertical violence changes to horizontal violence among the oppressed—these are the issues that Fanon examined with a brilliance that led Jean-Paul Sartre to state (Fanon, 1968, p. 14): "If you set aside Sorel's fascist utterances, you will find that Fanon is the first since Engels to bring the process of history into the clear light of day."

Pivotal to Fanon's theory is the notion that a Manichean psychology underlies human violence and oppression. A Manichean view is one that divides the world into compartments and people into different "species." This division is based not on reciprocal affirmations, but rather on irreconcilable opposites cast into good versus evil, beautiful versus ugly, intelligent versus stupid, white versus black, human versus subhuman modes. This duality of opposites is not dialectical and hence not an attempt toward a higher synthesis. Its logic is a categorical *either/or*, in which one of the terms is considered superfluous and unacceptable. Yet in reality, this duality of opposites in the Manichean outlook are interdependent. Each is defined in terms of its opposite and each derives its identity in opposition to the other. Yet in such a perspective, it is necessary to keep the line of demarcation quite clear or else the Manichean psychology collapses. Oppression creates and requires such a psychology whereas at the same time violence too emerges from and reinforces the Manichean psychology.

In a situation of oppression, the Manichean psychology permeates everyday living. The environment and how it is structured reflect it. There is, on the one hand, the district or town in which the oppressor resides. The houses are spacious and grand. The streets are brightly lit, the trees are well-manicured, and litter is seldom seen. Indeed how objects are put together reflect peace, order, organization, and fastidious care. Neither in the huge boulevards nor in the spacious houses does one feel hemmed in or crowded. The well-fed and well-dressed people are well disposed to each other so long as everyone possesses the characteristics—racial or otherwise—that identify the species on this side of the world. The police too are cordial and helpful to all but those intruders who may cross the color and class boundary. Indeed their job is to keep these "born" criminals and unredeemable scum out of sight. If by chance they find a member of the other species, their cordiality vanishes and they act like hounds ready to pounce on their prey.

There is, on the other hand, the ghetto in which the oppressed live on top of each other in dilapidated tenement houses, hovels, and shacks. The streets, if they are paved, are rough and full of potholes. They are poorly lit and dark and forbidding once the sun sets. Garbage collection is sporadic. And since there are no garbage cans, one finds bottles and litter everywhere. The ill-fed and badly dressed inhabitants of this district are well disposed to only a few people they know and trust. The way their world is put together betrays the ravages of an undeclared but ongoing war. And so long as the inhabitants deny this fact, their behavior and the objects around them reflect disorganization, apathy, and neglect. The police here are invariably hostile and suspicious. Their headquarters are huge, fortified installations. They reach for their batons and pistols upon the slightest suspicious act. On this side of the world, everyone is frequently on edge—the police and the soldiers more so.

The Manichean psychology also permeates the prevailing values and beliefs. The oppressor identifies himself in terms of the sublime and beauty while depicting the oppresssed in terms of absolute evil and ugliness.

> In fact, the terms the [white] settler uses when he mentions the native are zoological terms. He speaks of the yellow man's reptilean motions, of the stink of the native quarters, of the breeding swarms, of foulness, of spawns, of gesticulation. (Fanon, 1968, p. 42)

Civilization and high values are used to characterize the oppressor. His skin color, habits, and all else that identifies him are considered superior, whereas those features of the oppressed are despised as if they personify filth and evil. Indeed the oppressed is depicted as lacking any values or ethics—he is the quintessence of evil. He can be neutralized only by spraying with DDT and by conversion to Christianity. In short, the oppressor puts himself beyond human attributes and reduces the oppressed as subhuman.

On his part, the oppressed assumes his role in the Manichean psychology thrust upon him. But he does so with much ambivalence and smoldering rage. He defines the oppressor as "the other" who personifies all that he despises and also envies. He is depicted as an animal and devoid of intelligence—characterizations he may not publicly dispute until he is ready to reverse the Manichean equation. Secretly and in the privacy of his group, the oppressed knows and jokes about the fact that his pretenses and feigned smiles fool his tormentor. Nonetheless, the ignominious role in which he is cast does not leave him unscathed. For to the extent that the oppressor gains, to that extent does the oppressed lose. To the degree that the oppressor is jubilant, to that degree is the oppressed mournful. Inasmuch as the former is content, in the same intensity is the latter unhappy and enraged. These are the imperatives of the Manichean psychology. And so long as this psychology prevails, the oppressed is in a state of permanent tension. His immediate dream is that of changing roles: "to sit at the settler's table, to sleep in his bed, with his wife if possible" (Fanon, 1968, p. 32).

This way of dividing the world into compartments and people into species derives from and reinforces violence. The disparaging characterizations, the military barracks, the towering statues of conquering generals, the rampant police brutality, the imposed national anthem, the alienating history lessons, and the racist glances all constitute expressions of violence. Once the Manichean psychology takes root in people's heart and mind, it becomes remarkably easy to embark on pogroms, pillage, rape, and every other conceivable crime. Indeed it is difficult to abuse and murder another in the absence of the Manichean psychology. That is why American soldiers referred to the Vietnamese as "gooks," the racists to blacks as "niggers," the blacks to whites as "honkies," and the protestors to the police as "pigs." These labels are categorical and permit no individual differentiation. Once so labeled—an act that itself is violent, the ground is prepared for more violence and victimization.

The Manichean psychology is hard to counteract once it takes root in people, the environment, and the culture. Those who live it rely on it for their individual and collective identity. On the surface, the oppressor benefits in the continuation of the Manichean psychology. His identity is more secure; his self-respect is maintained; his confidence seems firm; and he enjoys a relatively harmonious bond with his kind. He has a sense of history, a measure of control over his destiny. All this is however founded on the wreckage and dehumanization of the other. Thus the oppressed is full of self-doubt; he is made to feel inferior; his self-worth is undermined; his confidence and bond with others are weakened. His history is obliterated; he cannot control what happens to him; he feels victorious if he escapes an ever-present peril. One question of significant import is this: What does the oppressed do with the smoldering rage engendered by the Manichean psychology?

Fanon provides some rare insights into the dynamics and self-destructive consequences of violence imposed on the oppressed: The victim of oppression feels "hemmed in" when he internalizes the self-negating prohibitions of the oppressor. He initially adopts avoidance reactions. His dreams are violent and of muscular prowess. He dreams of being chased by motorcars, of jumping, swimming, climbing, and bursting into laughter. At the collective level, this repressed counterviolence exhausts itself through vigorous dances, sexual escapades, symbolic killings, and exaggerated beliefs in terrifying myth and magic. Such acts, Fanon (1968, p. 57) suggested, "may be deciphered as in an open book the huge effort of a community to exorcise itself, to liberate itself, to explain itself." Fanon also detected an aggressive component even in the very propensity to imitate the oppressor and be assimilated into his culture—an interesting insight recalling the well-known psychological process of "identification with aggressor."

But when the repressed counterviolence finds neither sublimated canalization nor conscious social praxis, one observes an appalling incidence of crime, and particularly of homicide, among the oppressed (Fanon, 1968, p. 52):

> The colonized man will manifest this aggressiveness which has been deposited in his bones against his own people. This is the period when the niggers beat each other up, and police and magistrates do not know which way to turn when faced with astonishing waves of crime.

The victim of prolonged oppression, once he submits to bondage, learns to take the violent assaults and dictates of his oppressor patiently, even with a feigned smile. He may obsequiously obey orders, seek assimilation into the dominant culture, develop a knack for minor sabotages through passive resistance, and refine his own means of vicarious retaliation. Yet the violent assaults and everyday abuses are too much to bear. His demeaning public behaviors of submission and compliance are at the same time ego-dystonic. Thus under the cumulative impact of this impossible situation, he turns his anger as well as his frustration against himself and his own people. The result is a higher incidence of alcoholism, psychiatric disorder, hypertension, and homicide (Fanon, 1968, p. 54).

> When the [white] settler or the policeman has the right the livelong day to strike the native, to insult him and make him crawl to them, you will see the native reaching out for his knife at the slightest hostile or aggressive glance cast on him by another native: *for the last resort of the native is to defend his personality vis-à-vis his brother.*

Homicide in an oppressed community has its own psychodynamic and social dialectic. The oppressed knows that any effort to defend against the assault on his personality and dignity produces only further abuse. The numerous armed police around him, the disproportionately high number of prisoners of his class and color, the all-pervasive media and institutions of social control engender in him a heightened sense of vulnerability, on the one hand, and a muscular tonicity, on the other. Now if he cannot defend his personality in the larger social arena, he must by all means defend what is left of it in his last refuge—namely, in the circle of his family and friends. That is why the slightest challenge, rejection, or offense by those worthy of his love or respect (thereby of his high expectations) pushes him to a volcanic eruption of a repressed aggression, a welling-up of an accumulated anger, and a long-delayed but now reflexive action of dead finality. Indeed for homicide under such conditions, one can even postulate an unconscious wish to eliminate an intimate covictim of oppression who but mirrors what one hates in oneself—namely, the internalized cupidity of the oppressor and the inculcated cowardice of submission.

Interestingly, Fanon did not view such fratricidal assaults as permanent characteristics of oppressed communities. He observed that when political consciousness takes hold and the struggle for freedom is well under way, the rate and character of this violence are strikingly modified. The oppressor's violence, which has been internalized and institutionalized among the oppressed, is henceforth externalized and redirected in the service of personal and collective liberation. Horizontal violence thus changes into vertical counterviolence. Avoidance reactions expressed in dreams, violent fantasies, and autodestructive behaviors give way to a proactive, revolutionary praxis. Pent-up anger and tension, previously repressed and somatized, now find appropriate targets and constructive avenues of discharge. The hostility that had permeated most relationships among the oppressed is markedly reduced and the community adopts such affiliative terms as "brother, sister, and friend."

Fanon suggested that it is also precisely during this revolutionary period of self-affirmation and objectification that new identities unfold, creative energies long repressed are revitalized, and stagnant traditions transformed into dynamic cultures. An act of violence against the unrelenting oppressor, an irrevocable action against his world strewn with prohibitions—decisive measures such as these take on a new significance during this period. These, according to Fanon, demystify the power of the oppressor, detoxify all negative accumulations of oppression, restore self- as well as group-confidence, and promote strong social cohesion among the oppressed. Indeed such acts may serve as a communal pardon allowing "strayed and outlawed members of the group to come back and to find their place once more, to be integrated" (Fanon, 1968, p. 86).

In short, Fanon began with the belief that reason and goodwill were potent means to resolve the situation of oppression. Experience led him to reformulate the problem as well as the solution. The question of violence became the focus of his interest and he began his classic and last book on that topic. He described a particular type of psychology—the Manichean psychology—which underlies human oppression and violence. He also concluded that those who profit by violence can be made to change only through greater violence. The oppressed who are dehumanized by the violence of the oppressor also turn that violence against themselves when they lack the consciousness and organization to fight back. But they regain their identity, reclaim their history, reconstitute their bonding, and forge their future through violence. Through violence, they remove the primary barrier to their humanity *and* they rehabilitate themselves. By killing the oppressor, as Jean-Paul Sartre summarized in the preface to Fanon's book (1968, p. 22), the oppressed "kill two birds with one stone . . . there remains a dead man and a free man" (Fanon, p. 86).

FANON AND VIOLENCE REVISITED

Not surprisingly, Fanon was severely criticized for his theory of violence. Because of it, he has been characterized as an "apostle of violence" and denounced as a "prisoner of hate." His book, *The Wretched of the Earth*, was compared to Hitler's *Mein Kampf.* Others invoked Georges Sorel whose *Reflections On Violence* is said to have influenced Fanon. Sorel's flirtation with fascism is well known and Mussolini himself declared: "I owe most to Georges Sorel. This master of syndicalism by his rough theories or revolutionary tactics has contributed most to form the discipline, energy and power of the fascist cohorts" (Sorel, 1970, p. 24).

The association of Fanon with hate, Hitler, and Sorel is actually a blatant and curious distortion of the facts. It is an association that viciously maligns Fanon and puts down his insights into a crucial but neglected problem in human affairs. Leaving aside unsubstantiated charges the effect of which is character assassination, three important questions require answers. First, Was Fanon an apologist of violence for violence's sake? Second, Was he influenced by Georges Sorel? Third, Why is Fanon's theory of violence so readily misconstrued? We will briefly comment on these three questions and explore their implications.

There are two major critiques of Fanon's theory of violence. The harshest and best known is by Hannah Arendt (1970) who evaluated Fanon essentially from a staunchly Eurocentric vantage point. The second is by Nguyen Nghe (1963) who examined Fanon's ideas in the light of the revolutionary experience in Vietnam. The two critiques are drastically different in purpose, approach, and affective content. Hannah Arendt's critique is hysterical, combative, and contemptuous. She seems determined to search for flaws and manages to find them, but only on flimsy and unsubstantiated grounds. Indeed her critique of Fanon is part of a broader attack on black Americans in particular and the Third World in general. Nguyen Nghe's critique is more sober and sympathetic and merits careful consideration. He shares with Fanon similar concerns over the plight of the colonized and oppressed, but takes issue with Fanon's tactics and analysis. Woddis (1972) used Nghe's critique and elaborated on it by using data from Africa.

One significant charge Arendt (1970, p. 65) made was that Fanon glorified violence for violence's sake. Thus Fanon is equated with Sorel and Pareto:

> Not many authors of rank glorified violence for violence sake; but these few—Sorel, Pareto, Fanon—were motivated by a much deeper hatred of bourgeois society—than the Conventional Left, which was inspired by compassion and a burning desire for justice.

Arendt not only places Fanon in close affinity with Sorel and Pareto, but she also claims that "Fanon, who had an infinitely greater intimacy with the practice of violence than either, was greatly influenced by Sorel and used his categories even when his own experiences spoke clearly against them" (Arendt, 1970, p. 71). These two contentions—that Fanon glorified violence for its own sake and that he was influenced by Sorel—are presented along with a sweeping and disdainful attack of the Black Power movement in the United States, black students on American campuses, and the Third World which, in her words, "is not a reality but an ideology."

Arendt traced the violence that flared on some college campuses during the sixties to the influences of Frantz Fanon, the black students, and the black

American community. Thus we are told that the student rebellion during the sixties was nonviolent and principled until the Black Power movement and black students entered the scene.

> Serious violence entered the scene only with the appearance of the Black Power movement on the campus. Negro students, the majority of them admitted without academic qualification, regarded and organized themselves as an interest group, the representatives of the black community.

What, in Arendt's view, did the black student really want? Her answer (Arendt, 1970, p. 18): "Their interest was to lower academic standards."

We are further informed that not only were white students nonviolent, but also that their communities never condoned violence on campus. In contrast, Arendt accused not only black students, but also "the Negro community (which stands) behind the verbal and actual violence of the black students." Arendt (1970, p. 19) is enraged at the academic establishment for "its curious tendency to yield to Negro demands, even if they are clearly *silly* and *outrageous*, than to the *disinterested* and usually highly moral claims of white rebels. . . ." Equally, she derided black students desire to learn Swahili, African literature, and "other nonexistent subjects [which in a few years] will be interpreted as another trap of the white man to prevent Negroes from acquiring an adequate education" (Arendt, 1970, p. 96). And so goes Arendt's tirade and racism masquerading as intellectual discourse.

The claim that compassion and a burning desire for justice inspired the Conventional Left more than did Fanon, or that troublesome blacks dragged highly moral whites into mediocrity and violence, could be discarded as problems of personal bias and idiosyncracy. But the charge that Fanon glorified violence for violence's sake and that he was influenced by Sorel requires evidence that indeed Arendt did not present. Keeping her personal biases from clouding the issues, and a closer look at Fanon's life and work, would have led Arendt to a different conclusion. Fanon believed that everyone has a sacred right to life, freedom, and dignity and that none of us—least of all Fanon himself—should enjoy this right while somewhere others are persecuted, exploited, and dehumanized. By his choice of profession, he committed himself to heal troubled and tormented psyches. In his early years he ardently believed in the potency of reason to resolve human problems—whether public or private. But life and work in colonial Algeria infused his humanism with unswerving resolve and militancy. His observations there underscored the fact that colonialism and the men who run that violent machine were impervious to appeals to reason. Established clinical practice too became untenable when those who govern willfully thwarted the life, freedom, and dignity of the governed. It became clear to Fanon and to the Algerian people that, when all peaceful measures failed, there remained only one recourse—and that was to *fight*. Fanon's goal of healing tormented psyches thereby moved from the consulting room to the larger societal arena, from a concern with private and personal problems to an emphasis on public and collective well-being, and from curative and institution-based to preventive and mass-participatory measures. Taking up arms was for him never an end in itself but only a last recourse—and a perilous one at that.

A related issue that others have unjustly emphasized and taken out of context is Fanon's assertion that, at the individual level, revolutionary violence "disintoxifies" the oppressed. This assertion has given rise to rabid criticism of Fanon by nonclinicians who could not differentiate between "disintoxification" and catharsis. Gendzier (1973, pp. 198–205) in particular has made too much out of the common misinterpretation that Fanon's assertion was a justification for "catharsis" through violence. In discussing Fanon's theory of violence, she dwelt on what she referred to as Fanon's "notion of the cathartic effect of violence" only to condemn it to be "considerably less convincing as a policy." This interpretation actually misses Fanon's point. The confusion derives partly from Farrington's translation of "la violence desintoxique" into "violence is a cleansing force." There is also a frequent tendency to take the remark out of context and suggest, however indirectly, that Fanon glorified violence for its own sake.

Here as elsewhere, Fanon was actually concerned with how the oppressed could free themselves from the legacy of an inferiority complex, reclaim their identity, reconstitute their bonding, and take control of their destiny. Avoidance behavior with respect to the structural and institutional violence of the oppressor or obsequious pleas for denied justice are not only impractical but also intensify the dehumanization of the oppressed. Fanon's argument was that conscious and determined confrontation of the oppressed was unavoidable if the oppressed are to rehabilitate themselves and that this confrontation was necessarily collective and goal directed.

Fanon was of course well aware that violent actions have residual effects on perpetrators and their families. The clinical cases reviewed in Chapter 9 show his keen realization that catharsis in itself is not therapeutic—least of all when one's actions directly injure and dehumanize others. But the stubborn refusal and violence of the oppressor leaves no option but to fight him. And in fighting him, the oppressed is collectively and individually "disintoxified." In other words, the recovery of the alcoholic begins in his detoxification; the cure of the phobic lies in confronting the very object of his fears; and the self-rehabilitation of the oppressed begins in directly confronting the source of his dehumanization. This—not simply a recommendation of wanton violence—is Fanon's point. That he did not celebrate violence for its own sake is illustrated by his following remark (Fanon, 1967c, p. 25):

> Because we want a democratic and renovated Algeria, we believe we cannot rise and liberate ourself in one area and sink in another. We condemn with pain in our hearts, those brothers who have flung themselves into revolutionary action with the almost psychological brutality that centuries of oppression give rise to and feed.

On the question of whether Sorel influenced Fanon, there is simply no evidence to support that contention and no indication that Fanon ever read Sorel. The two men in fact approached the question of violence from drastically different vantage points and with opposing goals. Sorel, a conservative moralist, saw life in terms of a fundamental conflict between "decadence" and "renascence." He combined this staunchly moralist outlook with some aspects of Marxism, particularly the theory of class struggle. An incurable pessimist, he believed that the possibility of deliverance was narrowly conditioned. He saw the bourgeoisie, politicians, and intellectuals as the epitome of decadence and thought that only the practice of violence promised any possibility of deliverance. His goal was not to restore justice and equality, but rather to attain moral superiority, heroism, and glory through violence and some cataclysmic showdown.

Sorel was least concerned with the poverty and material distress of the oppressed who, in any case, he viewed with much scorn. The dissolution of traditional morality disturbed him; the growing dominance of rationality and hedonism appalled him; compromise and cowardice enraged him. The Sorelean vanguard was a small, dedicated, and disciplined elite who embraced violence as an end, cared nothing about consequences, and were guided by a social "myth"—a combination of unrefutable claims, remote goals, and a belief in apocalyptic success. Taking up arms for Sorel was not a last resort, but rather the beginning of an engulfing and redeeming violence. Clearly, Sorel and Fanon were worlds apart, even antithetical, and any claim that one influenced the other is a sheer distortion of the facts.

Nghe's discussion of Fanon was based on a careful reading, a statement of some fundamental areas of agreement, and a critique on certain key issues—mainly, the role of violence, the significance of the peasantry, and the centrality of the working class in revolutionary change. Unlike Arendt, Nghe emphasized his shared sense of outrage about the atrocious misery and humiliation imposed on colonized peoples. He also concedes Fanon's ability to articulate that outrage with moving and appropriate language, his undeniable insights into oppression, and his relentless commitment to social justice. He regretted the premature death of Fanon who doubtless would have revised some of his ideas in light of subsequent developments in Algeria and the world. Having paid due respect to the man who contributed so much, Nghe proceeded to correct flaws he found in the book Fanon left behind.

On the question of violence—the question that concerns us here, Nghe pointed out that armed struggle, however crucial, is only a phase, a passing moment, in the revolutionary struggle of a people. Underlying the resolve to take up arms and guiding the armed struggle must be a well-defined political struggle. Nghe accused Fanon of confusing, or at least not differentiating, the political essence of armed struggle from its existential side effects. He traced this "flaw" to past influences of French existentialism on Fanon. Nghe claimed that, although Fanon had overcome the *a*political orientation of his existentialist influences, he nonetheless remained an "individualistic intellectual" who emphasized psychology over politics. Nghe further argued that to emphasize the existential over the political aspects of armed struggle is to risk oversimplification of complex social problems, romanticism of the spectacular, and lack of preparedness when peace at last prevails and the task of national reconstruction begins. So long as the political consciousness of people is left undeveloped and only martial arts are emphasized, Nghe warned, the very political goals for which arms were taken up are lost. Nghe illustrated this point with early experiences in Vietnam where, because the people's political confidence was shaken, veterans who fought for nine years once again took up opium and peasants who fought guerrilla wars once again became scared of ghosts.

Nghe's critique of Fanon is one of the most informative yet. The power of this critique lies not only in the analytical acumen of its author, but also in his ability to draw on the experiences gained from the revolutionary struggle in Vietnam. Moreover, it is a constructive critique with the aim of correcting perceived flaws while recognizing essential contributions. There is certainly much in Nghe's critique that can serve as cautionary markers to aspects of Fanon's ideas. But the accusation that Fanon did not emphasize ideology or political struggle—which indeed he did—actually boils down to a regret that Fanon deviated from traditional Marxist dogma. Thus for instance, Fanon's contention that the most authentically revolutionary class in Africa is the peasantry, not the working class, and that the *lumpenproletariat*—the idlers, pimps, prostitutes, and petty criminals—can play significant roles in revolutionary struggle, has brought him much criticism from Marxist writers, including Nghe (1963) and Woddis (1972).

Some of Nghe's criticism of Fanon seems to be justified. Fanon indeed overgeneralized from the Algerian experience and drew categorical conclusions from one historical moment in Algerian history. He provided little data to support his claims regarding the attributes, problems, and prospects of social classes in Africa. His style of writing, which was aphoristic, graphic, and moving, also tended to be imprecise with respect to time and place and the actual and the ideal. One is sometimes hard pressed to figure out if Fanon is referring to the past or the present or the Algerian situation specifically or the African predicament generally and if statements are based on data or yet unconfirmed hypotheses. Fanon also tended to fix certain attributes to one or another social class and to define them in categorical affirmations or negations, and he seldom delved into their dynamic relation to one another and the importance of each class during a given stage in the struggle for liberation. As Amilcar Cabral (1979) has so well demonstrated, it is crucial to delineate when and under what circumstances a particular class can advance or hinder revolutionary change and what conditions foster alliance and conflict among classes.

Other aspects of Nghe's criticism are indeed quite unjustified. One of these is the claim that Fanon failed to consider ideology or political struggle. Fanon (1967b, p. 186) himself said, "For my part, the deeper I enter into the cultures and the political circles, the surer I am that the great danger that threatens Africa is the absence of ideology." In his later works particularly, Fanon emphasized the role of ideology as he underscored the necessity of political struggle. The importance he attached to careful organization, social mobilization, effective leadership, and political education is quite obvious from a careful reading of his works. The accusation that whoever deviates from traditional Marxist dogma therefore does not appreciate ideology or political struggle is actually counterproductive. Indeed two of the new dangers facing the oppressed today are the degeneration of "progressive" precepts to religious dogma and the inquisitions of high priests residing in alien academic ivory towers or in capitals like Moscow. Equally counterproductive is the neglect of psychological considerations by Marxists like Nghe and the reflexive rejection of matters scornfully labeled as "subjective." Any political thought which prides itself to be nothing but "objective" not only risks self-delusion, but also condemns itself to irrelevance by neglecting human and therefore subjective factors in history. Fanon was a pioneer precisely because he combined a commitment to social transformation with the psychological liberation of individuals.

Of course, one must realize that *The Wretched of the Earth* in which Fanon elaborated his theory of violence was written in haste and at a time when Fanon, then a victim of leukemia, knew that his days were numbered. Efforts to treat him in Tunisia and the Soviet Union proved unsuccessful. A period of respite from the disease permitted him to embark on what was to become a classic. The major part of the work was writtten in about three months and Fanon read the proofs in Washington, D. C., only a few days before his death. This fact is not only remarkable in itself, but it should suggest a measure of modesty in critiques usually written in better health, with more resources, and at a more leisurely pace. The point here is not to decry criticism of Fanon's ideas, but, rather to suggest the need to place them in proper perspective.

The fact that he wrote on violence while the Algerian revolution was in progress also had distinct advantages although it imposed serious problems. It is one thing to speculate from an academic ivory tower about the upheavals of revolution, view the gigantic machinery of war from a distance in time and space, maintain emotional detachment in manipulating lifeless statistics, and reduce the immense travails of anonymous victims into convenient intellectual paradigms. It is quite another to be totally immersed in the social upheaval, to commit one's life to a cause now looming larger than everything else, to rub shoulders with living persons in the din of battle, and to fully identify with them in victory as well as in defeat. In the first situation, one merely intellectualizes an immensely complex and emotionally-laden experience, groping to at best capture its profile and common denominator. In the second situation, best exemplified by Fanon, one is so totally submerged in that reality that consideration of it becomes less a cerebral excercise and more a visceral onslaught. Fanon wrote about violence from a personal and intimate vantage point. Deeply involved in the Algerian war of independence, he wrote with the passion and insight that come from an existential immersion. At the same time, this existential immersion and his total identification imposed some problems. Thus it is often difficult to separate what Fanon intended as a statement of fact from a justification of the Algerian Revolution and what he intended as merely descriptive from the prescriptive.

In spite of these problems, Fanon presented a fresh perspective on violence hardly matched in its depth, insight, and courage. Many who studied the problem demonstrated their unwillingness to break out of the narrow and sanctioned conceptions of violence that every social order imposes by focusing only on illegitimate violence. By focusing on criminology, they simply mistook the tip of the iceberg for the whole iceberg. Others sought to go beyond the superficial, delved into the realm of instincts, and unwittingly further mystified human violence. Their contention of primordial causes diffused the ideas of where human responsibility, and the human capacity to avert man-made disasters lie. Either approach reduces the salience of human oppression and the violence it entails. In the end, both justify, defend, and bolster the *status quo*.

Charles Pinderhughes (1972, p. 111), a black American psychoanalyst, has offered a wealth of theoretical and clinical insights that confirm and elaborate the significance of Manichean psychology in all violent interactions. He demonstrated that it is not possible to act violently against another person, group, or object without narcissism and self-aggrandizement of the perpetrator, on the one hand, and denigration and devaluation of the victim, on the other. In every violent action, there is a paranoid process and content prior to, concurrent with, or subsequent to the violent action. Projective mechanisms and their attendant false belief systems justify the violent action and attenuate guilt. This is so for all violent actions occurring in intimate circles as well as in larger groups. "In every case of marital conflict which I have explored," wrote Pinderhughes (1972, p. 113), "such violence as occurred took place when the party taking violent action perceived the marital partner as an embodiment of evil." Thus for instance, a husband perceived his wife as a "witch" at the very moment when he was swinging a fist at her and she in turn thought of him as a "monster" while she was aiming her car at his.

The perpetrator perceives the victim as an enemy threatening his existence. The destructive action becomes rationalized as a way of bringing him to justice, correcting a defect, and improving his person or behavior. There may indeed be an aspect of the victim that is actually threatening, provocative, and troublesome. But more often than not, the external "enemy" represents a renounced, unacceptable, and projected part of the self.

> Violence to another cannot occur in a moment of introjective relationship, when the would-be victim is perceived as an acknowledged and valued part of the self. Violence can only occur under circumstances of projective relationship. (Pinderhughes, 1972, p.111)

Introjective identification is the process by which we take as our own the acknowledged part of others, bond with them, and develop a trusting relationship. *Projective identification* is the process by which we renounce unacceptable impulses and attributes, cast them on safe objects, and define boundaries between the valued self and devalued objects.

Paranoia is by no means a monopoly of pathological persons. It is also a characteristic feature in the psychology of "normal" persons. Individuals identified as pathological are those who fail to align their paranoid processes and content with the paranoia prevalent in their community or society. They are also persons who fail to develop introjective, affectionate, and trusting relationships. Each society offers its members a set of beliefs, values, and institutions around which to align their paranoia. Each individual thus comes to view the world as a member of a given faith, political affiliation, professional association, social class, nationality, race, sex, etc. Of course not all group beliefs are paranoid, but they often contain a measure of shared paranoia with projective processes and contents. A racist society elaborates paranoia and false belief systems into cultural and institutional reality. Socialization in turn conditions members, including the primary victims, to align their conditioned paranoia.

One characteristic feature of paranoid patterns, shared or idiosyncratic, is that they are obvious to others but not to those persons caught up in them. Indeed reason itself loses ground and comes to serve paranoid, exploitative, and violent interests. Hence, once enlisted into a system of exploitation, scholars, researchers, and otherwise reasonable persons use their intellect and knowledge in the service of the prevailing paranoia and elaborated false beliefs. Another characteristic is that confrontation tactics offer educational, therapeutic, and corrective measures to paranoid processes. Traditional psychotherapy has tended to favor alliance tactics and positive transference in effecting change. Pinderhughes (1972) and Fanon (1961) show that confrontation tactics, used appropriately and at strategic moments, are most effective means of effecting change.

When a Manichean psychology dominates group relations and the social organization, collective paranoia permeates everyday living. There is, on the one hand, the self-aggrandizing, more privileged, and more powerful "elites" or "masters" and, on the other hand, the devalued, less privileged, and less powerful "non-elites" or "slaves." The dominant group relate to the dominated primarily by means of projection, whereas the dominated relate to the dominant by means of introjection and identification with the aggressor. The dominant group controls the ruling ideas, values, and institutions that not only confirm and reinforce their narcissism, sense of superiority, and privileged status, but also devalue the attributes of the dominated and use them as receptacles for their own renounced and unacceptable aspects.

The non-elites, the slaves, the oppressed depend on and share the paranoia and false beliefs of their oppressors. But since they ordinarily lack safe and convenient objects on which to project these beliefs, they project on themselves the negative attributes cast on them and those emanating from their condition. This further compounds their experience of depression, disorganization, and an inferiority complex. It also reinforces and "validates" the false beliefs and narcissism of the dominant group. The oppressed therefore become victims of others and of themselves. For instance, centuries of slavery and racism have inculcated and institutionalized what Pinderhughes calls "pro-white and anti-black" paranoia among black Americans and adversely affected black identity and mental health. These remained intact until blacks began to confront directly the prevailing pro-white and anti-black paranoia on two fronts: in themselves and among whites. The Black Power movement of the 1960s began to unmask and undo the corrosive consequences of pro-white and anti-black paranoia. Confrontations of this sort may be predictably decried by those who have a stake in the *status quo* of oppression. But one thing is quite certain: the Black Power movement has been the most effective mass therapy for black Americans yet.

In short, violence is a pivotal aspect of oppression. Establishment scholars define the concept and study violence in ways that limit an understanding of its role and significance in situations of oppression. Underlying an act of violence is often a Manichean psychology; a degree of paranoia; and the associated processes of projection, rationalization, and dehumanization. A Manichean psychology and paranoia, whether shared or idiosyncratic, are fertile grounds for violence. Their associated processes of projection, dumping, and victimization occur vertically: from top to bottom, from the powerful to the powerless. Structural violence and collective paranoia are embedded in the culture and the social structure. Having "official" and sanctioned status, they are difficult to discern and dismantle. They are reinforced by institutions, belief systems, the ordering of the environment, and the ritualistic behavior of members.

The oppressed are the primary victims of structural violence and the prevailing paranoia. So long as they lack consciousness and a will to take control of their destiny, they remain victims of others and of themselves. They join in complicity with their oppressors in a manner akin to *folie à deux*, except they suffer more in consequence. Periods of heightened consciousness and social change bring forth an awareness of objective grievances, a determination to change, but also the open declaration or elaboration of *reversal paranoia* whereby projective processes and content flow from bottom to top. This reversed paranoia combines with legitimate grievances to cement the oppressed into a cohesive group with the passion and mission necessary to detoxify members from past humiliations and to effect change. It is in this sense that the struggle for freedom is also a struggle against a well-entrenched Manichean psychology and sedimented paranonia. Chapter 8 provides data showing the immense suffering and loss of human resources resulting from such a deeply entrenched Manichean psychology and collective paranoia. We will later see that it is more difficult to effect change in who owns what or who controls whom than to give birth to and sustain a world without Manichean psychology and collective paranoia.

8

STRUCTURAL VIOLENCE
AND PREMATURE DEATH

The well-being and the progress of Europe have been built up with the sweat and dead bodies of Negroes, Arabs, Indians, and the yellow races. We have decided not to overlook this any longer.
—Fanon, *The Wretched of the Earth*

Structural violence is the most lethal form of violence because it is the least discernible; it causes premature deaths in the largest number of persons; and it presents itself as the natural order of things. A situation of oppression rests primarily on structural violence which in turn fosters institutional, interpersonal, and intrapersonal violence. Structural violence pervades the prevailing values, the environment, social relations, and individual psyches. The most visible indicators of structural violence are differential rates of mortality, morbidity, and incarceration among groups in the *same* society. In particular, a situation of oppression increases the infant mortality rate and lowers the life expectancy for the oppressed. Disparity on these dimensions is greater the more intense the socioeconomic and structural violence.

This chapter examines aspects of violence from the perspective of the oppressed. Violence considered from the perspective of victim and consequence provides a far better conceptual schema to study many seemingly disparate phenomena among the oppressed than is violence studied from the perspective of the perpetrator and intent. This chapter provides empirical and historical data on the structural, institutional, and personal violence imposed on oppressed blacks. It also highlights the ubiquity of autodestructive violence among blacks in the United States and South Africa. The relation of structural, institutional, and personal violence to premature deaths among blacks will be underscored. We hope to show that these extensive data confirm the relevance of a Fanonian perspective to violence.

VIOLENCE AND BLACK AMERICA

The experiences of black Americans offer glaring examples of violence in its different forms. Earlier chapters have already detailed the ruthless violence of the slave trade and plantation slavery. The consideration of these colossal undertakings casts doubt on narrow definitions of violence and underscores the human capacity for destruction. It also becomes clear that more was actually involved than a question of personal intent to do harm or of mass suffering by default. Slavery in fact reeked with violence in its crudest forms. A society founded on the exploitation of slaves was the crudest form of *structural violence.* The use of white militia to search out runaway black slaves exemplifies undisguised *institutional* violence. The omnipresent whip not only symbolized authority, but also ritualized *interpersonal violence.* The countless Africans who flung themselves from ships into the Atlantic Ocean or who committed suicide on plantations also emphasize the desperation underlying *intrapersonal violence.*

Violence against blacks did not end with the abolition of slavery. In fact, the abolition of slavery renewed the efforts to ensure white supremacy. It is not surprising that fears of black reprisal and white hysteria were prevalent even during the heyday of chattel slavery. The end of slavery and its associated legal systems of social control brought forth informal and extralegal measures to maintain white supremacy. Urban race riots, Ku Klux Klan violence, and lynching became common means of terrorizing blacks and keeping them in "their place." Thus from 1825 to 1960, the real or imagined white *perception* that blacks were unwilling to keep "their place" in the physical environment, action, or mood quickly triggered violent white reprisal. These violent reprisals reaffirmed a shared paranoia and attempted to prevent any blurring of boundaries defined according to well-entrenched Manichean psychology. Cementing whites into a compact group, these violent reprisals were often directed at any effort or institution that promised black self-improvement and community development. Thus a 1842 document stated that

> all the mobs by which the people of color have been hunted and persecuted, have been directed against their efforts and means of improvement. A negro brothel, or a dance house, might have stood . . . without being mobbed by the populace, or torn down as a nuisance. . . . But a negro church or school house, or a temperance hall, is not to be tolerated at all. (Brown, 1975, p. 206)

Race riots and associated pogroms were numerous and bloody, but the ritual of lynching underscores the sadism and celebration of the violence ordinary people are capable of in a climate of shared paranoia. There is no accurate record of how many blacks were lynched but estimates are that, between 1882 and 1951, at least 3,437 blacks were lynched (Brown, 1975). There is evidence that this total is highly conservative. That lynching of blacks rarely occurred before emancipation is not an enigma. That the majority of lynchings occurred in former slave states is also not surprising. Nor indeed should one find it difficult to believe that lynchable offenses included not only alleged crimes of murder and rape, but also trivial "cases" of black pushiness, insubordination, or some perception of an inclination, a comportment, or a mood deemed threatening to white supremacy. But what is certainly hard to fathom is the ritual of sadism and mass celebration of violence associated with the lynching of a black person. Clinicians have of course considered sadism long ago, but only as an isolated individual problem, not as a collective social phenomenon exemplified in the lynching ritual.

Brown (1975) described the macabre details of the "typical lynching" ritual. Once a person was condemned, public notices were circulated a day or two in advance to whites in the locality and neighboring areas. Sometimes, the notices were sent to distant white communities. Trains made special trips, adding extra cars to meet the demands of crowds wishing to watch the gruesome spectacle of a man being lynched. The number of spectators sometimes reached 15,000. The lynching was preceded by torture and mutilation, climaxed by what was euphemistically called "surgery below the belt." Parts of the victim's body were dismembered and photographed for picture postcards, which were sold as souvenirs. The remains were then burned. The leaders of this macabre proceeding were often well known to and seen by thousands of spectators. But everybody, including law enforcement officers, joined in a conspiracy of silence and the coroner declared that the lynching was commited by unknown persons. This in short was the ultimate of historical white justice and black death. It was also the most blatant amalgam of structured, institutional, and personal violence.

Much has changed in the intensity and pattern of racial violence in the United States. The change has surely been for the better. During the past several decades, black Americans have been extended an increasing measure of social justice and legal protection. These changes did not come easily, or without struggle. Yet racial equality before the law and in society is to this day a project of the future in the United States. Black Americans remain entrapped in a cycle of violence and death. They still suffer more unemployment, more fatalities, more disabilities, more incarcerations, and more indignities than white Americans.

By almost every measure of social or individual well-being, black Americans are at a marked disadvantage when compared with their white counterparts. This is so in economics as in other arenas of life. The median income of black families has always lagged behind that of white families. The median income of both has steadily increased over time, but white families continue to earn almost twice as much as blacks. This is shown in Table 1, which compares median income for the two races since 1950. More recently, the

TABLE 1. Median Family Income by Race in Constant 1980 Dollars: 1950–1980

	1950	1960	1970	1975	1979	1980
All races	11,361	15,637	20,939	21,004	22,320	21,023
Black families[a]	6,398	8,987	13,325	13,441	13,219	12,674
White families	11,792	16,235	21,722	21,845	23,275	21,904
Black to white ratio	54	55	61	62	57	58

Note: From "Money Income and Poverty Status of Families and Persons in the United States: 1980," Current Population Reports, Consumer Income, Series P-60, No.127, August 1981. (See McGee's 1983 article in The Status of Black America, National Urban League.)
[a]Prior to 1970, black families were not counted separately but were included in the category "Black and Others."

black–white income ratio has been somewhat stable without significant improvement. In fact, the median income of black families has decreased since 1979, showing that blacks are hardest hit during recessions (McGhee, 1983).

The per capita income of the black American community in 1980 was $4,804; it was $8,233 for a white person during the same year. In other words, for each $58 available to a black person, there was $100 available to a white person. In the same year, one out of three black persons but only one out of ten whites were below the official poverty level. The recent recessions have fast eroded what gains blacks have made since the 1960s and pushed them back to grinding poverty (Swinton, 1983). The unemployment rate of blacks has consistently remained at least twice that of whites in the postwar years. This observation has given rise to the well-known 2:1 rule of thumb that states that the unemployment rate of blacks will remain double that of whites. Looking at unemployment rates spanning 30 years, Swinton (1983, p. 66) concluded: "This rule holds for blacks of all ages, both sexes, all educational levels, in all regions of the country, center cities and in suburbs." Shocking as this may be, the unemployment rate of blacks has risen in recent years. Hardest hit by the recession are blacks under age 35 whose current unemployment rate is the highest in postwar years.

Brenner (1973, 1977, 1982) has shown quantitatively the social, physical, and psychological effects of unemployment. Based on the 1970 census data, Brenner estimated that a 1% increase in unemployment in the United States leads to at least 36,887 deaths, mostly from heart disease, 920 suicides, 684 homicides, 495 deaths from alcohol-related diseases, and 4,227 admissions to state hospitals. More recently, Brenner (1982) calculated that every 1% rise in the unemployment rate increases the mortality rate and cardiovascular death by 2%, homicides and incarcerations by almost 6%, the infant mortality rate by about 5%, and mental hospital admission by almost 4%. Yet the unemployment rate of blacks is now above 20%, the unemployment rate of black youth soars above 45%.

Infant mortality rate is generally considered to be a sensitive indicator of a nation's health ranking. Infant mortality rate for black Americans was 23.6 deaths per 1,000 live births in 1977. During the same year, the infant mortality rate for white Americans was 12.3 deaths—almost one-half that of blacks. These rates changed over the years, but as Table 2 shows, the infant mortality rate of blacks remained consistently about twice as high as that of whites. Similar differentials are also indicated for neonatal and postneonatal mortality rates. It is clear that, from the very beginning, society places the black infant at a greater risk of death than his white counterpart.

The inequities of death rates go hand in hand with inequities in the major causes of death. Black infants are three times more likely to die of disorders related to short gestations and unspecified low birth weight, 2.7 times more of pneumonia and influenza, and 2.3 times more of causes associated with maternal complications. Moreover, a black baby is four times more likely to lose his mother due to causes associated with pregnancy, childbirth, and postpartum complications. He is also twice more likely to be born to a mother who re-

TABLE 2. Infant, Neonatal, and Postneonatal Mortality Rates, According
to Race: United States, Selected Years 1950–1977

Mortality Rate and Year	Black	American Indian	White
Infant[a]	Number of Deaths per 1,000 Live Births		
1950	43.9	82.1	26.8
1960	44.3	49.3	22.9
1970[b]	32.4	22.0	17.8
1977[b]	23.6	15.6	12.3
Neonatal			
1970[c]	22.8	10.6	13.8
1977	16.1	8.3	8.7
Postnatal			
1970[d]	9.9	11.4	4.0
1977[d]	7.6	7.3	3.6

Note: From U.S. Department of Health and Human Services. "The Status of Children, Youth and
Families," 1979, August, 1980 (see Poussaint's 1983 article in The Status of Black America, the
National Urban League).
[a]Infant mortality rate, number of deaths for infants under 1 year of age per 1,000 live births.
[b]Excludes deaths of nonresidents of the United States.
[c]Neonatal mortality rate, number of deaths for infants within 28 days of birth per 1,000 live
births.
[d]Postneonatal mortality, number of deaths for infants within 28 days to 365 days of birth per
1,000 live births.

ceived little or no prenatal care. When a black child is spared early death, he is
still more likely than a white baby his age to suffer inadequate nutrition,
mental retardation, learning disability, and educational disadvantages (Pouissaint, 1983).

This racial inequity is also reflected in life expectancy. In 1979, the life
expectancy for blacks and whites in the United States were 68.3 and 74.4 years,
respectively, a difference of 6 years. The life expectancy for both blacks and
whites changed over the years, but the differences in expectancy remained
almost the same. Thus for instance, the life expectancy for white American
males was 67.4 years in 1960. In the same year, the life expectancy for nonwhite males was 61.1. The ratio of nonwhite to white was .91. Ten years later,
life expectancy was 68.0 years for white males and 61.3 for nonwhite males.
Again, the ratio of nonwhite to white was .90. Indeed it is instructive to note
that life expectancy for nonwhite males in 1977 was about the same as what it
was for white males in 1945. Lawrence Gary (1981, p. 51) estimated that if we

assume that life expectancy rate for white men will remain the same while that of
black men continues to increase at the present rate, it will take about 70 years before
the two groups are at parity with respect to this measure.

Not surprisingly, overall mortality rates also show racial disparity as do
infant mortality and life expectancy. In 1977, the mortality rates for black
males and white males were, respectively, 1,046 and 782 deaths per 100,000.
This mortality rate of black males exceeded that of white males by 34%. In the
same year, the mortality rates of black females and white females were, respectively, 621 and 428 deaths per 100,000. Thus the mortality rate of black

females was 45% greater than that of white females (Cooper *et al.*, 1981). When the two races are compared on major causes of death, one also finds differences that underscore sedimented inequities in the American society. In particular, blacks die at higher rates of heart disease, cancer, stroke, and homicide.

Cardiovascular disease has become a major cause of death in industrialized countries. In the United States, for instance, it accounts for one-half of the 2 million deaths each year (Cooper *et al.*, 1981). Some have mistakenly called it a "disease of affluence." The term had meaning in the past when it primarily affected the well-to-do in developed countries. Then as now, the fact remains that infectious diseases prevail in underdeveloped countries. However, recent data show that cardiovascular disease is also a major cause of death among black Americans. For instance, in 1977 black males between the ages of 1 to 39 were at least twice as likely to die of heart disease than white males in the same age group. In particular, coronary heart disease, hypertensive heart disease, and stroke are major killers of black Americans. The integration of blacks into the "consumer economy" and into industrial, urban centers has brought about significant changes in diet, level of stress, cigarette smoking, and exposure to pollution. The tragedy is that blacks became integrated faster into the so-called "diseases of the affluent" than into affluent America.

Coronary heart disease is a leading cause of death among blacks generally and black women in particular. The white mortality rate from this disease far exceeded that of blacks until a few decades ago. Gradually, the rate for blacks began to approach and in some cases outstrip that of whites. Black men between the ages of 45 and 64 have now a higher death rate for coronary heart disease than matched white males. Worse, black women between the ages 45 to 75 have a far higher death rate from coronary heart disease than white women in the same age group. This fact is not sufficiently appreciated. Public health measures involving early detection, treatment, and above all, prevention are urgently needed to reduce the massive toll exacted by coronary heart disease in the black community.

The prevalence of hypertensive heart disease and stroke in the black community today is well recognized. A number of studies (Akinkugbe & Bertrand, 1976; Seedat *et al.*, 1978; Vaughn & Miall, 1979) have shown that high blood pressure is common among American blacks, South African blacks, West Indians, and urbanized Africans, but infrequent among rural Africans. In addition, it is known that blacks in poor areas of central Mississippi have three to four times more high blood pressure than middle-class whites in the suburbs (Cooper *et al.*, 1981). Whatever the role of genetic predisposition, excessive sodium intake, or smoking, the etiological significance of stress in high blood pressure and related diseases cannot be doubted. Remarkable advances have been made with regard to the treatment and control of these diseases. Yet blacks are less likely to benefit from these advances because of inequities in the health care system in the United States.

A higher cancer death rate is also found among black Americans. Data comparing cancer death rates for 1950 and 1977 show a dramatic increase of cancer deaths for black males. There was a decline in rates for women of both races, an increase of 22% for white men, and a shocking increase of 63% for black men (Cooper *et al.*, 1981). A major portion of those cancer deaths among blacks involves cancer of the respiratory tract. Lung cancer deaths have been steadily increasingly since the 1930s with black rates trailing those of whites until 1960 when black cancer death rates came to exceed those of whites. The differential is now more alarming not only because it is much higher, but also because it is highest among younger blacks. What is more, studies have shown that black males are less likely to survive cancer, once detected, than white males (Gary, 1981). Again, inequities in health care account for lower survival rates of black cancer patients. Because of this, cancer in many blacks also remains undetected or is diagnosed at a much later stage.

Three explanations are offered to account for the astounding rate of lung cancer among black males. First, studies have indicated that black males above 20 years are now more likely to smoke cigarettes than are white males. This is a significant break with the past. A national survey in 1956 indicated that blacks smoked less than whites (Cooper *et al.*, 1981; Gary, 1981). Second, migration of blacks to urban centers with highly polluted air increase their risk of lung cancer. Indeed as blacks migrated into these high-risk urban centers, whites moved out of them in large numbers. Third, black males who find employment in industry are more likely to be hired for occupations in which they are exposed to high levels of carcinogens and given the most dangerous assignments. This was demonstrated by Lloyd's (1971) study of steel workers. The study had shown that, among other disturbing inequities, 325 out of 496 steel workers assigned to jobs involving carcinogenic smokes and fumes were black. It was therefore not accidental that nearly 50% of the deaths due to lung cancer occurred among the black employees. The gravity of this structural violence becomes clear when it is considered that less than 4% of the American population dies of lung cancer.

Such inequities in occupational hazards are by no means confined to a few industries. The American labor market as a whole partakes in the acceleration of death and disability of blacks. It does so in one of two ways: by *exclusion*, hence relegating blacks into a chronic and corrosive unemployment, or by *inclusion* through job assignments that undermine the health and dignity of blacks. For instance, it has been shown (Davis, 1977) that blacks have a 37% greater chance than whites of suffering personal injury on the job and 20% chance of dying from a job-related injury. A national survey also indicated that, compared to whites, black men have 45% more "bed disability days" in which the entire work day is lost due to illness or injury and 27% "restricted activity day" in which the person reduces his usual activities for the whole day due to illness or injury (U.S. Department of Health and Human Services, 1980).

Selection of blacks for higher risk assignments has also been observed in the armed services of the United States (Hope, 1979; Schexnider, 1983). Black Americans have often gravitated to the military for the economic opportunities and social recognition they could not find in the larger society, and the contribution of blacks in the U.S. military has a long history. The black community has time and again sacrificed more than its share to the nation during periods of war at home and abroad. The military was legally desegregated in 1948 and has since attracted many young black males. Yet this institution is also a microcosm of the society it serves. Blacks are overrepresented in high-risk combat units and in nontechnical, unrewarding occupations. In both cases, the acquisition of marketable skills is lower for blacks and hence, unable to find appropriate jobs in society, they tend to reenlist. In the early years of the Vietnam War, black combat deaths were excessive, peaking to over 20% of all combat deaths by 1966. Following public reaction at home, the Department of Defense ordered a reduction in the number of deaths of blacks in combat (Schexnider, 1983).

More blatant examples of structural and institutional violence against blacks are the disproportionate representation of blacks in prisons and on death rows. Townsey (1981, p. 223) who studied the incarceration of blacks in this country concluded that "the incarceration of Black men throughout the United States is extreme, harsh, and brutal." Currently, black men account for 46.6% of all male prisoners in the United States. This is a total of 136,893 black males, mostly in the prime of life. In 18 states, blacks comprise 50 to 75% of the prison population. Since 1930, a total of 3,861 persons were executed in the United States and 53.6% (2,051) of them were black men. There are now 443 persons sentenced to death in the United States and 43.8% (194) of them are black men. Since 1930, 455 men have been executed for rape and 89% (405) of them were black. Further, black men comprise 76% (23) of persons executed for armed robbery and 100% (11) of those executed for burglary. Currently, blacks comprise nearly 58% of those on death row. The death penalty was ruled unconstitutional in 1972, but some states are now reversing this ruling with grim prospects for blacks in this country.

These inequities are not confined to blacks in prisons and on death rows. The pattern of arrest and judicial proceedings have consistently shown a bias against blacks. The Scottsboro Boys, Marcus Garvey, George Jackson of the Soledad Brothers, Malcolm X, the Wilmington Ten, and countless others demonstrate a sordid history of unjust arrests or severe sentences meted out for blacks whose misfortune or offenses brought them into the criminal justice system. For instance, George Jackson, the brilliant, self-educated martyr, was sentenced from "one year to life" for stealing $70 from a gas station. He spent eleven years of his life in prison, eight and one-half in solitary confinement. He was later shot by prison guards allegedly for attempting to escape. There are worse examples, like the man in Dallas, Texas who was sentenced to 1,000 years in prison for stealing $73.10 whereas white executives convicted of a price conspiracy involving over $1 billion were sentenced to 30 days in prison (Townsey, 1981).

Such blatant miscarriages of justice may be infrequent, but unjust arrests, harsh sentences, mistreatment in prisons, and lack of rehabilitation into society are quite common for blacks, compared to whites. As is often the case in other social arenas, this sedimented inequality in the criminal justice system is based not only on racial, but also on class grounds. Poverty also predisposes whites to injustice, but it further intensifies injustice for blacks. Moreover, some studies (Robin, 1963, p. 54; Takagi, 1979) show that in "justifiable homicide" whereby a policeman on duty kills a civilian, blacks are killed at a rate six to twenty times higher than whites. Yet rarely are policemen prosecuted for this legitimized violence against civilians of any race or sex. Worse, even white civilians have historically gotten away with every form of crime against blacks. It is indeed instructive to note that "in the history of the United States, no white person has ever been executed for murder, rape, or other capital crimes against a Black person "(Gary, 1981, p. 234).That blacks are punished harshly for offenses—minor or serious, proven or suspected—and that whites get away with gross and substantiated crimes against blacks are only further indications of structural and institutional violence.

It would of course be wrong to assume that blacks on their part are simply passive victims. Far from it. Blacks do engage in violent and destructive action. Violence and crimes of all types are indeed rampant in the black community. Homicide, rape and attempted rape, robbery, aggravated and simple assaults, purse-snatching, and pocket-picking are all too frequent occurrences exacting immeasurable toll among blacks. Most of these crimes are not interracial; they involve perpetrators and victims who are black. But these forms of interpersonal violence cannot be explained apart from the prevailing structural and institutional violence in society. Moreover, such acts of violence against persons and property constitute expressions of misdirected rebellion and collective autodestruction. Homicide among blacks best illustrates how victims of oppression turn on each other the systemic violence imposed on them.[1]

A growing body of literature on homicide among black Americans supports three unmistakable and disconcerting conclusions. First, there is a far higher incidence of homicide among blacks than any other ethnic group in the United States. Second, black males between the ages of 20 and 35 are the most common victims of as well as the most convicted offenders for homicide. Third, homicide typically occurs within a familial, intimate, interpersonal context. These conclusions and the data from which they are drawn confirm the view that violence breeds more violence and that a community of victims, unaware of its history and unable to control its destiny, tends to victimize itself viciously. The following studies underscore the point.

One of the most extensive epidemiological studies on homicide was conducted by Klebba (1975). The study covered a period of seven decades, 1900–1970. The findings were revealing. The total and adjusted rates of homicide for all ethnic groups in the United States increased from 1900 to about 1933. There was then a gradual decline through the 1940s and 1950s, with a noticeable drop during World War II. Homicide rates remained almost constant from 1955 to the mid-1960s. But the national trend soon turned upward from a total of 4.7 deaths per 100,000 in 1960 to 9.8 deaths in 1973. Though this was a sizable increase, the national trend actually obscures the appalling dimensions of the problem among black Americans.

---

[1]H. A. Bulhan, *Violence and Psychopathology among Blacks: A Theory of Auto-destruction,* unpublished.

During these seven decades, black males had the highest homicide rates. Black females maintained the same trend as black males when compared to white females. By 1973, the age-adjusted rate for black males reached 77.1 deaths compared to a rate of 8.7 per 100,000 for whites. Black females had a rate of 16.0 deaths compared to 2.8 deaths for white females. The problem is even more appalling when specific age groups are compared. By 1970, urban centers like Chicago recorded rates of 298.1 deaths for black males between the ages of 15 to 24 years, compared to 10.9 deaths for white males in the same age range. Black females 15 to 24 years old had 24.6 deaths compared to 0.7 deaths for white females in the same age range.

It is interesting to note that, from 1900 to 1970, there were only two periods in which the escalating national rates of homicide declined in the United States. The first was during World War II. A drop of 55.5 deaths per 100,000 in 1940 to 44.1 deaths in 1944 was recorded for black males. This decline was partly due to the recruitment of many black males in the war effort and partly because the war economy offered employment for those who remained at home. But the trend soon turned upward as the veterans of the war returned home to once again face chronic unemployment. The second period of decline was from 1955 to 1961. We have suggested elsewhere (Bulhan, 1983) that the legal injunction against segregation, notably the *Brown vs. Topeka Board of Education* decision, and the Korean War contributed to this second decline. Legal and economic changes created a climate of hope, expectations, and solidarity among blacks. The Korean War also put many U.S. black males into battlefields abroad. But the hopes and expectation of the 1950s were hardly matched by tangible changes in living conditions.

By 1960, homicide among blacks began to escalate. Social reforms and the black consciousness movement during the sixties had, no doubt, calming and integretive effects in the black community. But the educational and socioeconomic benefits that ensued were largely confined to a burgeoning black middle class. The so-called "Black Underclass," given only tantalizing promises of change, was to remain in worse poverty and the ghettoes of urban centers. With the assassination of Dr. Martin Luther King, black America went up in flames. The outrage of this sad incident ignited an accumulated, festering rage. The subsequent autodestructive reactions were both collective and costly. Massive riots, widespread vandalism, and black-on-black crime became desperate reactions to a dream long deferred and also to the assassination of an acclaimed leader. Herein lie some of the most tragic ironies of history: A community of victims, in total outrage, turns to victimize itself after the most committed black advocate of nonviolence, a Nobel Peace Prize winner, died from the bullets of a white assassin.

If riots have since become rare or sporadic, homicide among blacks did not decline. Indeed the homicide rate among blacks continued to outstrip that of whites by an astonishing margin. By 1977, homicide was the fifth leading cause of death for black males, but it was not even among the top ten causes of death for white males. For males between the ages of 25 and 44 years, homicide was the number one cause of death for black men, but number five for white males. In that year alone, more blacks (5,734) were killed than all the blacks (5,711) who died in the entire nine years of the Vietnam War. This fact should underscore that there has been an undeclared war on black Americans and that many blacks have become agents of their autodestruction.

The pervasiveness of intrapersonal violence can be shown by the growing menace of suicide, alcoholism, and drug abuse. Suicide has not been a leading cause of death among black Americans. Traditionally, white men had the highest rate of suicide in the United States and their rate increased with advancing age. However, there are indications (Davis, 1981; Seiden et al., 1980) that the rate of suicide among young black males has increased during the past decade. The increase has been highest among black males between 20 to 29 years. From 1947 to 1977, the suicide rate increased 195% from 7.3 to 21.5 per 100,000 for black males in the age group 20–24 and 250% from 8.2 to 28.5 per 100,000 for black males 25–29 years old. For the age-group 15–24, suicide has become the third leading cause of death for black males and the second leading cause of death of white males. Though there are some disturbing indications of an increase in rates, the suicide rate among blacks still lags behind that of whites. But when suicide is reconsidered beyond its legal definition, thereby taking into account "accidents" and victim-precipitated homicides, the rate for blacks increases dramatically.

The prevalence of alcoholism in the black community is less ambiguous than suicide. Harper (1976b), who studied the problem extensively, declared alcohol abuse the number one health and social problem in the black American community. We have earlier outlined the tortuous and scandalous role of alcohol in the slave trade particularly and the imperialism of Europe generally. That alcoholism remains a serious problem in the black community suggests both a continuity with the past and the depth of frustration in the black community. Not surprisingly, alcoholism has had a long and stubborn presence among black Americans. There are indications that alcoholism is a growing menace among black Americans. A rapid increase is reported for 18 to 25 year olds and women under the age of 45. Moreover, one-third of all black adults and one-half of all black youth are users and abusers of alcohol (Harper, 1976a,b; King, 1982).

The problem is not only alcoholism per se, it is also its effects on health and social well-being. It is estimated that alcohol abuse is the primary or secondary cause of at least one out of ten deaths in the United States. More than 50% of murders and 50% of deaths from accidents in the black American community involve alcohol (Gary, 1981; Pouissaint, 1983). Blacks die at three times the rate of whites from alcohol-related diseases. Data from 1950 to 1975 indicate that the age-adjusted rate for cirrhosis of the liver—a disease often associated with alcoholism—has increased 50% for whites and 200% for non-whites in the United States.

Alcoholism is indeed one of those self-inflicted human problems that has wide repercussions in a community. Not only does every alcoholic bring upon himself preventable disease and premature death, but also every alcoholic is a serious menace to at least five to seven persons around him. Usually, the victims are his loved ones and his friends. The economic cost to a community in terms of sick leave, accidents, and disability is equally staggering. And as in the past, many profit from the sale and distribution of alcohol. Thus, for instance, the National Institute of Alcoholism and Alcohol Abuse estimated that, in one year alone, the alcohol industry collected more than six and one-half billion dollars from the sale of alcohol to blacks in the United States (Harper, 1976a).

In short, violence and premature death have been persistent features among black Americans. Comparing blacks to whites in most indices of health and social well-being reveals that black America carries an inordinate burden of the violence in society. The structural, institutional, and interpersonal violence imposed on it exact an immense toll and in turn predisposes to various forms of autodestruction. Each premature death is a loss of human potential for the community. Not only is every black American at greater risk of preventable disease and death, but also blacks between the ages of 15 and 35—the most energetic and promising members of the community—are targets of violence in its various forms. It is impossible to estimate the person-years and potential work-years lost due to premature deaths, incarceration, alcoholism, drug abuse, and mental illness. Each premature death also brings grief, pain, and a chain of victims. Thus data on Black America shows that the community of the oppressed suffers not only excess physical deaths, but also excess social and psychological deaths. And yet, bad as conditions are for black Americans, there are countries today where people live in a worse inferno. South Africa is a good case in point.

VIOLENCE IN SOUTH AFRICA

It is increasingly recognized that South Africa is a society of opulence for a minority of whites and a consuming inferno for a majority of blacks. There is perhaps no society in the world today that better illustrates the results of a violent compartmentalization of people into races and the calculated fortification of a Manichean psychology. South Africa is a country in which the ruling authority relentlessly strives to divide its population into, as it were, four distinct "species" differentiated on the basis of race. Wealth, power, and privilege are distributed accordingly and so are rates of preventable death and disability. Apartheid is indeed structural violence in its crudest form.

Various estimates are given for the population and racial composition of South Africa. Substantial agreement exists as to how many are white, but there is a marked variability in the population estimates of blacks. One obvious problem is how one defines "black" when the term refers more to political and social characteristics than to actual racial attributes. There are four legal groupings in South Africa: Whites, Coloreds, Asians, and Africans. The 1980 census estimated that Africans, excluding residents of the so-called "homelands," comprise 67% whites 19%, coloreds 11%, and Asians 3%.[2]

[2]In *Survey of Race Relations In South Africa*, Johannesburg: South African Institute of Race Relations, South Africa, 1981, p. 54.

Since residents of the homelands are excluded from official estimates, these percentages significantly underestimate the size of the black population. Uncertainty about the size of the black population is often explained by claims that Africans fail to report births and deaths. The 1980 census was severely criticized, particularly by those whites worried about the "black menace" they sense lurking everywhere. Thus a representative in the all-white parliament, unhappy about the 1980 census, complained: "Without offending the Department of Statistics, I want to say that we do not know how many black people there are in South Africa. There are many more black people than our statistics report."

If an accurate census on blacks in South Africa is not available, the systemic violence meted out to them is well known. The national obsession on race classification is part of an elaborate scheme to enhance the wealth and well-being of whites at the expense of nonwhites. This fact is borne out by stark economic, social, and health inequities among the races. In 1975, the average per capita income for whites was almost 15 times greater than that of blacks. Two years later, blacks comprised 83% of the entire South African population, but received less than one-third the nation's income. In a country of expanding economy and soaring profits, 75% of African families live below the Poverty Datum Line—that is, the bare subsistence poverty level. Meanwhile, white families enjoy a standard of life comparable to and often better than many in Western Europe and the United States.

White workers in South Africa are virtually guaranteed full employment, higher salaries, better compensation for accidents and illness, and better old age benefits (Harsch, 1980). They and their families also enjoy better housing, nutrition, and health care. Thus for instance, there was in 1972 one doctor for every 400 whites and only one doctor for every 144,000 blacks. Five times more whites than blacks live in homes for the aged, even though the population of blacks is greater and they are taxed at a higher rate than whites. Blacks suffer from a serious housing shortage, excessive crowding, and frequent dislocations. Social services for them are almost nonexistent and, when they do exist, they are mediocre. Chronic malnutrition and diseases are rife. Thus for instance, the incidence of tuberculosis is 20 times higher for blacks than for whites. In 1971, infant mortality was 19.4 deaths per 1,000 live births for whites and peaked at about 250 deaths per 1,000 live births for blacks. A year earlier, life expectancy was 68 years for whites, 62 years for Asians, 55 years for Africans, and 53 years for Coloreds. Evidently under the structural violence of apartheid, how one lives and for what length of time depend on the value assigned to one's "racial" attributes.

The pillars of apartheid are numerous institutions and harshly enforced laws that control and regulate black labor—after of course the largest and best portions of the land have been expropriated. The pillars of apartheid include the migratory labor system, the pass laws, influx control, the police, the prisons, and even the educational system. All these institutions and laws are designed to uproot blacks, subject them to absolute control, and turn them into insecure, obedient, underpaid laborers. The migratory labor system is actually a modern-day system of slavery. Historically, South Africa depended on slave labor to work the mines and farms. The migratory labor system is today's counterpart to the "peculiar institution" of yesteryear and a major contributor to the fallout profits that have made South Africa a "treasure house" for a minority of whites.

Typically, the black migrant workers sign a contract for a specified period, usually a year, without any choice of job assignment or negotiating power on salary. They are strictly prohibited from bringing their families to the environs of their employment and thus are forced to leave them behind. These migrant workers are usually cut off from their families for a good part of their adult working life. The institution of the family is thereby disrupted with significant consequences for the laborers, their spouses and children, and ultimately, their community. The circumstances under which they work only deepens their alienation. At the end of each day's hard labor, they go "home" to hostels fenced with barbed wire. These barren hostels are invariably crowded and control is absolute. They have few amenities, no visitors' rooms, no recreation facilities, and no privacy. Visitors, particularly of the opposite sex, are not permitted. The laborers are also grouped by tribe to prevent the development of class or national consciousness.

Work in the mines is both arduous and dangerous. The excavated and deep mines are cramped and roasting hot. Ear-shattering noise from drilling, rock-falls, and accidents are constant. "In the three decades from 1936 to 1966, no less than nineteen thousand miners, more than nine-tenths of them Black, were killed in the gold-mines, an average of three per shift."[3] And yet the wages earned by black mine workers are nowhere commensurate with this hard and perilous labor. The ratio of white to black wages in the mines is very high, sometimes reaching 20:1 (Harsch, 1980). Wages for black miners have gone up since 1970, but they still trail far behind those of white workers. Thus in 1978, the average wage per month was R119 for African miners and R840 for white miners.

African migrant laborers working on white-owned farms are paid even less than mine workers and are more badly treated. They are kept in hostels or shacks on the farm. Not only are they underpaid for the 14 hours per day and seven days per week they work, they also suffer abuses that hark back to the time of undisguised slavery. Their movements are severely restricted and they are flogged with the *sjambok*, a whip made of ox hide, for any behavior, word, or attitude their *baas* (master) finds unacceptable. And as can be readily expected, a whip in hand finds many pretexts for ensuring many bodies on which to land. The physical and psychological scars of these cruelties can be easily surmised.

The "homelands" or "Bantustans" are actually concentration camps in which thousands of Africans are kept against their will. The notion of "native reserves" has been on the books for decades. It has been legislated through successive land acts, most recently by the Bantu Homelands Citizenship Act

[3]Ernest Harsch (1980, p. 84).

of 1970. The scheme behind these acts has been to strip blacks of all rights to South African citizenship, push them out as "undesirables" from the "white areas," and ensure the availability of well-controlled, desperate cheap laborers. Thus all Africans in South Africa—that is, over 80% of the total population—are arbitrarily classified as "citizens" of one or another homeland that, together, comprise only 13.7% of South Africa's land mass. These homelands are not only tiny areas, they are also located in the poorest lands where farming or mining is difficult if not impossible.

The obsession to remove "black spots" from the so-called white areas has led to large-scale, compulsory uprooting of blacks from their homes and land. Thus for instance, the South African authorities removed 1.9 million blacks between 1960 and 1970. Since this callous bulldozing of homes and forced resettlement began, at least 6 million blacks were pushed to native reserves without jobs, schools, hospitals, a water supply, and roads. Another 7.7 million more were slated for such removal. The primary victims of this policy are the aged, the infirm, widows, and children whom official documents refer to as "unproductive," "idle," "superfluous," and "undesirable." The former Minister of Bantu Administration and Development, Mr. M. C. Botha, stated in no uncertain terms the intention behind this resettlement of blacks *en masse:*

> Bantu individuals can be present in the white areas solely for their labor. . . . There is a wall, a roof, and one cannot get past that. . . . The Bantu cannot strive towards the top on equal footing with whites in our policies, social matters, labor, economy and education in South Africa.[4]

The all-white government of South Africa forces millions of Africans into homelands, even though studies have shown that the majority of urban blacks have at best tenuous links with these parcels of land. Thus a survey conducted in 1978 showed that, among Africans in "white areas," 57% were born there and 80% had not visited the native reserves to which they were forced. For those Africans who have already been pushed into homelands, life is a nightmare replete with the sight of malnourished children, frequent death, and daily burials in the makeshift cemeteries that dot the landscape. These homelands, with no economy of their own, are also dumping grounds for aged laborers who no longer are useful in the white areas. In effect, the so-called "homelands" are mass graveyards for *living* millions who legally have been pronounced *dead.*

Those who still remain in urban areas must live in crowded ghettoes and shantytowns where squalor, eviction, poverty, disease, and crime are rampant. Soweto—an acronym for *South West Township*—is the best-known and largest ghetto in the continent of Africa. Joyce Sikakane's *A Window on Soweto* provides a personal and harrowing account of life in this segregated township. Soweto lies only a few miles from Johannesburg. Nowhere is the Manichean world of which Fanon wrote more starkly evident as in the contrasts and relations between Soweto and Johannesburg. The Manichean psychology and the violence that nurtures it are here unambiguously reflected in

---

[4]Quoted in A. Sachs (1969).

all manners of things, action, and attitudes. Both are evident in the contrasting arrangement of the environment, the unequal distribution of economic resources, the rates of death, and of course, in the relation each of these "cities" has to the legitimized violence of the state. And yet, true to the Manichean logic, Soweto and Johannesburg are as intimately interdependent as they are irreconcilably opposite.

Johannesburg, where the whites reside and work, is a prosperous urban center and the financial capital of "white" South Africa. It is a bustling city of skyscrapers, luxury hotels, modern apartments, plush homes, and all the modern conveniences of any developed European or American city. Its residents include old tycoons, the nouveaux riche, and professionals whose umbilical cord extends to London, Amsterdam, Paris, New York, and Tel Aviv. Public facilities bear signs ostensibly inviting "Europeans Only"—meaning of course that only *whites*, of any nationality, are welcome. Jo'burgians exemplify that vociferous species relishing expensive consumer goods and enjoying all the technological advances—except, perhaps, vacuum cleaners, and dishwashers long made superfluous by the abundance of black domestic workers. They freely buy, own, and sell any property they can afford. Whites here have an unmistakable air of omnipotence and a shared sense that each of them is *somebody* with rights, dignity, and legal protection. They walk, eat, and rest with confidence that the awesome machinery of state violence exists on their behalf so long as they permit their conscience to be numbed and never commit themselves to the cause of justice. In short, Johannesburg is a hub of industrial magnates, international commerce, banking concerns, medical and educational institutions, museums, art galleries, cultural centers, and of course the dreaded John Vorster Square, the main police headquarters where hundreds of handcuffed blacks are daily rushed to interrogation or torture.

Soweto, in contrast, is a depressing urban ghetto extending over a flat terrain of 33 miles. The physical ordering of this ramshackle urban concentration betrays the real intent of the ruling white authorities, the daily humiliation of its black residents. The monotonous row of cubicles, the unpaved roads, the huge potholes, the litter, the lack of sidewalks, the absence of public amenities—all are in violent contrast with Johannesburg, grandly located only a few miles away. The streets of Soweto are narrow, dusty, and dimly lit, except those leading to police stations, administrative offices, and big stores. Although Johannesburg has modern communication facilities, Soweto had only 39 public phones in 1976, which suggests a plan to force a cloak of silence and isolation on its residents. Only 15% of the houses in Soweto have bathrooms. For a black person to own land here involves political and economic complications only a few can overcome. Poverty and disease are rife. Freedom of speech and of assembly is nonexistent. Movement is restricted. A permit is needed for everything, including when and if one can welcome a guest to stay overnight. Police raids are common; doors are kicked open at dawn and naked and panicked blacks herded into vans. Blacks are evicted for failing to pay bribes or for no reason at all, and a host of other abuses, all of which are designed to humiliate, torment, and exploit blacks, occur. The message echoed by things, persons, and institutions permeated by the ideology of apartheid is that one who by birth is black has absolutely no rights, no dignity, and no claim to human status. The emptiness, rootlessness, and purposelessness this pervasive assault engenders is suggested by the way Sowetans sardonically refer to their bleak ghetto as "So-Where-To."

And yet Johannesburg and Soweto would not be what each is if the other did not exist. Johannesburg owes its origin to the opening of gold fields and to cheap black labor. By 1910, it overshadowed Cape Town and Kimberly, soon to become the largest city in South Africa. To this day, in spite of a policy to quarantine blacks like lepers, Johannesburg cannot do without the hard and cheap labor of the nonwhite residents of townships like Soweto. Its factories, offices, homes, kitchens, and even segregated bathrooms depend on that labor. The sons and daughters of Jo'burgians too rely on the care and nurturance of "black nannies" who have no choice but to leave their own children in ghettoes like Soweto or in a distant homeland so they can earn a pittance to keep them alive. The 411 or more intensely crowded trains running daily between Soweto and Johannesburg and the more than 200,000 black passengers they transport around the clock attest to the fact that apartheid is an official delusion contradicted by the practical exigencies of everyday living in South Africa.

Among the most humiliating and tormenting consequences of this delusion are the pass laws, which date back to the years of undisguised slavery. The pass laws are the key to apartheid. All Africans over 16 must carry, at all times, the hated "pass" or "reference book," which Africans usually call the "stinker" or *dom pass* (stupid pass). This document contains all identifying particulars, including a Polaroid photograph, personal and ethnic identity, tax receipts, work record, employer's current address, and the employer's signature that is valid for only a month. The police, or any government official, can stop an African and demand to examine the pass at any time and anywhere. The inability to produce a valid pass is an offense punishable by imprisonment or a fine. Pass offenders comprise about 40% of the daily prison population.

Frequent raids are undertaken to catch pass offenders. These raids, which always involve an element of surprise and terror, are conducted on the streets, at the places of work, and even at homes when all are fast asleep. The shock of being suddenly awakened late at night by the clamor of boots, the blinding flood of flashlights beamed at one's half-dazed eyes, the sight of terrified parents scurrying to cover their naked bodies and find their pass book, the force and insults with which a relative is snatched away—these are some of the common traumas that initiate a black child into the obscenities of apartheid. Another ritual of degradation to which one never becomes accustomed is the spectacle, every morning, of long files of pass offenders, handcuffed to each other and herded from one street to another until officers decide they have enough of a catch to take to police headquarters. Each file of handcuffed offenders and the ceremony of humiliation associated with it hark back to the days of open slavery. Indeed a Professor A. G. Middleton, a member of the Hoexter

Commission of Inquiry, sought to improve on this practice when he recently suggested that "Africans be made to wear a disc around their neck instead of carrying a pass book."[5]

To be arrested for a pass offense, not an uncommon experience for any black adult, is to be taken out of circulation in a society that is itself a prison-without-walls and to be plunged into a mass of humanity held captive by iron bars and callous guards. A 1980 report by the Institute of Criminology at the University of Cape Town showed that South Africa has the highest prisoner per population rate in the Western world. The rate per 100,000 was 440 for South Africa, 189 for the United States, 75 for the United Kingdom, and 52 for France. The rate for South Africa remained the highest even when offenses against influx control, which comprised 40% of the black prison population, were excluded. South African prisons are extremely crowded. They can accommodate no more than a total of 70,606 prisoners, but the daily prison population approached one-half a million in 1980. What is more, torture and mysterious "suicides" are common in these prisons. Harold Strachan, a white political prisoner, exposed the horrors of South African prisons. He reported that "the most terrible and prolonged screams you ever heard" came from the African section of the prison. He also reported that African prisoners were forced to stand naked in the cold winter: "They had to stand with frost thick on the ground, barefoot, clutching each other to try to keep warm. Shivering."[6]

It should come as no surprise that South Africa also has the highest execution rate in the world. The rate of execution in South Africa has at times accounted for 50% of all the legal executions in the world. From 1942 to 1967, at least 1,300 persons were hanged in South Africa. Indeed the pace of executions in South Africa has increased over the past half-century. The annual rate was about 16 persons executed in the early 1940s, 60 in the 1950s, 100 in the 1960s, and 130 in 1980. In the first six months of 1981 alone, at least 57 persons were hanged. Most of those executed of course were Africans and coloreds. In 1967, for instance, 81 Africans, 14 coloreds, and 2 whites were executed. In 1980, 85 Africans, 43 coloreds, 1 Indian, and 1 white were executed. Not included in these numbers are the many deaths that occur during detention, the mysterious "suicides" of those under arrest, and frequent gang-murders in prison. When the South African Minister of Justice was asked in a 1981 session of Parliament about details, such as if condemned persons were sedated before execution, he refused to answer these questions because these matters were "too gruesome" to discuss. What he failed to realize is that the whole policy of apartheid and the "justice" over which he presides are no less gruesome.

Health data also reflect the destructive consequences of apartheid. However, before we highlight some epidemiological findings, one caveat is in order. Until recently, the South African Department of Statistics provided no infor-

[5]*Survey of Race Relations, op. cit.* p. 68.
[6]Quoted by Harsh (1980, p. 131).

mation on the vital statistics of blacks. The data it has traditionally reported on whites, coloreds, and Asians is indeed quite impressive—certainly the most systematic for the continent of Africa. It is as if blacks have never existed in South Africa. The information currently provided about blacks is limited and scanty, involving at best "select" magisterial districts that comprise less than one-fifth of the black population. Moreover, such essential information as size of population and age structure is not provided for these select districts. This limits the chances for a valid epidemiological comparison among the races in South Africa. Nonetheless, a number of epidemiological studies based on the select districts have been made.

Wyndham and his colleagues at the University of Witwatersrand have lately published some impressive surveys in South Africa. For instance, Wyndham and Irwig (1979) compared the age-adjusted mortality rates of the four racial groupings in South Africa for a four-year period (1968–1971). The data on blacks, from the select districts, showed a remarkable similarity to that on coloreds. The black and colored death rates far exceeded those of whites. Asians had intermediary levels of mortality. Thus for instance, the infant mortality rates of blacks and coloreds were six times as high as that of whites. The death rates for one- to four-year-olds were 13 times higher for coloreds and blacks than for whites of the same age group. Indeed 50% of all colored and black deaths and only 7% of white deaths occurred among children 0 to 4 years of age. Comparisons on causes of death among coloreds and whites for which data existed was also revealing: 28 to 45 more colored children in the age groups 0 to 4 and 1 to 4 died of infective/parasitic diseases than their white counterparts. Similar patterns were observed for other ages and causes of death. The authors explain this excessive and differential pattern of death among colored and blacks in terms of preventable environmental and nutritional insults.

Wyndham (1981a) compared death rates and the leading causes of death in the economically active age groups, 16–64 years. He found a marked contrast in the pattern and rates of death among the four racial groups. Whites and blacks showed the greatest differences in both respects. In 1970, the black and colored rates were 1.8 times greater than that of whites. The five leading causes of death for whites were ischemic heart disease, motor vehicle accidents, cerebrovascular disease, cancer of the digestive system, and bronchitis, with associated respiratory complications. This pattern of death for whites in South Africa is similar to that in a "developed Western community"—namely, whites in North America and Western Europe. In contrast, the five leading causes of death for blacks in 1970 were "ill-defined causes," pneumonia, tuberculosis, cerebrovascular disease, and homicide. The Asians and colored held intermediary positions. The pattern of Asians was more similar to that of whites and the pattern of coloreds was more similar to that of blacks. Turberculosis ranked third in the five leading causes of death among blacks and coloreds. Comparison on the basis of the 1976 data showed similar patterns except for homicide, which was the second leading cause of death for blacks and the fifth leading cause of death for coloreds. Homicide was not among the ten leading causes of death for whites and Asians. This pattern of death among blacks and coloreds was similar to those in other oppressed communities.

Even more revealing were examinations of the 1970 rates and patterns of death for the different age groups. For the ages 15 to 34 years, the death rate for blacks was 2.5 times greater than that of whites. In this age group, the first leading cause of death for whites, Asians, and coloreds was motor vehicle accidents. Homicide was the first leading cause of death for blacks, second for coloreds, and did not figure at all in the five leading causes of death for whites and Asians. For blacks in this age group, the second, third, fourth, and fifth causes of death were motor vehicle accidents, "ill-defined diseases," tuberculosis, and "unspecified violence," which included mine accidents. Tuberculosis was the third cause of death for coloreds, but did not figure at all in the five leading causes of death for whites and Asians. In short, whites and Asians tend to die of causes related to "destructive life-styles" having to do, for instance, with dietary excess and cigarette smoking. Behavioral and attitudinal changes are recommended to reduce rates for these two groups. Blacks and coloreds, on the other hand, die of causes having to do with structural inequities and frustrations engendered under apartheid. A radical restructuring of society, along with changes in health priorities, is a precondition for reducing the death rate for blacks and coloreds.

The victimization of blacks and coloreds is also evident in the workplace. Not only are both groups underpaid, they also have higher risks of dying due to occupational accidents and exposure to carcinogens. This is illustrated by Myers (1981) who examined the pattern of asbestos-related diseases in South Africa. South Africa is the third biggest producer of asbestos in the world. It is also the only producer of blue asbestos (crocidolite) and brown asbestos (amosite). Asbestos production plays a key role in South Africa's economy. It is well known that asbestos is a carcinogen that causes various lethal diseases and that, for instance, asbestos workers have a 10 times higher risk of death due to lung cancer. Data for 1977–78 show that 92% of asbestos workers suffer greater exposure and die more frequently from asbestos-related diseases. Exposed whites receive appropriate compensation, but black workers and their survivors do not. As in other industries, a black worker who is ill, aged, or no longer productive is dumped in one of those homelands.

As suggested, and documented, earlier, violence breeds more violence and a community of victims, unaware of its history and unable to control its destiny, engages in much autodestructive behavior. The rate of homicide in Soweto supports this. In 1979, the average rate of homicide in Soweto was 27.7 per 100,000 compared to 9.7 per 100,000 in the United States. In 1980, there were 1,221 victims of homicide among a population of about one and one-half million in Soweto compared to 1,733 persons out of 7.4 million residents in New York City. Thus, if a Sowetan escapes "justifiable homicide" by the police, he is at high risk of being murdered by another Sowetan. Sikakane writes that each morning "it is very rare for any worker to board a bus, a taxi, or a train without having stumbled across a corpse lying in a street." This has become so common that each corpse found but not recognized brings a sigh of relief. A family missing a member for one night searches in panic through police stations, hospitals, and finally the government mortuary. "The search is done at a sacrifice, jobwise, because invariably (white) employers are not sympathetic to absenteeism."[7] Being terminated from your job entails not only the loss of sorely needed salary, but also the loss of the legally required validation of one's pass.

Although a high death rate for blacks and coloreds is well documented, it is impossible to quantify accurately the psychological and social toll of each premature death on the survivors and the community. There are now methods of estimating the man-years lost to a community as a result of premature deaths. For instance, Wyndham (1981b) discussed the implications of premature deaths in terms of lost-man years for the four races in South Africa. An examination of the 1970 mortality data showed that the man-years lost among whites was 33% due to circulatory disease, mainly ischemic heart disease, and 34% due to accidents, mainly motor vehicle accidents. The patterns for Asians and whites were similar. The man-years lost for blacks was 34% due to violence, mainly homicide, 11% due to infective diseases, mainly tuberculosis, 14% due to circulatory diseases, and 11% due to "ill-defined diseases." The pattern for coloreds was similar to that of blacks. The 1976 data confirmed similar patterns for the four races. If the high death rates of coloreds and blacks were lowered, the annual savings in man-years would be remarkable. Reducing the death rate of coloreds and blacks to that of whites would save *annually* at least 50,000 man-years for coloreds and well over one-half million man-years for blacks. And this estimate for blacks is based on the better-off select magisterial districts. To consider the lost man-years each year for the *total* black population in South Africa is indeed mind boggling.

Premature Death: Inevitable or Preventable?

The empirical data we presented on blacks in the United States and in South Africa underscore the relevance of Fanon as well as the need to reconsider violence in terms of its structural, institutional, interpersonal, and intrapersonal manifestations. Fanon did not define violence nor did he offer a way of classifying its different features. But the definition and taxonomy of violence suggested in the previous chapter are implied in his discourse on violence. Fanon's thesis that a Manichean psychology underlies violence and oppression is confirmed by the extensive data we reviewed in this chapter. The ordering of the environment, prevailing values, the pattern of human relations, and the structure of psyches all reflect Manichean features in a situation of oppression.

It is also clear from the above that the emphasis on personal *intent*, and hence the perspective of the perpetrator, limits our conceptions of violence and masks its ubiquity in society. Emphasis on *consequence*, and hence the perspective of the victim, widens the range of our perceptions and permits a

[7]Sikakane (1977, p. 22).

consideration of the data on the immense toll borne by the oppressed. One has to be clear and careful here. It is not a question of considering *either* intent *or* consequence. Personal or collective intent is very important and relevant to violence and oppression. The victim, perpetrator, or witness invariably infers, asserts, and justifies intent. Human action cannot be divorced from intent. The intent could be inferred or declared, conscious or unconscious, magnanimous or malicious, intrinsic or attributive, determinative or justificatory. Assessment and knowledge of these aspects are useful and necessary. The point here is not to minimize the significance of intent in human relations, but rather to underscore the fact that the consideration of consequences provides a different vantage point from which to study violence and oppression.

Every social order of course dispenses rights and privileges unequally. An oppressive social order deepens this inequality in how it dispenses life and death to its citizens. Data on the United States and South Africa show that blacks carry an inordinate burden. By almost every measure of social and individual well-being, they are at a marked disadvantage, compared to whites. They die earlier. They suffer greater poverty, disease, and dislocation. They have higher rates of incarceration, execution, and industrial accidents. Their space, time, energy, mobility, and bonding are curtailed, exploited, and abused. The consequence of this structural, institutional, and personal violence is a greater rate of physical, social, and psychological death. To claim that all these happen accidentally or simply by default is to distort reality and, worse, to hinder the prevention of suffering and premature death.

Disease and physical death are inevitable. Both define the limits and possibilities of the human condition. Realization of this fact—a realization that is most often repressed—has profound consequences for what and how we live. The oppressor searches for unhindered pleasure and immortality, but unable to achieve this, creates circumstances in which he finds confirmation in the ostensible wreckage and frequent death of the oppressed. A situation of oppression is inherently one of comparison and contrasts. The well-being and worth of the oppressor depends on the suffering and despair of the oppressed. The power and affirmation of the former rests on the powerlessness and negation of the latter. Things, actions, people, life—all these lose intrinsic meaning. Thus, everyone within the orbit of oppression looks at the misfortune and despondence of his neighbors, colleagues, and acquaintances to measure his fortune and feeling of satisfaction.

Disease and physical death are also integral to living. The best of technology and social privileges can only postpone, never do away with, the ravages of disease and the physical death of *individuals*. People everywhere attempt to transcend physical death through creation and procreation. Human labor and social bonding hold a most critical place in this attempt to overcome the finality of physical death. Not only do both satisfy immediate and basic human needs, they also offer opportunities to objectify one's personality, identity, values, and social commitments. A people whose labor is expropriated and whose social bonding is ruptured are therefore doomed to psychological and social death. And since neither human labor nor social bonding can have reality and meaning without land, since a culture and an economy cannot effectively survive without land, a people whose land is expropriated, or a people who are given no fair share of what land is available, are condemned to a life of eternal rootlessness, insecurity, dependence, and premature death—physically, socially, and psychologically.

One of the tragic ironies in situations of oppression is that the oppressed submit to subjugation for fear of physical death, yet they die more frequently and at an earlier age than their oppressors. What is more, as we have shown in this chapter, the most promising and energetic members of the oppressed are at higher risk of being incarcerated, executed, unemployed, murdered, and disabled. These premature deaths and higher morbidity rates are of course preventable, as is obvious from the lower rate of mortality and quality of life achieved by others in the same society. It so happens that most communities with higher mortality rates attempt to compensate for this by higher rates of birth, as the "survival hypothesis" in public health indicates. The so-called family planning programs are indeed suspect so long as they fail to take into account structural violence and the various forms of premature deaths it fosters.

A problem worth considering is also the reflexive bias and contempt that are conjured up by such terms as *antisocial* and *lumpenproletariat*—the former used by mental health professionals and the latter by traditional Marxists. Anyone who has worked clinically with a prison population knows that there do exist persons who are indeed *antisocial* and that such persons, who are profoundly disturbed and incapable of genuine relationships, cannot be relied on or trusted. Yet the value judgment that mental health professionals and most traditional Marxists make by the use of labels must be reconsidered in light of the fact that a situation of oppression blurs who is antisocial and who is prosocial. Thus for instance, how many of those confined in prisons today are really "criminals" or "political prisoners?" Clearly, the prevailing definitions and biases need to be reevaluated by the oppressed and replaced by new definitions, new criteria, and new rewards consistent with their values and goals. The claim that the *lumpenproletariat* is *ipso facto* unreliable, dangerous, or unredeemable is belied by the remarkable transformations in countless persons, of whom Malcolm X is most exemplar. The early interventions of the Black Muslims in United States prisons also show that few among those labeled antisocial or *lumpenproletariat* are actually lost and unredeemable "cases."

It was Amilcar Cabral who made the point that, once colonialism arrived in Africa, it forced Africans to leave their history and made it an appendage to European history. Actually it is not only the history of the collective, but also the biographies of individuals that have become appendages. One could also say that the very life and death of blacks became the springboard from which Europeans and their descendants vainly hoped to affirm their accustomed feelings of omnipotence, superiority, and immortality. No people can of course be made an appendage to other peoples and lives without the practice of structural, institutional, and personal violence. The question then as now is this: How can the oppressed reclaim their *history, biographies,* and *lives* and thereby avoid premature social, psychological, and physical death?

9

PSYCHOPATHOLOGY AND OPPRESSION

Mental illness . . . presents itself as a veritable pathology of liberty.
—Fanon, *Day Hospitalization*

Psychopathology is indeed a highly contested and controversial topic. The literature on psychopathology is replete with efforts to isolate reified causes *in* the patient and attempts, often by violent means, to effect a cure through the modification of the person, his brain, his attitude, and/or his behavior. Debates abound on whether psychopathology is a "medical problem" or a "moral verdict" and how much of it can be explained in terms of "nature" or "nurture." Often forgotten, however, is that coercion and victimization characterize the experience of those labeled "abnormal" and that a central feature of psychiatric patienthood is the denial and/or abdication of liberty.

This chapter highlights the problem of psychopathology among blacks in the United States, where extensive data exist. The obvious pattern of overdiagnosis and overinstitutionalization, for instance, underscores the extent to which psychopathology—notwithstanding scientific or medical jargon—is actually a form of violence and oppression. This chapter also reviews the concept of alienation inasmuch as this important concept bridges personal-subjective and socio-historical domains. Fanon's reformulation of the concept will be discussed, along with a theory of identity change derived from his writings and personal evolution. Moreover, to underscore the relationship of psychopathology to oppression, I will present Fanon's sociogenetic perspective to psychopathology, his implicit contention that madness is organically linked to a situation of oppression, and his work with the victims as well as the perpetrators of torture.

PSYCHOPATHOLOGY AMONG BLACK AMERICANS

Leaving aside for the moment the thorny problems of definition and valid diagnosis of psychopathology, it is widely acknowledged that mental disorders are not randomly distributed in populations. It is often found that these disorders are more frequent and severe among certain groups than others. In particular, there is an extensive literature indicating significant association of mental disorders with social class, migration, and ethnicity (Dohrenwend & Dohrenwend, 1969; Faris & Dunham, 1939; Fried, 1969; Hollingshead & Redlich, 1958; Leighton *et al.*, 1963; Rabkin & Struening, 1976; Srole *et al.*, 1962—to cite only a few examples). Reviews of the literature concerning the influence of social and cultural factors on psychopathology are provided by Dohrenwend and Dohrenwend (1974), Draguns (1980), and King (1978).

An extensive literature also compares the prevalence of mental disorder among blacks and whites in the United States (Banfield, Kramer *et al.*, 1973; Cohen, 1934; Fischer, 1969; Kleiner *et al.*, 1973; Lemku *et al.*, 1942; Ozarin & Taube, 1974; Passamanick, 1963; Rosanoff, 1917; Roth & Linton, 1944; Rowntree *et al.*, 1945; Sharpley, 1977, among others). Although the findings are not always consistent, most of the works on psychiatric epidemiology tend to agree that the rate and severity of mental disorders among blacks far exceed those of whites. What this corroborated finding means is still a matter of controversy and speculation. There are strong indications that social class is a more primary etiological factor than race (Dohrenwend & Dohrenwend, 1969; King, 1978). But since black Americans are predominantly poor or working class, the question of how much of this diagnosed psychopathology can be accounted for by social class or race is at least partly academic. In reality, blacks in the United States suffer the double jeopardy of belonging to a denigrated race and a dominated social class. The following studies underscore the point.

Studying nationwide point prevalence rates for a six-year period, Pugh and MacMahon (1962) found that psychiatric hospitalization rates were higher for blacks than for whites. This was the case not only when black rates were compared to the rates for whites born in this country, but also to the rates for foreign-born whites. By 1950, the overall rates for blacks exceeded those of whites in all geographic areas, for both sexes and all age groups. The racial discrepancy was greater for black males between 15 and 24 years old. These rates exceeded those of whites within the same age group by 300% in 1950. Pugh and MacMahon suggest that these higher rates reflect higher rates of first admission and a longer period of hospitalization for blacks.

Fried (1969) reviewed 21 studies of racial differences in mental disorders. Fifteen of the studies showed higher rates for blacks than for whites. Two were ambiguous and four indicated higher rates for whites when community surveys were included. An important consideration in these findings relates to the differential rates of hospitalization. Since 1922, mental disorder rates have risen more rapidly for blacks than for whites. Passamanick (1963) also found that blacks had a 75% higher hospitalization rate than whites in Baltimore. Fischer (1969), Pokorny and Overall (1970), and Pettigrew (1964, 1974) also corroborated the findings that blacks are overrepresented in public mental hospitals.

A number of studies attempted to measure incidence rates for mental disorders among different racial groups. But for reasons to be outlined later, these attempts were not successful. Most studies are based on prevalence rates, which are a more ambiguous and uncertain measure than incidence.[1] What is more, the estimates of prevalence usually derive from data on first admission to psychiatric hospitals—which itself raises problems concerning accessibility of services, selection, and institutional variability. Earlier studies looked mainly at admission rates to public psychiatric facilities. More recently, estimates of prevalence have been made from first admissions into mental hospitals and various institutions delivering some kind of health care. There also exist a few community-based surveys on psychopathology among blacks in the United States.

Particularly noteworthy is Malzberg's (1959) intensive study of first admissions into New York State Hospital. For 1914, first admission rate for blacks was about 126 per 100,000. By 1940, the annual admission rate for blacks increased to 203 per 100,000. The corresponding rates for whites during these two periods were 64 and 92 per 100,000. A marked increase in average annual rates was noted for the period between 1930 and 1940. By 1950, the rate jumped to 246 for 15- to 19-year-old black males and to 82.6 for white males of the same age group. In general, the increase in rates was higher for black males in the 10 to 34 and the over 55 year age groups.

Kramer et al. (1973) also reported the 1969 national admission rates for psychiatric hospitals in the United States. Age-adjusted rates per 100,000 for schizophrenia were 266.6 for nonwhites and 132.2 for whites. The admission rate for schizophrenia was thus twice that of whites. The same difference was found in rates for alcoholism and drug addiction. The alcoholism rate was 90.9 for nonwhite males compared to 27.6 per 100,000 for white males. The drug addiction rate was 30.7 for black males and 5.6 for white males. The rate of personality disorders remained comparable for the two groups. The finding on neuroses was particularly interesting. The highest rate per 100,000 was found for nonwhite females (113.7), the second highest for white females (109.1), and the third highest for white males (55.3); the rate was lowest for nonwhite males (38.4).

Schwab et al. (1973) conducted a community survey involving 318 persons in Florida. Blacks were found to have a psychiatric "impairment" more frequently than whites. The racial discrepancy was most striking among the youngest and oldest of those surveyed. Other researchers focused on mental retardation or milder forms of psychopathology. In both community surveys and studies of institutionalized retardates, the rates were higher for blacks than for whites (Passamanick, 1963). It was also found that 80% of those diagnosed as being mentally retarded were poor, with blacks being overrepresented in the category "environmentally deprived" (Hurley, 1969).

An interesting study focusing on the differential manifestation of distress

---

[1]Prevalence rate is the number of cases of a disorder "existing" in a given population at a specified point in or during an interval of time. Incidence rate is the number of "new" cases of a disorder in a population during a given interval of time. The first measure includes all cases of the disorder (new and chronic), the latter only the "new" cases.

was that of Derogatis *et al.* (1971). Studying 1,000 black and white neurotic outpatients, they found an inverse linear correlation between distress levels and social class for whites, but not for blacks. For blacks, however, the highest distress levels were exhibited by middle-class patients. This suggests that blacks in a racist society have to contend with more than economic inequity. In other words, socioeconomic advancement alone for a small minority of blacks in a racist society may not necessarily diminish, but may even intensify the degree of personal distress.

Also informative are the *Task Panel Reports* (1978) submitted to the President's Commission on Mental Health. These were summary reports of findings and recommendations on the mental health of various ethnic groups in the United States. The report on the mental health of blacks notes that in 1975 blacks constituted 25.5% of all persons arrested for criminal offense, 54% of those arrested for murder, 47% of victims of murder, and 42% of those in jail. The alarming amount of black victimization becomes clear when one considers that, in that year, blacks comprised only 11.4% of the population of the United States.

The findings on mental disorders and demographic disparity are equally grim. National data on inpatient admissions to state and county mental hospitals show that the age-adjusted rate per 100,000 is 509.4 for black males and 213.2 for white males. The rates for black females and white females were 248.5 and 110.0, respectively. When age-specific rates are compared, black admission rates are at least twice those of whites in all age groups. Particularly noteworthy is the fact that the admission rates for blacks under 44 years far exceed (by about three times) those of whites in the same age group. The most striking differences between rates are for the 18–24 and 25–44 age groups. For the 18–24 age group, the rates are 892.1 for black males and 343.9 for white males. For the 25–44 age group, the rates are 1,032.7 for black males and 349.3 for white males.

The similarities of these findings to the data we discussed in the chapters on violence are striking and certainly not unrelated. Indeed this should suggest that psychiatric disorders among the oppressed are better conceptualized in terms of structural, institutional, and personal violence. Data on inpatient admission rates for outpatient clinics corroborate the same pattern. Black males have higher rates than white males, black females than white females. In the 25–44 age group, black females have the highest admission rates for outpatient clinics than any age and sex group. It would seem that black males tend to be hopsitalized most for severe psychiatric problems, whereas black females in crisis tend to require no more than one or two hours of therapy per week. Another way of interpreting the same data is that black males are forced to "therapy" by incarceration, whereas black females seek it on their own.

Such considerations make sense only when rates within races are compared. Actually, the plight of black females is best discerned by comparing their rates with those of white females. Thus for instance, when five leading diagnoses for admission to state and county hospitals are compared, black females had higher rates than white females in all except depressive disorders.

The rates for schizophrenia were 118.2 for black females and 42.8 for white females. The alcoholic disorder rates for black and white females were 50.1 and 12.4, respectively. Similar differences for organic brain syndromes and personality disorders are noted, although by less of a margin than for schizophrenia and alcoholism.

National data on rate of institutionalization are equally revealing. Between 1950 and 1970, the rate of institutionalization *increased* by 56% for nonwhite men and 14% for nonwhite women. For the same period, the institutionalization rate *decreased* for white men by 21% and for white women by 39%. The rates for institutionalization in mental health facilities decreased for all sex–race groups, but the relative decrease (in percent) was largest in the following order: white women (53), white men (46), black women (42), and black men (25). Further, estimates of professional representation in the mental health professions show that blacks comprise at best 2.0% of American psychiatrists, 4.0% of American psychologists, and about 7.6% of American social workers. Thus blacks are overrepresented in the mental health industry as patients and markedly underrepresented as professionals. This discrepancy also raises questions about appropriate diagnosis and treatment.

There is a growing body of literature on diagnosis and treatment. Much of the research in this area emphasizes social class. But what is true for whites in the lower socioeconomic status is all too often true for most blacks as well. An individual's social class and racial background correspond with the severity of his or her diagnosis, what treatment is offered to him or her, by whom and where, length of hospital stay, and outcome of therapy (Jones, 1978; Luborsky, 1971). Persons with a lower socioeconomic status tend to be diagnosed as severely impaired. This is so not only after diagnostic interviews, but also when psychological tests are employed.

For instance, Haase (1964) found different diagnoses for identical Rorschach protocols for different levels of income and occupation. Rorschach protocols identical in every respect were attached with contrived differences in occupational and income histories. Seventy-five psychologists were then asked for their diagnostic and prognostic evaluations. There was a clear indication that psychologists prefer a diagnosis of character disorder or psychosis for lower socioeconomic status clients and a diagnosis of normal or neurosis for middle-class clients. Others (Baldwin, 1975; Deragotis, 1975; Wilkinson, 1975) have shown the association of serious diagnosis with social class and racial background. How much of an ordinary diagnosis reflects valid psychopathology or simply the cultural imperialism of diagnosing agents thus remains problematic.

The diagnosis of psychopathology is certainly a highly judgmental, value-laden, imprecise venture. In his comprehensive review of the literature, King (1978) indicated that a "satisfactory level" of interpsychiatrist agreement exists only for the diagnosis of mental retardation, organic brain syndrome, and alcoholism. Agreement is only "fair" for the diagnosis of psychosis as well as schizophrenia and "fairly poor" for all other categories. At the same time, however, there is a great deal of evidence that a black person is more likely to be diagnosed as schizophrenic, psychotic, or borderline. In contrast, whites have a greater likelihood of being diagnosed as obsessive-compulsive or depressed (Baldwin, 1975; Blake, 1973; Jones, 1978; Kaplan & Warheit, 1975; Rome, 1974).

Furthermore, once having received a diagnosis of a psychosis or character disorder, lower socioeconomic status patients are also more likely to be either rejected for therapy or given inexperienced therapists. Schaffer *et al.* (1954), in a study of an outpatient psychiatric clinic, found that well-to-do clients were provided the best available treatment, whereas the poor were given little or none. Using Hollingshead's Social Index Scale, it was found that 64% of Class II and 55% of Class III patients were offered individual psychotherapy. Only 34% of Class IV and 3% of Class V patients were offered such treatment. The senior staff often treated patients in Class II and III, whereas residents were assigned to treat patients in Class III and IV. Medical students were assigned to treat patients in class IV and V, the lowest socioeconomic groups.

Rosenthal and Frank (1958) found that blacks were more likely to refuse or drop out of therapy. They found that although 60% of whites had six hours of treatment or more, only 30% of blacks made themselves available for the same number of therapy hours. Other researchers have found that there is a significant correlation between low socioeconomic status and inability to keep initial appointment (Yamamoto & Goin, 1966). Significantly, more blacks than whites refuse therapy after an initial diagnostic interview (Gibby *et al.*, 1953; Lager *et al.*, 1980; Lorion, 1978). Upon hospitalization, length of stay is longer and discharge rates lower for black than for white patients. All too often, treatment for the poor never begins and, if it does, it is terminated too early. Therapists and diagnosticians alike readily impute greater hostility, suspicion, and aggression to these patients. An assigned therapist may act on his or her self-vindicating belief that such patients lack motivations for therapy, are incapable of insight, fail to establish rapport, and are low in empathy. In other words, if therapy works, it is readily explained as reflecting the competence of the therapist; if it fails, as it often does for the poor, it is said to show the inability of the patient.

In short, a body of data on mental disorders shows that blacks, in comparison to whites, are more frequently institutionalized and for more severe disorders. They are also kept longer, given less therapy and more drugs, and assigned less qualified therapists. Consistent with the data on violence, black males between the ages of 18 and 44 are the most ostensible casualties of social inequity, incarcerative abuse, and professional bias. It is unclear whether the excessive admission rates for blacks indicate actual psychopathology, misdiagnosis, therapeutic inequity, or systemic gerrymandering of blacks with the help of the mental health establishment. It seems reasonable to assume that these rates reflect a combination of these, and more fundamentally, the social oppression that is the bedrock of greater stress, ethnocentrism, and professional bias.

Yet while the grave implications of these studies are considerable, it is important to realize that most studies on psychopathology are bedeviled by a host of conceptual and methodological problems. The intractable problems of research on diagnosis and studies on therapy outcome are well known. What constitutes a "case" and the criteria for identifying one lack standardization and universality. The value premise of diagnosing agents and their judgmental assessment of unwanted conduct make it difficult to distinguish between actual psychopathology and the results of cultural imperialism.

Even psychiatric epidemiology, which has a longer and more developed research tradition than any other area of research on psychopathology, still has many conceptual and methodological problems. Major impediments include problems of precise definition for mental disorders, the absence of standardized case finding, unreliable instruments, biased differential diagnoses, an inability to determine the actual onset and termination of mental illness, population differences in accessibility and utilization of mental health services, and variations in community tolerance to deviance.

Incidence studies are very rare in psychopathology for these reasons. Most studies in psychiatric epidemiology are based on prevalence, and even then this measure is often derived from available records on admission rates to public psychiatric institutions. We therefore know more about the diagnosis and institutionalization of the poor and less about the epidemiology of the well-to-do who utilize private services and whose confidentiality is protected. Most epidemiological studies use point prevalence rates that reflect only a census of patients hospitalized at a particular *point* in time. Few use interval prevalence and fewer still employ life-time prevalence (Kramer, 1973). Prevalence rates in any case are imprecise and complex. They combine incidence and duration. Thus it is possible to have an equal incidence of a disorder in two groups, but lower prevalence rates in one group because of a higher mortality or "cure" rate. For instance, whites could have an equal incidence of a disorder as blacks but less prevalence because they take advantage of earlier detection and treatment whereas blacks do not.

In spite of these problems, one can draw a few conclusions. The studies we reviewed underscore the intimate association of psychopathology with poverty and powerlessness. If contradictions and inconsistencies abound in the literature, this association is widely corroborated and must be taken seriously. The complex pathway through which psychopathology is induced in society, whether a given person is selected for "patienthood," a diagnosis made, the degree of severity determined, hospitalization or lack of it imposed, and subsequent rehabilitative programs instituted are still subject to one or another form of inequity and injustice. Blacks in the United States and generally the poor suffer greater stress in society, a greater likelihood of misdiagnosis, longer periods of incarceration, and greater therapeutic inequity. The need for a theory to make sense of all this has never been more acute.

ALIENATION: THE MARXIAN AND FANONIAN FORMULATIONS

The concept of alienation has been extensively discussed and debated. Geyer (1972, 1974) compiled a bibliography on the topic and found more than

1,800 books, articles, and dissertations on alienation. There is reason to believe that this bibliography, which covers works written prior to 1974, is nowhere exhaustive. In addition, a great deal more has been written on alienation since 1974. Few concepts have been so readily invoked in common parlance and serious works as the concept of alienation to refer to various conditions, processes, and experiences.

Frequently, the concept is used for purposes of description and social criticism, and with prescriptive implications. Indeed alienation has become an omnibus diagnosis for economic, social, psychological, and existential malaise. Various disciplines have appropriated the concept for their own ends, defined it according to their specialized language, and attempted to verify it with their particular methods. The concept has thus acquired numerous meanings and has been invoked for so many "evils" that some have suggested discarding it altogether.[2]

The fact is, however, there is hardly a concept as pertinent to the situation of oppression as alienation. Contrary to some claims, its value actually rests in its synthesizing power. Being a dynamic concept, it not only relates experiences to social conditions, it also entails a critique. The critique also implies a solution. But this assumes, first, the avoidance of a glib application of the concept and, second, an appreciation of its historical as well as its conceptual foundation. The concept has a long past and had gone through many reformulations, most notably by Rousseau, Hegel, and Marx. Fanon too used alienation as a descriptive, diagnostic, and prescriptive guide. His application of the concept had a Marxian influence, even though he chose to emphasize some aspects (i.e., psychological and cultural) more than others (i.e., economic and class).

Meszaros (1970) presented perhaps the most careful and informative review of Marx's theory of alienation. There are four major aspects to alienation in the Marxian formulation: (a) man's alienation from *nature*, (b) man's alienation from *himself*, (c) man's alienation from his *species-being*, and (d) man's alienation from *man*. The first aspect Marx referred to as "estrangement from the thing," which means the alienation of the worker from the *product* of his labor—that is, the alienation of that which mediates his relation to the "sensual external world" and hence to the objects of nature. What the worker produces is not his own, but rather someone else's; it meets not his but alien needs; it is a commodity he sells to eke out a bare existence. The more he produces, the more his product and hence the objects of nature stand opposed to him.[3]

The second aspect Marx referred to as "self-estrangement," which emphasizes the worker's relation to the *act of production* itself. The process by which he produces permits him no intrinsic satisfaction. His "life-activity," which

---

[2] Among the most widely known writings on alienation from a psychological perspective are those of Melvin Seeman (1959, 1975). He delineated six forms of alienation and used a version of Rotter's Internal-External Locus of Control Scale to measure powerlessness.

[3] A most informative discussion of this and other aspects of alienation is found in Karl Marx (1964, 1973).

should be spontaneous, free, and creative is coerced, controlled, and regimented. He engages in work not for its own sake, as an expression of his essential *being* or of his natural activity, but for a wage to permit him only animal existence—eating, drinking, sleeping, etc. In consequence, the worker is alienated from his own activity, which also is alienation from his body, cognition, and affect. He is alienated from himself.

The third aspect refers to the negation of human essence inasmuch as the worker is denied actualization of his inherent human potentials through activity. That is, man expresses, objectifies, and duplicates his "species-being," his human essence, through his labor, affirming not only his personality, but also the humanity he shares with others. Without his life-activity, everything about him remains implicit, unrealized, and unrecognized. When his labor is alienated, so too is his "humanness." Through activity, he leaves his mark in the world, transforming objects around him, which in turn transform him. Because of alienated labor, his being remains alien to him and to all others.

Finally, the fourth aspect refers to the estrangement of man from other men. Although the third aspect emphasizes alienation from mankind in general, the fourth aspect concerns alienation from specific others by virtue of class contradictions. It should be stressed that at the conceptual kernel of the Marxian formulation is a dialectical reciprocity between man, productive activity, and nature. A threefold interaction permeates these constituent parts. Man is part of nature, but he also humanizes nature. With his activity, he creates and is created. Capitalism divides society into private property and owner, on the one hand, and wage labor and worker, on the other. It is to this antagonistic opposition of man against man, with the violence and degradation it entails, that the fourth aspect of alienation refers.

One can see from the preceding that, in the Marxian formulation, all four aspects of alienation reduce to characteristics of "alienated labor." For according to Marx, the root causes of alienation reside in the substructure of society—in particular, the alienation of productive labor engendered by a capitalist mode of production. Contrary to vulgar materialist claims, however, the Marxian formulation is dialectical, showing the reverberation of "alienated labor" in all domains of social and psychological life.

Alienation was also a central and synthesizing concept for Fanon. There is no doubt that Fanon was greatly influenced by the Marxian formulation on alienation. The influence was partly direct, since there is an indication that Fanon studied Marx, and partly indirect, since the writers he avidly read (Césaire and Sartre included) were themselves influenced by Marxism. At the same time, Fanon was a psychiatrist and hence interested in the exposition of alienation from a psychological perspective. His exposure to existentialism, phenomenology, and psychoanalysis further enriched his perspective on alienation. As pointed out earlier, Fanon was a personal friend of Sartre; moreover, he attended some lectures of Merleau-Ponty during his student days in Lyons.[4]

---

[4]Simone de Beauvoir in *Force of Circumstance*, Vol. II, wrote: "Fanon had attended Merleau-Ponty's philosophy classes without ever speaking to him; he found him distant."

Above all, however, his personal experiences and observations among the oppressed gave poignancy and relevance to his exposition on alienation.

Zahar (1974), as noted earlier, presented a detailed discussion on Fanon's
perpective on alienation. Rather than merely recapitulating Zahar, it seems
more appropriate here to "reconstruct" Fanon's formulation from his various
works in order to present a developmental perspective. But before embarking
on such a developmental presentation, it must be emphasized that Fanon's
perspective on alienation continuously changed in substance and accent.

Fanon's first book, *Black Skin, White Masks*, had primarily a psycho-
existential thrust. He thus focused on the prejudice of whites and the feeling of
inferiority of blacks. Relying heavily on case studies and personal accounts,
Fanon articulated the dynamics of interpersonal problems and experiential
anguish in the midst of a European society and in the thoroughly colonized
Antilles. Though his critique and analysis were poignant, his early solution to
alienation was ambiguous. At best, two solutions were offered—one for the
"Negro intellectual" and another for the "Negro laborer." For the former, it
was implied to be a question of rediscovering one's lost identity through self-
analysis and the study of black history. For the latter, it was said that nothing
is left but to fight.

Life and work in Algeria brought to the fore much that was implicit
earlier, and enriched Fanon's conception of alienation. The psycho-existential
emphasis was supplanted by a psycho-historical perspective. Psychological
considerations of course persisted, but interpersonal difficulties and existential
crises were subsumed under a more comprehensive and clearer view of social
structural and cultural problems evident in colonial Algeria. Clinical data were
thus used to complement and concretize the critique of colonial violence and
collective victimization. Substructural problems involving social practice, institutions, and mode of production were emphasized. The consideration of
culture, no longer marred by reactive and metaphysical assertions as in
negritude, with which Fanon briefly flirted, became directly linked to the
realities of the *nation*. What is more, the solution to alienation was articulated
as nothing short of total war—a coordinated, and collective counterviolence
against the violence of the oppressor. We have already seen Fanon's formulation on violence.

Taken together, Fanon's works suggest five aspects of alienation: (a) alienation from the *self*, (b) alienation from the *significant other*, (c) alienation from
the *general other*, (d) alienation from one's *culture*, and (e) alienation from
creative *social praxis*. The first aspect involves alienation from one's corpo-
rality and personal identity. The second emphasizes estrangement from one's
family and group. The third is best shown by the violence and paranoia characterizing the relation between whites and blacks. The fourth involves estrangement from one's language and history. The fifth concerns the denial and/or
abdication of self-determining, socialized, and organized activity—the very
foundation of the realization of human potential.

These five aspects are implicit and integrated in Fanon's works. They are
delineated here for the purpose of summary and clarification. As would be

expected, Fanon's immersion in clinical work and his pained awareness of deracination led him to emphasize alienation from the self and from culture. The following brief discussion of Fannon's formulation on alienation begins where he himself began.

Fanon began *Black Skin, White Masks* (1967a, p. 38) with the theme of cultural alienation, exemplified by the imposition of a European language on blacks in the diaspora. "To speak a language," he wrote, "is to take on a world, a culture. The Antilles Negro who wants to be white will be whiter as he gains greater mastery of the cultural tool that language is."[5] In the case of the Martinquean, the culture and language imposed were French. One took pains to speak "the French of France, the Frenchman's French, French French," all the while avoiding Creole, except to give orders to servants. The fact of having to speak nothing but the other's language when this other was the conqueror, ruler, and oppressor was at once an affirmation of him, his worldview, and his values; a concession to his framework; and an estrangement from one's history, values, and outlook.

As we have seen earlier, the imposition of European culture and language on blacks in the diaspora was realized through massive violence, forcing the history, culture, and genealogy of blacks into oblivion. Culture always has had an intimate, dialectical link with the prevailing mode of production and the prevalent mode of psychological existence. Economic exploitation becomes possible to the extent that the culture, and hence the history and biography, of the dominated is sequestered, stunted, or obliterated. Cultural deracination of blacks was but the intellectual and emotional counterpart of economic enslavement. The Middle Passage uprooted *bodies,* transporting them to alien lands. Cultural deracination dislocated *psyches,* imposing an alien worldview.

One can thus speak of a cognitive and affective "Middle Passage" in the cultural deracination of blacks. Like the historic Middle Passage involving the movement of bodies across the Atlantic Ocean, from one continent to another, so too the uprooting of psyches from their culture to their insertion into another, in which the basic values were prowhite and antiblack, elicited a victimization difficult to quantify but very massive. What Fanon thus emphasized was that to acquiesce to and embrace the oppressor's culture, leaving behind what is left of one's own, is to plunge oneself into profound alienation in all its varieties and anguish.

Fanon elaborated on cultural alienation and its consequences elsewhere. In the stable societies of Europe, he argued, there is a continuity and synchrony among three main domains: the nation, the family, and the identity of members. The family and the nation turn on the same axis. The family is in fact a miniature of the nation. Both are governed by essentially the same values, laws, and principles. Both observe similar rituals, resort to common admonitions, and take the same punitive measures to ensure conformity and to exert control. A basic interdependence exists between them because the nation is but the sum of its families. Even the very structure of authority-relation in the

---

[5]See, in particular, Chapter Six of Fanon's *Black Skin, White Masks,* pp. 141–209.

nation corresponds to the authority-relation in the family. Thus a militaristic nation fosters greater father dominance. An autocratic and centralized nation promotes strict discipline and obedience in the family. Where goes the nation, so follows the family. How the family socializes a member also prepares the citizen of the nation. The continuity and synchrony existing between the nation and the family ultimately give rise to a national culture, a collective bond, and a sense of common destiny.[6]

An analogous continuity and synchrony also exists between the family and the identity of its members. The child growing up in a stable European society grows in a relatively stable family constellation. The values he internalizes, the parental rules he observes, the forms of self-expression he is permitted—all these prepare and guide him along a normative course of socialization. The childhood stories he is told and the family members after whom he models himself also impart to him acceptable modes of catharsis, an ego-syntonic view of himself, and a shared sense of belonging. The child grows in this stable family constellation and later emerges from that intimate circle to encounter a wider social world governed by similar values, laws, and principles. The result is that a normal child who grows up in a normal family will be a normal adult. If and when some abnormality occurs under these conditions, the clinician searches for defects in the individual or, at best, in his family circumstance. The social structure, readily vindicated, recedes in the background. A psychology of individual differences gains theoretical prominence and individual therapy becomes one treatment of choice.

The colonial situation, in contrast, fosters neither continuity between the nation and family nor synchrony between the family and the identity of its members. The social structure exists primarily for the purpose of exploitation. Violence, crude and subtle, brought it into existence and maintains it. This violence, pervading the social order, in time affects the life of the colonized in a most fundamental way. The indigenous social structure is dislocated. The family institution subsequently is disrupted. The identity of members also is constantly assaulted. In situations of prolonged oppression, as found among blacks in the diaspora, the oppressor had long obliterated the culture, language, and history of the oppressed. It is here less a question of discontinuity of the social structure and the family or the family and personal identity than of a massive swamping of the family and a profound intrusion into the psyche.

The black child in Martinique is taught to sing songs of praise about "our ancestors, the Gauls." At home and in school, he is taught to scorn Creole and the values it represents. How he talks, dresses, eats, and lives meticulously conforms to the rules laid down by the dominant group. This is so particularly among those whose economic and class standing permit dreams of greater assimilation into the white world. By crude and subtle means, the development of personal biography and the reckoning of collective history, apart from the biographies and history of whites, are discouraged. As suggested earlier,

[6]Fanon was not indeed the first to offer this formulation of psychopathology. Earlier writers, including members of the Ey School in French psychiatry, had used such a formulation.

what make this process of negation so insidious and so difficult to overcome is the fact that one's loved ones along with the family hearth in which one was socialized have unwittingly been enlisted as instruments of the prevailing social order. Memories of harsh punishment meted out for resistors of the past are still fresh in the collective psyche. And one needs no more convincing admonition about the "wisdom" of capitulating than to observe the countless unemployed, imprisoned, and deprived.

Even if the family remains relatively intact or little tarnished by this violent social order, the attack on the self is merely postponed until one moves away from the intimate circle of the family to the ubiquitous violence of the wider social world. Thus black children who grow up in a healthy family environment sooner or later come up against massive social forces that undermine and sometimes overwhelm their development. Since the values, laws, and principles enforced in the social order are largely discordant with those governing life in the family, profound contradictions are inevitable. Since the love of the family is incongruous with the violence of the social order, the transition from childhood to adulthood, from the intimate circle of the family to the violent social order, involves inordinate personal conflicts and turmoil.

The school, the history books, the comic strips, the theatre halls—all these also enforce cognitive dissonance and even self-hate. The psychic suffocation increases with each progressive step in colonial education. The closer the schoolboy gets to the social circle of the oppressor, the more he learns to disparage what he is by birth and race. On the one hand, he is assimilated into the dominant culture, and on the other, he is made to break away from his own culture. As he moves through various stages of colonial education, he progressively reduces his contact with his relatives and the indigenous culture. As the bond with family members grows more tenuous, he increasingly enters the social orbit of the oppressors. Then comes the stage when he must choose *either* his own group and culture *or* the ruling group and its alien outlook. For many, the "choice," made long ago, follows an Aristotelian logic: There is no middle ground. Acceptance of one entails rejection of the other; a gain in some respects involves a loss in others.

In this process of assimilation, the oppressors win an auxiliary, an indigenous defector, who by this time feels he has arrived. The oppressed community loses a member, suffers brain-drain, and risks betrayal by one of its own. The family too loses a loved one who, having embraced an alien outlook, returns on occasions only to criticize its traditional ways of living and of being. Fanon illustrated this by recounting the feigned amnesia and pretended mutation of the young Martiniquean returning to his village after a few months in France. No sooner did he arrive home than he proceeded to act as if he were a European tourist—and a foolish one at that. Pretending that he knew nothing about farm implements, he turned to his father and asked, "Tell me, what does one call that apparatus?" Fanon (1967a, pp. 23–24) informs us that the father responded by dropping the tool on the boy's feet. The amnesia suddenly lifted.

For most, however, the amnesia of who they are or of their social origin persists, although their repudiation of tradition and their people is more subtle.

The simultaneous rejection of one's own and the uncritical acceptance of the alien nonetheless presents a fertile ground for psychopathology. The delusion of having arrived there, but the fact of having lost ground here, the fact of being a battleground for many social contradictions, the feeling of being torn between two opposing worlds—all these exact a cumulative and immeasurable toll. Of course even for the intensely oppressed, there do exist many social buffers protecting the individual in his own community. The recognition of these buffers and their reinforcement cannot be overemphasized, since without them there can be neither a protective shield nor the basis for a proactive response.

According to Fanon, it is particularly when the black person is cut off from his community and thrown into the white world that structural, institutional, and personal violence intensifies and the psycho-existential crisis unfolds with poignancy. The black person seeking his destiny in a country in which whites are the majority learns quickly that his self and most concretely his body are under constant assault. In his everyday interactions, even chance encounters, he is made to feel a stranger in this world and ultimately a stranger to himself. On the streets and in shopping centers, he is assailed by stares as tormenting as the remarks made to him and about his race. The white child, untutored yet in the hypocrisy of his parents, shouts: "Look, a Negro!" The black person initially finds this amusing; he smiles in return. Elsewhere and another child: "Look, a Negro!" Everywhere, the same alarm. The circle draws tighter and there is little room for escape. It is no longer amusing. "Mama, see the Negro! I'm frightened!" Now how could one find amusement in causing fear in children by his very *body* and *being*?

On trains, the black person is kept at a distance. Two or three seats next to his remain unoccupied. And one need not dwell on the anger, frustration, and desperation a search for an apartment involves. Besides the stares, the racial slurs, the distance kept, there are also elaborated cultural myths about the black person's body and sedimented stereotypes about his race. The Negro is ugly. The Negro smells. The Negro is a sexual beast. If not avoided, he is paternalized—talked to as a child or in pidgin French. Gradually, he is thrown back to reexamine his corporal schema and his very being. A self-concept that started developing in the first few years of life is shaken to its foundation.

Agreement with the verdict of this hostile other inevitably entails a profound psycho-existential crisis, a veritable amputation of the self. This is so particularly when the initial edifice of the self was itself tenuous and the family circle had long assimilated the corrosive values of the dominant other. Even as various defensive maneuvers are installed, the dialect between one's body and the world, between the self and the other, is nonetheless ruptured. Because of elaborated racial myths and the evident structure of dominance, whites on top and blacks at the bottom, his corporal schema is overlaid by a "racial epidermal" and "historico-racial" schema. What is more, he is personally held responsible not only for his body, but also for his ancestors and his whole race. It is not only a rejection of one's body and self, but also a verdict of eternal guilt.

In this respect, two primary questions arise: how are these assaults defended against and, if amputation of the self is realized, by what means are the
"pieces" pulled together or, better still, "another self" forged? I explored answers to these questions elsewhere (Bulan, 1979, 1980c) by proposing a theory
of identity development that is implicit in Fanon's writings and personal evolution. In brief, under conditions of prolonged oppression, there are three major
modes of psychological defense and identity development among the oppressed. The first involves a pattern of *compromise,* the second *flight,* and the
third *fight.* Each mode has profound implications for the development of identity, experience of psychopathology, reconstitution of the self, and relationship
to other people. Each represents a mode of existence and of action in a world in
which a hostile other elicits organic reactions and responses. Each also entails
its own distinct risks of alienation and social rewards under conditions of
oppression.

To go into the details of the proposed theory here would take us far beyond
what space and priorities of this chapter permit, even though the theory clarifies much about Fanon's thought and personal evolution. Suffice it to point
out, however, that I discuss the three modes of psychological defense and
identity development as "stages." The first stage, based on the defensive
mechanism of identification with the aggressor, involves increased assimilation into the dominant culture while simultaneously rejecting one's own
culture. I call this the stage of *capitulation.* The second stage, exemplified by
the literature of negritude, is characterized by a reactive repudiation of the
dominant culture and by an equally defensive romanticism of the indigenous
culture. I call this the stage of *revitalization.* The third phase is a stage of
synthesis and unambiguous commitment toward radical change. I call this the
stage of *radicalization.*

These three stages are best understood within the framework of the historical and cultural confrontations in which they occur. Figure 1 shows three
intersecting Venn diagrams representing the dominated culture (A), the dominant culture (B), and a third culture, which is *in statu nascendi* (C). The
dominated culture comprises the values, beliefs, norms, and outlook that historically prevailed among the oppressed. The dominant culture is that imposed
on the oppressed by personal, institutional, and/or systemic violence. The
degree of cultural imposition and hence overlap between A and B varies from
one place to another and from one type of oppression to another. Frequently, it
is less a question of overlap of cultures than the obliteration of one and the
supplantation of the other. The culture *in statu nascendi* is partly a synthesis
of aspects of the dominant and dominated cultures. The other part, shown by
broken lines, represents the emergent and unique aspects of the culture that is
in the process of formation.

The shaded area is the region of cultural contact, confrontation, and mutual influence. It is also the zone of "cultural in-betweenity," in which the black
elite reside with aspects of the "new" and the "old," the "modern" and the
"indigenous." Here the dominant and dominated cultures coalesce with considerable regularity and intensity, one modifying the other and each losing in

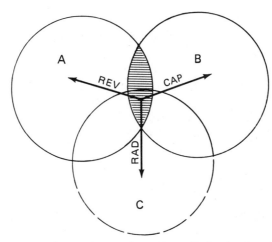

FIGURE 1. Culture contact, domination, and reactions of the dominated; (a) The dominated culture; (B) the dominant culture: (C) the emerging culture. The shaded area is the region of contact, confrontation, and mutual influence—the zone of "cultural in-betweenity" for the dominated. → = predominant tendencies, patterns of reaction, or stages of adaptation. CAP = Capitulation; REV = Revitalization: RAD = Radicalization.

consequence its original character. The dominant culture is propagated by the ruling group and buttressed by institutions of social control, as well as by existing patterns of reward. Imposed aspects of the dominant culture may be religious precepts, a mode of thought, a set of values, a pattern of social behavior, and frequently a combination of these. The mediating institutions are usually the oppressor's churches, schools, mass media, hospitals, courts, and other institutions.

The arrows in Figure 1 indicate the three major directions open to those inhabiting the zone of cultural in-betweenity. It should be emphasized that one can talk of these not only as stages, but also as tendencies or patterns, depending on whether one considers them longitudinally or cross sectionally. But whether considered as stages, tendencies, or patterns, it is important to note that none of them exists in a "pure state" nor is any one in a way exclusive of the others. All three coexist in each individual and among each generation of the oppressed, with one or another being dominant at a given moment, era, or situation. We have seen in Chapter 2 that Fanon traversed all three phases in his development. A similar progression of stages, but at a different pace and intensity, can also be found, for instance, in the development of Kwame Nkrumah, Patrice Lumumba, Amilcar Cabral, W. E. B. Du-Bois, and Malcolm X.

Frequently it happens that ordinary persons remain in one or another phase that is prevalent in their time and social milieu. Thus, for instance, some individuals and even their generation may remain fixated in the stage of capitulation. Others may go beyond this and enter the stage of revitalization with all its charged affect, vehement denouncement of the present, and marked romanticism of the past. Still others may attain the stage of radicalization on their own or find themselves in a revolutionary era with potent influences they cannot resist. As I have shown previously (Bulhan, 1980c), these three modes of psychological defense and identity development have significant implications for the degree and form of alienation among the oppressed and more generally the orientation one adopts toward the self, others, one's culture, and social praxis.

FANNON'S RADICAL SOCIOGENY

To Fanon, psychology was essentially social psychology and psychiatry, too, was fundamentally social psychiatry. Thus unlike other theorists, Fanon did not seek to discover human psychology through instinctual, genetic, or intrapsychic reductionism. According to him, all human problems must be cast in a definite socio-historical and cultural context. The press and gravity of lived human travails imbued in him a keen sense of urgency and passion. Rare among students of psychopathology who boast of their neutrality and detachment, this feeling of urgency and passion is crucial in understanding the theory and practice of Fanon.

Not only did he personally experience the massive weight of an oppressive social structure, he also observed its effects on those in his social milieu. The question for him was therefore neither academic nor abstract. Living beings around him were abused, mutilated, dehumanized. The victims were indeed none other than his brother, his sister, himself. Personal experience and observation convinced him that the source of their shared anguish was not bad genes or poor heredity, but rather a specific social structure. What is more, it is only the social order—not genes or heredity—that is most amenable to *just* resolve and human intervention.

Thus to Fanon the social structure is most crucial in a way other psychologists have rarely appreciated. It is true that some establishment theorists occasionally concede the significance of the social order. But that concession is often half-hearted and tends to treat the social order as if inert like a fixed background, as a canvas to a painting. Fanon, in contrast, viewed the social structure as a dynamic and potent force, which at once is a determinant of human psychology and a result of collective praxis. He was convinced that psychological theories that ignore the central role of the social order tend to blame the victim and also negate the human capacity to transform both the social order and human psychology.

This Fanonion perspective indeed suggests a re-definition of primary tasks for psychology and psychiatry. According to him, the paramount tasks of psychology and psychiatry are to unravel the relation of the psyche to the social structure, to rehabilitate the alienated, and to help transform social structures that thwart human needs. As we shall see later, this redefinition recognizes the role of biological substrates of human psychology without underestimating the crucial significance of the social order.

Insisting on a dialectical conception, Fanon sketched the outline of a sociogenetic perspective. Central to his radical approach was his conviction that seemingly private, individual pathology is actually a socially induced pathology of liberty. Moreover Fanon articulated a dialectical and materialist underpinning for his sociogenetic perspective. He emphasized this fact early in the introduction of his first book. *Black Skin, White Masks* (1967a, pp. 10–11):

> The analysis that I am undertaking is psychological. In spite of this, it is apparent to me that the effective disalienation of the black man entails an immediate recognition of social and economic realities. If there is an inferiority complex, it is the outcome of a double process:
> —primarily, economic
> —secondarily, the internalization—or better, the epidermalization—of this inferiority.

This quotation in fact contains two concepts that, I believe, are crucial to an understanding of Fanon's sociogenetic approach to psychology. These are the concepts of *internalization* and *objectification*. Internalization refers to the process by which external, socio-historical reality is assimilated into "internal" and subjective reality. Objectification is the reverse process in which man, through praxis and particularly labor, actualizes himself and his personality in the world around him. Taken together, internalization and objectification refer to a double process mediating the dialectic between the human psyche and the socio-environmental world. As the quotation indicates, Fanon explicitly referred to the notion of internalization. He even used the term *epidermalization* to underscore the profound transformation of economic inferiority to subjective inferiority. The concept of objectification was never explicitly formulated by Fanon, but such a concept is implicit in his works.

Fanon was acutely aware of how an oppressive social structure at once thwarts self-objectification and fosters the internalization of negative identities. There is here a double jeopardy. The oppressed is robbed of his labor—the very labor by which he could actualize himself. He also falls victim to the oppressor's damaging assaults and psychic mutilation. Earlier chapters elaborated the psychological consequences of this double jeopardy. It is sufficient to stress here that Fanon recognized the intimate relation between the psyche and the social order. He was also well aware that such a relation is invariably mediated by social institutions and significant others.

Fanon's sociogenetic perspective is best appreciated from the aggregate of his contributions. We will select here for discussion only three areas having to do with his definition of "abnormality," his suggestion of an integrative etiological theory superseding the nature versus nurture debate, and his clinical illustrations of colonially induced mental disorders. How he defines "abnormality" is of course a crucial first step in comprehending Fanon's revolutionary view of psychopathology. His seminal ideas for an integrative theory suggest a way of overcoming the stalemated predicaments in theory imposed by the either/or debate hindering a constructive response to urgent human problems. Moreover, his clinical illustrations underscore the crucial significance of an oppressive social structure for psychopathology.

Obviously, the definition of *abnormal* is fundamental to the discussion of psychopathology. Yet the concept itself and the criteria by which abnormality is identified are subject to various definitions and interpretations. Commonly used are one or a combination of five approaches. First, there is the statistical approach that identifies normality with conformity to the behaviors and characteristics of the majority in a given society. Deviation from the established norm would thus be identified as "abnormal" according to this approach. Second, there is the subjective discomfort approach that relies on personal accounts of distress for which the person seeks professional help. Third, there is the medical approach that literally or metaphorically invokes the notion of "disease," thereby emphasizing an imbalance in biochemical processes and an organic defect. Fourth, there is the cultural relativist approach that emphasizes the variability of definition, criterion, and symptom expression from one culture to another. Fifth, there is the approach that assumes ideal states that everyone is expected to embody or approximate; a marked inability to do so is then identified as "abnormal." A famous example of this is Marie Jahoda's (1958) criteria for mental health.

These approaches are often used in different combinations and emphases by various schools in the field of mental health. Each approach has many advantages attested to by their enduring use in professional and lay circles. At the same time, each approach has its own limitations. Thus for instance, the statistical approach vindicates the majority against the minority, even though the history of slavery and of Nazi era in Germany warn us that there is nothing sacrosanct about the tyranny of the majority. The subjective discomfort approach is useful inasmuch as it takes into account personal experience, but it also has its own serious limitations, as a hypochondriac well illustrates. The problems of the medical model have been sufficiently exposed during the past two decades. It has been argued that what is called "mental illness" is neither mental nor illness and that much of psychiatric diagnosis is but a moral verdict (Sarbin & Mancuso, 1982; Szaz, 1970, 1974). In reality, the cultural relativist and idealist approaches are variants of the statistical approach inasmuch as the norms and ideals of the majority, whatever it may be, are assumed to be the defining foundation of normality.

It seems obvious that no single, universally relevant approach can be delineated to incorporate the complex ways in which unwanted conduct is defined as "abnormal," then graded according to severity, a prognosis suggested, and appropriate interventions undertaken. The desire to come up with absolute and universal definitions or criteria for psychopathology is inevitably frustrated precisely because so much of what is labeled "abnormal" has value, judgmental, and subjective content. Although Fanon does not offer a decisive resolution of these problems, it is significant that he defined abnormality in a way that singularly emphasized the salience of human relations and liberty. Such a definition is, as we shall see in subsequent chapters, consistent and integral to his overall clinical perspective and practice.

Earlier in *Black Skin, White Masks* (1967a, p. 142), Fanon defined the abnormal as one "who demands, who appeals, who begs." At first glance, this is a curious definition indeed. Fanon did not elaborate on what he meant by this definition and in fact relegates it to a footnote. But judging from the context in which he mentioned this definition in passing and from his overall perspective, it seems to us that Fanon, convinced of the relational essence of psychopathology, viewed the putative patient as one who lives a ruptured relation with others and fails to harness his human potentials.

One can demand, appeal, beg, and hence be pathological only in the presence of another. The isolated patient with a purely personal pathology is a myth. It takes at least two for a demand, an appeal, a begging, and thus psychopathology to occur. Often it involves more persons: the patient's family and larger groups. To demand, appeal, and beg is to acquiesce to a prior condition of nonreciprocity and perpetuate it by demanding, appealing, and begging. We have already seen the centrality of reciprocal recognition and mutual affirmation of one to another in Fanon's perspective. Demanding, appealing, and begging demonstrate the lack or violation of the mutual give-and-take and reciprocal equality essential to a state of normalcy in human relations. One demands, appeals, and begs in a context in which the other is niggardly and stubborn. At the same time, demanding, appealing, and begging betray one's loss of personal dignity, autonomy, and resources.

Much later, when he became fully engaged in revolutionary practice, Fanon defined abnormality as a pathology of liberty. This latter definition entailed two intimately related meanings. First a patient is one whose "liberty, his will, and his desires are constantly broken down by obsessions, inhibitions, contradictions, and anxieties" (Fanon & Geronimi, 1959, p. 717). This is a person whose self is divided and at war with itself. Second, and this is very crucial in Fanon's sociogenetics, the obsessions, inhibitions, contradictions, and anxieties are not simply expressions of conflictual instincts, but rather the internalization of social conflict and imposed limitations of liberty. To occupy one's land entails occupation of one's psyche. To expropriate one's labor is equally to expropriate one's personality. The agent out there that monitors, punishes, and threatens becomes an introppressor, as we have earlier indicated. In the Fanonion perspective, loss of liberty is thus neither accidental nor secondary to psychopathology. Rather, the denial and/or abdication of liberty is definitional, etiological, and symptomatic for psychopathology.

A critical question is why some respond pathologically and others nonpathologically in situatons of shared oppression. There are usually two undialectic answers to this. One emphasizes individual difference at the expense of neglecting the commonality of shared social conditions and experiences. The other stresses the detrimental effects of shared social conditions and neglects individual differences. Fanon recognized the significance of individual differences in threshold for stress and conflict as he emphasized the potency of social conditions. For Fanon (1967a, p. 81), psychopathology is essentially a socio-historical and cultural conflict finding symptom crystallization in those with a low personal threshold; his view of the neuroses underscores the point:

> The neurotic structure of an individual is simply the elaboration, the formation, the eruption within the ego, of conflictual clusters arising in part out of the *environment* and in part out of the purely *personal* way in which the individual reacts to these influences.

What Fanon meant by the "environment" is quite obvious from his various works. Unfortunately, however, the second precondition—namely, "the purely personal way" of reacting to that environment—was never elaborated and this renders his psychological theory incomplete. His neglect of this aspect had do with the urgent press occasioned by the numerous casualties in a colonial situation. Fanon was thus engrossed in the exposition and transformation of that intolerable social condition and thus neglected also-needed studies on individual differences in response to the same situation of oppression. Fanon's suggestion that psychopathology is a result of a person-specific reaction to a pathogenetic environment nonetheless is a basis for elaborating a dialectic and holistic view. The consideration of a person-specific threshold, together with environmental insults, is thus what Fanon would fully endorse. He actually combined both aspects in his clinical illustration, but never explicitly elaborated this etiological integration. In the recent literature on etiology, the view that comes closest to Fanon's perspective is the proposed synthesis of Zubin and Spring (1977).

In their article, "Vulnerability: A New View of Schizophrenia," Zubin and Spring integrate previous theories and avoid reductionist conclusions. They argue that earlier descriptive and etiological approaches to schizophrenia have been theoretically and practically integrated. The search for common elements in these approaches led Zubin and Spring to formulate the vulnerability model. The model incorporates the role of the environment and a person-specific vulnerability to psychopathology. Zubin and Spring define their key concept of *vulnerability* as the empirical probability that a person will manifest an episode of psychiatric disorder. Vulnerability has both inborn and acquired components. The inborn component is determined by a person's genes whereas the acquired features arise due to perinatal insult, specific disease, traumatic experiences, and interpersonal conflict. An episode of schizophrenia is thus the joint result of one's vulnerability and encountered environmental "challengers," which can be either endogenous or exogenous. Endogenous challengers result from biochemical and neurophysicological process. Exogenous challengers are such environmental stressors as bereavement, divorce, and unemployment.

Everyone can therefore suffer a psychopathological episode, given suitable vulnerability and challengers. A highly vulnerable person becomes schizophrenic even under a small number or a low intensity of challengers. A demotion or even a promotion at work may trigger an episode of psychopathology in a highly vulnerable person. A less vulnerable individual would manifest similar reactions only under more stressful conditions—perhaps a catastrophic event involving the multiple loss of loved ones. What further distinguishes the more vulnerable from the less vulnerable is also the duration of the psychopathological episode. In the more vulnerable, the episode may last longer and have a formidable sequel. In the less vulnerable, the episode may be of shorter duration, with an earlier reconstitution to healthy and appropriate functioning.

Zubin and Spring also apply the concepts of accommodation and assimilation to explain the process by which one responds appropriately to life's exigencies. *Accommodation* refers to a temporary or permanent structural change in an organism to meet environmental demands. *Assimilation* refers to altering the environmental demands themselves to meet personal needs. A highly vulnerable person lacks to a higher degree both abilities, or uses them inappropriately. An episode of psychopathology may be further prolonged and complicated by the adverse effects of institutionalization and stigmatization.

The vulnerability model contains a number of insights and suggests an integrative perspective for the study of psychopathology. The model significantly departs from the nature versus nurture debate. According to it, every person is vulnerable to psychopathology. No specific population—poor or affluent, black or white—has a genetic susceptibility or immunity. Fanon would certainly find much to endorse in the model. He would probably shun its trait bias in the definition of vulnerability and also oppose its dilution of the "challengers" with endogenous features. Yet there seems to be a basic concurrence in what is implicit in Fanon's works with the model offered by Zubin and Spring.

To use Zubin and Spring's concepts, Fanon argued that an oppressive social order presents fewer "challengers" to its beneficiaries while it subjects the oppressed to greater and more treacherous assaults. Fanon was most impressed with the socioeconomic and cultural import of "challengers" on the oppressed, which so often exceeds the threshold of what is humanly tolerable. The economic life of the oppressed is disrupted; his culture disfigured; his history discredited. His social network is eroded and his family itself dislocated. Also denied him is self-objectification as his labor is expropriated. Much that he internalizes stands to testify and turn against him.

At the same time, Fanon was convinced that the neurotic, the alienated, is first a victim of others and later of himself. What is more, "the neurotic's fate remains in his hands." Obsession with individual differences is thus as counterproductive as denial of "personal ways" of reacting to the environment. According to Fanon, change must occur on both levels: The social conditions that fail to meet human needs must be replaced and, although social transformative action is taken, clinical work with casualties of the *status quo* remains indispensable. As we shall see, it is this combination of socially transformative action and clinically therapeutic practice that makes Fanon's ideas exceptional in the history of the behavioral sciences.

Illustrative of his sociogenetic perspective are some 14 clinical cases he presented in *The Wretched of the Earth*. His presentation and analysis of these cases do not, as Fanon himself admitted, have the aim of "producing a scientific work." Arguments about semiology, nosology, and therapeutic techniques are intentionally set aside in order to underscore the ravages of colonialism and the violence of the struggle for liberation. As we noted earlier, this work was written shortly before Fanon's death and one sees a measure of haste in the overall work and, particularly, the case histories.

Nonetheless, the clinical histories and illustrative symptoms are eloquent. His sketches and brief analyses attest to the fundamental humanism of Fanon and his pained awareness that violence can never be glorified for its own sake, as some of his detractors have accused him of doing. As discussed in

Chapter 8, these detractors failed to take into account the oppressor's consuming and ever-present violence, but expect the oppressed to eternally turn the other cheek. Fanon rejected this half-hearted, one-sided, and unjust pacificism. With respect to the oppressed who are left no recourse but to fight in defense, Fanon argued that revolutionary counterviolence offers a means of social reconstruction and psychological liberation. But in spite of this outlook and his efforts to justify the Algerian struggle, Fanon was deeply aware of how corrosive violence can be both to the perpetrator and victim, leaving behind devastating and sometimes lasting sequel.

Fanon's chapter, "Colonial War and Mental Disorders," is organized into four sections. A brief discussion of this chapter, such as we will present here, cannot, as we have tried elsewhere, do justice to the clinically rich cases Fanon offered.[7] Our intent here is simply to highlight some of the cases he chose to present and to underscore their obvious sociogenetic import. These psychological crises and personality decompensations are conditioned, precipitated, and/or exacerbated by one of the most violent and longest colonial wars. Some of the cases involve what we today would refer to as posttraumatic stress disorders, whereas others are so severe as to qualify as *reactive schizophrenia* in contradistinction to *process schizophrenia*. Each case history Fanon described demonstrates that the ruthless assaults of the oppressor exceeded the tolerance threshold of ordinary persons and that various psychiatric symptoms represent specifically "personal ways" of reacting to a violent condition of oppression Fanon referred to as "a veritable Apocalypse."

The first section, Series A, deals with five cases of *reactive* psychoses.[8] The second section, Series B, provides another five cases involving an assortment of issues with forensic and clinical import. The third section, Series C, discusses four cases demonstrating the debilitating effects and various techniques of torture. The fourth section, Series D, is the last section and groups together psychosomatic disorders and criminal behavior. No case illustrations are provided in this section, only characteristic symptoms are highlighted, with a short critique of traditional theories, particularly with respect to the Algiers School of Psychiatry and its explanation of crime among Algerians.[9]

The first section begins with the case of an Algerian liberation fighter, age 26, whose wife was tortured and raped by French authorities following the discovery of his guerrilla activities and their failure to apprehend him. Despite interrogation and torture, the wife refused to cooperate in providing information regarding her husband's friends and whereabouts. She was subsequently raped twice by French authorities and told: "If ever you see your filthy husband again don't forget to tell him what we did to you." As so often happens

[7]In Bulhan, *Fanon's Psychiatry Revisited: A Case of Benign Neglect or Selective Distortion*, unpublished.

[8]The English translator's rendering of "reactive" to "reactional" is misleading from a diagnostic perspective. Historically, psychodiagnosticians made a distinction between "reactive" and "process" psychoses; the former underscores the primacy of exogenic causes. Fanon, too, seems to have had such a distinction in mind.

[9]We shall examine in detail this critique of Fanon in Chapter 10.

with rape victims, the wife blamed herself for the rape and sent word to her husband, telling him what happened and requesting him to forget about her, begin a new life without her, because she was "dishonored." The rape and this reaction of the wife evoked overwhelming guilt, shame, and anger in the husband. He was treated for insomnia, headache, and impotence.

The second and third cases involved a 37-year-old survivor of a village massacre and a 19-year-old former student who turned nationalist guerrilla. The first escaped death miraculously during the mass murder in his village, suffered some bullet wounds, and was treated for paranoid reactions and undifferentiated homicidal impulses. The second was involved in the raid of the home of a settler who was known for his violent treatment of Algerians. The intended target of the raid happened to be away, but his defenseless, frightened wife, the only person present, was held hostage. In a sudden psychotic rage, this Algerian stabbed the European lady to death even though she pleaded to be spared for her children's sake. This brutal act came to haunt and torment him later. He was deeply depressed, he complained of persistent insomnia, and he twice attempted suicide. The patient's mother had been killed pointblank by French soldiers and his sisters taken to military headquarters.

The remaining two cases are of particular interest because they show the effects of the war in the other camp, so to speak. One involves a European policeman, age 28, whom Fanon treated while still at Blida, before his resignation as *chef de service*. This policeman was a witness to and active participant in many tortures of Algerian nationalists. The more often the victim answers "I don't know," thereby defeating the aim and person of the torturer, the more reason to intensify the torture. "Nowadays as soon as I hear someone shouting," the policeman reported, "I can tell you exactly at what stage of the questioning we've got to" (Fanon, 1968, p. 265).

Unfortunately for him, however, the screams of countless victims pursued him even to the privacy of his home, preventing him from sleeping. Each night he would close the windows in spite of the summer heat, to the chagrin of his wife. He would also stuff his ears with cotton and turn on the radio to avoid his tormenting "nocturnal uproar." One day while going to see Fanon for his regular therapy session, this torturer ran into one of his former victims who himself was now a patient. They recognized each other. The policeman found a living reminder of his sanctioned but unforgivable crimes. He was overcome by an acute anxiety crisis, trembling and drenched with sweat. The former torture victim thought that his tormentor had come for him once again. He was later discovered in a toilet trying to commit suicide.

The most telling example that violence begets violence is the case of the 30-year-old police inspector who smoked five packs a day, had lost his appetite, and was terrorized by nightmares. He was an accomplished torturer who, like many other torturers, equated tearing away information from a victim with "personal success." His violent ways of treating victims gradually generalized into a usual pattern of interaction with others, including strangers, friends, and family members. The slightest frustration in his daily living brought out the torturer in him. Everywhere and in each social encounter, he wanted to be the absolute "master" he was in the torture chamber. He wanted to strike at anyone upon the least frustration of his whims. He brutally beat his children with little or no provocation. It was finally the violent fury with which he fell upon his wife, following a mild criticism about his mistreatment of the children, that brought him to treatment. Although the first policeman wanted, and got, a discharge from his duties, this one asked for help to continue his practice of torture "without any pricking of conscience, without any behavior problems, and with complete equanimity" (Fanon, 1968, pp. 269–270). The former was a torturer who refused and repented; the latter embraced his profession and sought to do away with any residue of guilt.

Series B involves a mixed assortment of cases including child murder, the crisis of an Algerian youth overcome by identity-diffusion and guilt, the feelings of loss and intense ambivalence of a young Frenchwoman whose "highly placed" and ruthless father was killed by Algerians, and the multiple psychiatric reactions of Algerian war refugees. The most tragic illustration of the Manichean world and its senseless violence concerns two young Algerians, 13 and 14 years old, who killed their European friend and playmate. The interview with the 13-year-old Algerian shows the suggestibility of youth and the irrationality of violence (Fanon, 1968, pp. 270–271):

> "We weren't a bit cross with him. . . . He was a good friend of ours. . . . One day we decided to kill him, because the Europeans want to kill all Arabs. . . . So we got the knife from home and we killed him."
> "But why did you pick on him?"
> "Because he used to play with us. Another boy wouldn't have gone up the hill with us."
> "And yet you were pals?"
> "Well then, why do they want to kill us? His father is in the militia and he said we ought to have our throats cut. . . ."
> "Was it you that killed him?"
> "Yes."
> "Does having killed somebody worry you?"
> "No, since they want to kill us, so . . . ."
> "Do you mind being in prison?"
> "No."

The 14 year old is more developed, physically and mentally. To similar inquiries as the first, he retorted with indignation why it was always Algerians who were imprisoned and killed, never Frenchmen. He also talked about some of his relatives killed by the French in a mass murder (Fanon, 1968, p. 272).

> "But you are a a child and what is happening concerns grown-up people."
> "But they kill children too. . . ."
> "That is no reason for killing your friend."
> "Well, kill him I did. Now you can do what you like."
> "Had your friend done anything to harm you?"
> "Not a thing."
> "Well?"
> "Well, there you are. . . ."

The cases in Series C all involved the psychiatric reactions of torture victims. Also enumerated are the various techniques of torture including beatings, burning with cigarette butts, soapy water enemas given at high pressure, insertion of a bottle in the anus, electroshocks, and intravenous injections of pentothal. The psychiatric reactions included depression, phobia, anxiety reactions, and personality decompensation. Of particular interest is Fanon's (1968, p. 282) report that it is the mistakenly apprehended and tortured who frequently end up as psychiatric cases: "Being tortured night and day for nothing seemed to have broken something in these men." Those who "know something" tended to suffer with less sense of injustice and they were usually killed even if they confessed. A few among them who survived may be brought as patients with such stereotypic remarks as "I didn't tell them anything. You must believe me; I didn't talk" (Fanon, 1968, p. 285).

The last series deals with psychosomatic disorders common to veterans of other wars, but also some specific to Algerians. They also underscore the human ravages of colonialism and a war of liberation. In short, what is crucial about this chapter is not only that it dramatically shows the relevance of the sociogenetic perspective, but that it also demonstrates Fanon's fundamental doubts about violence even when practiced in self-defense. Perpetrators, as well as victims, continue to bear tragic wounds and the legacy, in their own person and also through their loved ones. The cases are hastily put together and could have been more effective if Fanon had had the time to explain them fully. But time was running out on him. A careful reading of these cases *and* the footnotes nonetheless impart the messages Fanon intended.

One of these messages is at once an assertion and a question. It appears in the discussion of an African nationalist who planted a bomb in a cafe frequented by the colonial officials for whom it was intended. Ten persons subsequently died in the blast. The nationalist had no personal contact with any of them and he harbored no personal grudge against any of the victims. Following independence, this nationalist became acquainted with persons from the formerly colonizing nation and found them to be nice, decent people. The realization that maybe some of the victims in that cafe incident were completely innocent or good-natured persons like his new acquaintances crystallized in him overwhelming guilt and "an attack of vertigo." Around the anniversary of that event, this nationalist would suffer prolonged insomnia, accompanied by anxiety and suicidal obsession. It is in this context that Fanon (1968, p. 253n) makes the assertion and poses the question:

> In other words, we are forever pursued by our actions. Their ordering, their circumstances, and their motivation may perfectly well come to be profoundly modified *a posteriori*. This is merely one of the snares that history and its various influences sets for us. But can we escape becoming dizzy? And who can affirm that vertigo does not haunt the whole of existence?

IV

PRAXIS AND SOCIAL THERAPY

10

FANON AND COLONIAL PSYCHIATRY

Have I not, because of what I have done or failed to do, contributed to an impoverishment of human reality.

—Fanon: *Toward the African Revolution*

To take up healing as a career assumes a degree of empathy with victims of disease if not with people. Among the crucial sources of empathy are first a recognition, conscious or unconscious, of one's vulnerability and second the kind of formative identifications—generally, the values—one has internalized. Yet empathy and regard for others are never absolute or dominant features in human relations. Like other qualities, they are contextually and historically determined. Group interests and shared biases inform to whom one may feel appropriately empathic, which may lead to projecting one's self into another's subjective state and appearing fused with the other, or to whom one may feel animosity, which can involve distancing, denigrating, and abusing. A situation of oppression not only imposes rigid boundaries between people, it also corrupts those who profess to heal.

Psychiatry—one of the specialities that deals with madness—ostensibly aims at the *improvement*, not the *impoverishment* of human reality. But stated goals are one thing, actual practices quite another. We have already seen how prevailing definitions of psychopathology, the process of diagnosis, and the pattern of confinement or overmedication are influenced by such realities of society as inequities of power, ethnocentrism, class bias, and racism. The French psychiatric establishment with which Fanon had to contend tellingly illustrates an oppressive psychiatry, and Fanon's attempt to reformulate it offers a valiant example of a struggle against such psychiatry.

This chapter discusses Fanon's quest for relevance, first in the land of his birth and later in Algeria. His search for an appropriate context was also a search for himself—what to live and die for. Psychiatry promised a means for making a living, and also a tool for correcting what he found amiss. However, learning its established theories and techniques proved insufficient. Fanon's Algerian experience underscored the need for a profound reevaluation in theories and practice, hence a direct confrontation of establishment psychiatry itself was inevitable. This chapter highlights Fanon's clinical reforms in a

207

colonial setting and his single-handed challenge of the French psychiatric establishment, particularly the so-called Algiers School of Psychiatry.

BEGINNING A CAREER IN PSYCHIATRY

Following the defense of his medical thesis on November 1951, Fanon left France with his brother, Joby, to return to Martinique. He soon took up medical practice in the island only to realize that the essential problems facing Martiniquans were political and economic. Most of the patients who came to see him suffered from maladies the primary causes of which were nutritional deficiency, poor sanitation, and poor public health practices. The possibilities of fundamental social reform seemed remote. French domination had long permeated every aspect of Martiniquan life. The economy, the culture, and the psyche were deeply penetrated. The *Békès*, a wealthy white aristocracy, was as powerful and hostile as ever. Poverty was rife, alienation rampant, and alcoholism pervasive. The latter, as Geismar (1971, p. 21) pointed out, served well as the opium of the masses:

> You could smell it in every laborer's sweat, in the air of the city's central square and narrow streets. . . . Rum was dispensed in cafes clustering the port area, in cafes surrounding the Savanne, in the cafes near the market place; it was sold by the bottle in stores near the Fanons' suburban home; it was available from a street car next to Fanon's office. Oblivion was never more than fifty feet away in any direction. Fanon wished to work toward the reform of this situation; but in 1952, he couldn't find a place to begin.

Fanon became a revolutionary several years later in Algeria and the Algerian liberation struggle had much to do with his becoming a revolutionary. Yet to argue that he accidently stumbled into revolutionary Algeria, or that he dissociated himself from Martinique and from politics for professional reasons, is to miss Fanon's deep and persistent commitment to the cause of social justice. One could very well imagine the personal anguish Fanon felt on his return to Martinique. The man who earlier wrote *Black Skin, White Masks* (1967a) would hardly have taken a complacent attitude to the poverty, alienation, and powerlessness rampant in Martinique.

Thirty years later, when I visited the island in 1982 on the occasion of the first international memorial for Fanon in Martinique, I could still sense what may have forced him away from the island. To this day the island is effectively under colonial domination; the black petty bourgeoisie and his revered teacher, Aimé Césaire, now a deputy-mayor of Fort-de-France, are in no mood for independence. Much of the population still identifies with France to such an extent that some Martiniquans consider Fanon a traitor for siding with the Algerians against France. And to this day, people consider a visit to France a mark of having "arrived" at where else but "la bas"—as if the only place, or only worthwhile place, beyond the island is France.

In any case Fanon left Martinique to specialize in psychiatry. In November 1951, he was admitted to the psychiatric residency program at the Hôpital de

Saint Alban in central France where Professor François Tosquelles had established a national reputation as a pioneer of *therapeutic institutionelle,* which was the equivalent of "milicu therapy." He supervised Fanon during his residency and, by 1953, presented three papers with Fanon at a professional conference for psychiatrists and neurologists of France and French-speaking countries.[1]

Tosquelles' innovations in psychiatric treatment are well summarized in one of these three papers (p. 546). The paper reflects its time, but it also anticipates changes that were to be incorporated into psychiatric care in various countries. The article is primarily concerned with the indications and contraindications of electroconvulsive therapy (ECT), which at the time was frequently used for diverse psychiatric disorders. The authors deplored the use of ECT merely "out of convenience" for the psychiatrist, but conceded that it is one of "the ultimate remedies in chronic, desperate, complicated cases, where the posttherapeutic deficit would be a minor problem in the face of progressive mental deterioration of the patient." Recommending the appropriate use of ECT, they also challenged the then-prevalent theoretical bias for biogenic explanations and the assumed "fixity" of character, constitution, and pathological development of personality. They further emphasized the role of psychological causation and the necessary role of ECT in the framework of institutional therapy (Tosquelles & Fanon, 1953, p. 549).

> We insist on the fact that for treating patients (with ECT) it is necessary, at the same time, to accord much importance to the hospital arrangement, to classification and grouping of the patients, and the establishment of concomitant group therapy. The coexistence of the ward for work and social life of the entire hospital is also as indispensible as the stage of active interventionist analysis that precedes the care. The Bini cure, without the possibility of an interventionist series of therapy, appears to us as nonsense.

Institutional therapy did not of course start at Saint Alban or with Tosquelles. Milieu therapy and the notion of a *therapeutic community* was first introduced during the 1930s and 1940s in England and the United States (Jones, 1953; Main, 1946; Sullivan, 1933). What was special with Tosquelles was his methodical, rigorous application of such an intervention at Saint Albans. The spontaneous, everyday experiences of patients within the institution were used therapeutically. Efforts were made to recreate ordinary experiences as they are lived in society and the patients were grouped into "life communities" consisting of no more than 10 or 12 persons. They regularly interacted with one another, sometimes in smaller groups, and with the larger community of patients in the institution through centralized and coordinated functions. Spontaneous interactions, put to maximum therapeutic value, were combined with structured group therapy, occupational therapy, and regular meetings.

At all times, patients were encouraged to confront one another and them-

[1]In F. Tosquelles and F. Fanon (1953): (a) *Sur quelques cas traités par la méthode de Bini.* (b) *Sur un essai de réadaptation chez une malade avec epilepsie morpheique et troubles de caractére grave.* (c) *Indications de thérapeutique de Bini dans le cadre des thérapeutiques institutionelles.*

selves to gain maximum "insight into their illness." Special care was taken to work with optimal numbers of patients and to group doctors into medical teams of two or three so that they could become intimately involved in a "life community." One doctor alone was said to hinder the resolution of oedipal and pre-oedipal conflicts of patients. The other two papers jointly authored by Tosquelles and Fanon (1953) provided case illustrations to underscore the efficacy of their approach to treatment.

After about two years of work with Tosquelles, Fanon left Saint Alban. He sat for *Le Médicat de hôpitaux psychiatrique*—the difficult, intensive examination that, if passed, confers upon one the coveted qualification to be *chef de service* in a major psychiatric institution in France or in one of its colonies. Fanon successfully completed this difficult examination in which less than one-third passed that year. He was subsequently offered the directorship of a hospital in Martinique. Fanon did not accept it, however. Geismar (1971, pp. 58–59) suggested that he declined because "there were no facilities there for psychiatric care or research." This is simplistic and unconvincing. We believe Fanon's refusal to accept the offer had to do with the stagnant sociopolitical condition that had previously made Martinique unattractive. The fact that he wrote to Leopold Senghor, President of Senegal and one of the advocates of negritude, and inquired about the possibilities of service in Senegal suggests that more was actually involved than the availability of "equipments for electroshock treatment, insulin therapy, and extensive *ergotherapie*," as Geismar claimed (1971, p. 59). Unfortunately, Senghor did not respond to Fanon's letter. Fanon then settled for a temporary assignment as *chef de service* in the psychiatric hospital of Pontorson, in Normandy.

Not surprisingly, his work in the eerie isolation of the psychiatric hospital at Pontorson was short-lived. The almost total absence of contact with the black world at Pontorson was not at all what Fanon wanted, even though his commitment to the psychiatric profession was intense. Then the opportunity to work in Algeria presented itself and Fanon immediately seized it. He applied for and was offered the position of *chef de service* at Blida-Joinville Hospital in Algeria. Geismar (1971, p. 60) surmised what the new assignment meant to Fanon: "It was a compromise: part of the Third World, but not Black Africa or the Antilles."

There are three questions worth asking at this point. First, Was going to Algeria a compromise as Geismar suggested? Second, Did Fanon opt out of political and social concerns during his residency and soon after its completion, as some, including Geismar, have claimed? Third, Was Tosquelles' influence so fundamental that Fanon simply followed in the footsteps of his teacher, as Gendzier emphasizes? Little exists by way of direct evidence to answer these questions. Fanon wrote no autobiography of his own and, as we pointed out earlier, he believed that those who write their memoirs have nothing else to do in the world. Thus the answers to these questions depend on who one had interviewed and, frankly, the interpretation to which one was predisposed. Geismar tended to view Fanon's involvement with politics and social issues as "interruptions" of his career in psychiatry. Gendzier (1973, p. 63), for her own reasons, emphasizes the towering stature of Tosquelles and the loyalty of his student to Tosquellean innovations, which, we are told, Fanon applied in a "mechanical fashion."

In our view, the choice of Algeria was not a compromise, Fanon did not opt out of social and political concerns, neither during his residency or at Pontorson; and the Tosquellean influence, though important in his formative years, was by no means the only guide or inspiration to Fanon's practice of rehabilitating alienated psyches. Support for these contentions is offered by one significant article Fanon wrote, "The 'North African Syndrome.'" It originally appeared in the February 1952 issue of *L'Esprit.* The article, written during his residency, shows that racism and oppression were central concerns for Fanon and that he also deeply empathized as well as identified with North Africans long before he became *chef de service* in Algeria. Moreover, it suggests that Fanon was never satisfied with prevailing medical practice with respect to the oppressed nor was he convinced that reformative tinkering with institutional milieus is sufficient while the question of social injustice remains. We will see later that Fanon significantly departed from Tosquelles in theory and practice.

The article "The 'North African Syndrome'" is an incisive critique of racism in society and in the medical establishment. In addition, it shows the depth of the psycho-existential crisis, diffuse malaise, and wandering syndromes of the oppressed. Underscored is the inability of the medical profession to comprehend the North African patient, as well as the failure of medical doctors to take a clear, responsible, and responsive position on racism and social injustice. Not only do they misdiagnose the profound and elusive afflictions of the oppressed, they also readily assume racist views and attitudes.

The article began with a question Fanon thought basic to all human problems and, no doubt, he frequently asked himself: "Have I not, because of what I have done or failed to do, contributed to an impoverishment of human reality?" In other words, Fanon (1967b, p. 3) asked: "Have I at all times demanded and brought the man that is in me?"

Fanon then proceeded to show the various expressions of racism, the pervasive malaise it produces, and the inability of standard medical practice to diagnose or treat the oppressed effectively. One remarkable facet of Fanon, here as elsewhere, was his capacity to adopt the perspectives of various protagonists, to delve into the affective particularity of each perspective, and to reveal the existential insularity of each group, oppressors and oppressed alike. In addition, there is his remarkable use of sarcasm and humor to show the tragicomical absurdities that characterize oppression. The issues discussed in this article were actually taken up years later in *A Dying Colonialism* and *The Wretched of the Earth.*

Fanon proposed three central theses in the 1952 article. The first states that North African patients in France often cause the medical staff to have doubts as to the reality of their illness. A patient comes to the physician with a great deal of pain, which is obvious from his words and comportment. But his vague complaints and wandering syndromes, illustrated in the following interview, do not fit standard etiological conceptions and diagnostic procedures.

The doctor inquires into the circumstance and experiences that preceded the ailment. But such inquires about the past is for the oppressed too painful to remember or talk about. Besides, he does not understand why he should be so interrogated when what he really needs is quick relief from his tormenting diffuse pain. The dialogue between patient and doctor recreates the tragicomical misunderstanding of the colonial situation (Fanon, 1967b, pp. 4–5):

"What's wrong, my friend?"
"I'm dying, *monsieur le docteur.*"
"Where does it hurt?"
"In my belly." (He then points to his thorax and abdomen.)
"When does it hurt?"
"All the time."
"Even at night?"
"Especially at night."
"It hurts more at night than in the daytime, does it?"
"No, all the time."
"But more at night than in the daytime."
"No, all the time."
"And where does it hurt most?"
"Here." (He then points to his thorax and abdomen.)

Meanwhile, other patients are waiting. The doctor, now impatient, seeks a way out of this frustrating impasse. He approximates a diagnosis and writes out a prescription. But the patient fails to follow the doctor's recommendations and, if he does take the prescribed medicine, he does not give it time to have the desired effect. Unable to attain immediate relief, the patient returns much earlier than instructed. He is indignant and suspicious because he believes that the doctor does not really want to help him. Or he may decide to seek treatment elsewhere, repeating time and again the same vague complaints, the same drama of mutual incomprehension and suspicion between doctor and patient. The pain of which the patient complains so often gradually becomes "his pain," and intensely cathectic. This pain comes to have a reality and social dynamic of its own and the patient shows that he jealously wants to protect whatever secondary gain he may derive from it.

An X-ray may show an ulcer or gastritis. Treatment in accordance to standard medical procedure may be provided. The doctor is now confident, he regains his sense of omnipotence, or at least feels relief in the knowledge that he can now get rid of this patient. But the patient soon returns, this time with a different complaint: "My heart seems to flutter inside here" or "my head is bursting" (Fanon, 1967b, p. 6). Instead of attempting to comprehend and treat the patient's specific affliction and the tormenting socio-historical conditions that produced it, the doctor resorts to ordinary stereotypes of the North African, calling the patient "a simulator, a liar, a malingerer, a sluggard, a thief" (Fanon, 1967b, p. 7).

The second and related thesis states that the racist tradition medical personnel have long internalized hinders appropriate diagnosis and treatment of the North African. There is, on the one hand, the medical dogma that a lesion underlies symptoms and, on the other, the cultural racism that stereotypes the

North African as a person who is lazy and inarticulate and who suffers from imaginary aliments. The doctor is urgently summoned to the home of a seriously ill North African immigrant. The relatives are ostensibly worried and distressed. They are weeping and screaming. The doctor carefully examines the patient. He asks questions, but gets only groans and vague responses in return. After considerable examination and thought, he refers the patient for surgery. To the surprise of the doctor, the patient with the "abdomen requiring surgery" turns up in his office with a grin three days later, completely cured. This of course deviates from standard medical tradition, conception, and procedure. The doctor henceforth quickly resorts to a diagnosis of "North African Syndrome," which implies malingering, lying, laziness, and all the other stereotypes. In short, in the conflict of oppressor and oppressed, the doctor sides with the former in outlook and practice. He at best patronizes the oppressed, but remains loyal to the prevailing cultural stereotypes. The North African patient, viewed no longer as an individual in his own right, is made to "bear the dead weight" of his despised group. Instead of properly diagnosing the disease and treating him for it, the whole group or race to which he belongs is "diagnosed" in accordance to prevailing stereotypes and "treated" as if they are indeed *the* disease.

The third and final thesis states that more is actually required than good intentions. The commitment to securing justice for all is everyone's responsibility. Such a personal commitment is also a precondition for healing and rehabilitating the oppressed. The vague and confusing aliments of the North African are neither imaginary nor insoluble. They are the afflictions of tormented, persecuted, and oppressed persons. The psycho-existential crises are a result of cultural dislocation, economic exploitation, and a web of dehumanizing stereotypes. It should not therefore be a question of looking only for lesions to diagnose the symptoms but also of making a "situational diagnosis" by examining the patient's social, economic, cultural, psychological, and biological circumstances. But prevailing stereotypes have it that the North African possesses no meaningful relations, no commitment to productive labor, no subjective life, no preoccupations other than those of sex, rape, and prostitution. As for his material condition, there is nothing but poverty, hunger, and overcrowding.

Fanon concluded that the North African can never be happier in Europe than he is in his home country. But contrary to what some have claimed, the answer is not repatriation so long as social and economic justice are not secured in his own land. What is more, Fanon emphasized, it is irresponsible and hypocritical to take the common view that one is neither part of the problem nor part of the solution. To young Fanon, who was then acquiring clinical skills at Saint Alban, the solution to alienation and disease was nothing short of fundamental social reconstruction (Fanon, 1967b, pp. 15–16):

> There are houses to be built, schools to be opened, roads to be laid out, slums to be torn down, cities to be made to spring from the earth, men and women, children and children to be adorned with smiles.

This means that there is work to be done over there, human work. That is, work
which is the meaning of a home. . . . There are tears to be wiped away, inhuman
attitudes to be fought, condescending ways of speech to be ruled out, men to be
humanized.

Fanon and Blida-Joinville Hospital

In November 1953 Fanon arrived in Algeria and soon proceeded to take
charge as *chef de service* at Blida-Joinville Hospital. This was the largest psychiatric hospital in Algeria. Geismar (1971) has described the medieval and
antitherapeutic conditions of the hospital when Fanon arrived. One of the
tasks Fanon accomplished in his first tour of inspection was to order the
release of all patients kept in straitjackets and chained to their beds. The staff
who for so long had taken straitjackets and chains for granted could not believe
what they heard. Fanon repeated the order and he himself began to unchain
inmates. The attending male nurses were shocked, others gathered around to
watch what they viewed as a brash and dangerous undertaking by the new
doctor. But their fears were not confirmed by the reactions of patients, some of
whom continued to lie as if they were still chained. Fanon then introduced
himself to the patients, assured them that they would no longer be kept in
straitjackets or chains, and informed them that he as well as the others were
henceforth available for consultation any time the patients wished it.

This event was historic and the male nurses who were present on that day
vividly recall the self-confidence of the new doctor and the deep respect he
inspired in them (Geismar, p. 65). These male nurses were later to become the
most loyal allies of Fanon and of his reforms in the psychiatric institution. It is
significant to note that these male nurses were all North African. Educational
opportunities denied them meant that psychiatrists had to be recruited from
France. But these nurses, though relegated to menial and low-paying tasks,
were in the most crucial line of contact and communication with patients. The
foreign psychiatrists did not speak Arabic and thus relied on these nurses to
translate conversations between doctor and patient. How a genuine dialogue
could transpire under these conditions is hard to imagine. But dialogue was not
really the *raison d'être* of colonialism or of such asylums. The fact of relying
on low-paid, demoralized, and exploited nurses for so essential a vehicle for
therapy as communication emphasizes also the low priority given to communication and therapy in this colonial institution. Significantly, Fanon did decide to learn Arabic and, what is more, later became an Algerian citizen.

The unchaining of inmates at Blida is reminiscent of Phillipe Pinel who,
soon after the first phase of the French Revolution, undertook the bold experiment of unchaining at La Bicetre. The same action in Algeria had to wait until
1953, ironically to be ordered by a descendent of Africans, taken away in
chains. The tragedy is that, to this day, many in the Third World remain
chained and straitjacketed in alien asylums mostly erected by the very Europeans who proclaim their mission as civilizing and humanizing the world.

When Fanon arrived at Blida-Joinville, there were six medical doctors and about 2,000 patients. The doctors were recruited from France and all except Fanon were European. A little more than one-half of the patients were also European and the rest were North African, primarily Algerian. The European and the "native" patients were segregated in separate wards and, as one would expect in the pervasive inequities of colonial rule, European patients were given preferential treatment and allowed more privileges. Nonetheless, conditions for both groups in the institution were dismal. The wards were overcrowded. The nonprofessional staff were overworked and underpaid. The doctors, as usual, were divided into the pack of profiteers who gained personally from human affliction, the eternal skeptics who were marking time while waiting for better posts elsewhere, and the few dedicated clinicians who far exceeded their call of duty.

The dismal conditions of the psychiatric institution at Blida and in Algeria generally was discussed by Fanon and his colleagues (Fanon *et al.*, 1955). In 1954, Algeria had a population of about 10 million of whom 8.5 million were Algerian and 1.5 million were European. For this population of 10 million, there were only eight psychiatrists and 2,500 beds. Five of the psychiatrists were in Blida Hospital; three psychiatrists were in three different hospitals in Algiers, Oran, and Constantine. The psychiatric hospital at Blida-Joinville, the largest in the country, was designed for 971 patients, but housed 2,000. Every available space was used to reduce the overcrowding. Nearly all the refractories and even the bathrooms were used as sleeping quarters. The chapel had to be used as an occupational therapy room, a classroom, and a movie theater. The mosque too had become a place other than for worship.

The understaffing and overcrowding at Blida also created a huge backlog of patients. In September 1954, there were at least 850 patients waiting for admission. The overwhelming majority of those kept on the waiting list were North Africans. Europeans were admitted earlier. Moreover, an already bad situation was made worse by pressure from colonial administrators who determined that certain types of patients be given early admission, even though others in more dire need had been waiting longer. The inability to admit promptly of course caused serious difficulties for the patients, their relatives, and the staff. Patients in acute crises, who would have benefited immensely from early intervention became worse as a result of the delay. The anger and frustration of relatives reduced their tolerance for the patient and their cooperation with the staff. Patients admitted after a long wait often were aggressive, a state that could have been avoided had they been admitted earlier. What is more, other hospitals referred their most difficult and chronic patients to Blida-Joinville Hospital, making it a psychiatric dumping ground.

It was easy for a young doctor to be discouraged with such dismal conditions or to join the ranks of older professionals who were comfortably settled into a pattern of indifference. But Fanon relentlessly devoted himself, learning to sleep only four hours each night, to the daunting task of reform at Blida. He endeavored to introduce reforms of the kind he saw practiced at Saint Alban. The Tosquellean influence was unmistakable, at least at the beginning. Fanon introduced occupational, group therapy and collective gatherings in an effort to create a therapeutic community. In addition, he organized a soccer team in the institution and arranged for matches with other teams in the community. Weekly outings to the beach, the serving of traditional dishes, and bus tours interrupted the crushing monotony of incarceration and also brought patients a measure of self-worth and social life. In addition, Fanon began a weekly periodical, appropriately called *Notre Journal*, in which patients and staff were to express their views and exchange information.

More politically controversial, Fanon desegregated his service and prohibited distinction or privileges on the basis of nationality or race. Fanon also allowed more freedom for patients who previously were kept in closed wards; the hospital grounds were mainly reserved for staff. Fanon introduced open wards, permitting free movement within the institution for all patients, except those who were violent. Those considered to present danger to others or to themselves were kept in closed wards, but incentives were introduced to "graduate" them into open wards. We will see later that Fanon had to reconsider the therapeutic value of this practice.

Not all these reforms were successful. In some cases, what seemed workable and appropriate from past experiences in Europe proved impractical or inappropriate in Algeria. One experience in particular drove home a lesson that proved a turning point in Fanon's psychiatric career. Fanon and Azoulay (1954) wrote about their attempt to introduce regular meetings and activities to create a therapeutic community in the Tosquellean tradition. Two separate sections, European women and Muslim men, of the hospital were followed. The 165 Europeans readily participated in the meetings and activities. The attitude of the women subsequently changed, their interactions improved, and a significant increase in rates of discharge was noted. In contrast, the 220 Muslim men failed to respond to the same reforms. The scheduled meetings of patients and service-providers failed mainly due to language barrier, since the doctors could not speak Arabic. These meetings were then abandoned. Activities involving music and drama were considered, but the nurses refused and this in turn was abandoned. Efforts to involve the patients in such activities as occupational therapy also proved unsuccessful. The marked success on the one hand and utter failure on the other necessitated some fundamental rethinking (Berthelier, 1979, p. 151):

> These rapid and relatively easy success [of sociotherapy introduced in the section for European women] only emphasized the total failure of the same methods, used in the section for Moslem men [for whom] . . . despite the multitude of attempts, no improvement took place. Little by little, it became clear that it could not be a question of laziness or of poor will: *We have taken the wrong road, it was necessary to re-examine the fundamental reasons for our failure so as to find a way out of the impasse.*

Fanon and Azoulay inquired as to why the reforms worked in one section and not in the other. Their conclusion was that they were imposing practices and methods that worked in Europe but were alien to the North African: "We naively . . . believed possible to adopt to a Moslem society the framework of a Western society . . . we have forgotten that the whole application . . . must be preceded by a tenacious and concrete interrogation of the organic base of native society." Fanon and Azoulay then asked: "Under the guise of what poor judgement had we believed possible a sociotherapy of Western inspiration to serve Muslim men?" (Berthelier, 1979, pp. 151–152.)

They offered two basic reasons. First, they unwittingly took for granted the prevailing colonial propaganda that the North African is French and thus they did not take the trouble to understand him in his own culture, history, and environment. As did others in the socio-political arena, the psychiatrist "automatically" assumed and attempted to implement an assimilationist policy. In actuality, the policy of assimilation negated reciprocity of perspectives. It imposed on the dominated party a greater burden to adapt, conform, and submit to an alien cultural outlook and normative behavior. This indeed was what the North African patients were resisting. It was Fanon and his student's conclusion that a "revolutionary attitude was indispensable" and that the assumption of cultural supremacy, which commonly undergirds clinical work, must give way to a cultural relativism. Otherwise, therapy and reform become worthless and even detrimental.

The second and even more important source of error was, they pointed out, the conceptual and cultural bias of the prevailing psychiatric thought. This was a critique of the dominant psychiatric establishment, particularly the so-called Algiers School of Psychiatry. The critique at this initial period was mild and cordial; later it changed in intensity and tone. Nonetheless, the point was made with unmistakable clarity:

> Finally and above all, it is necessary to say that those who preceded us in the exposition of the North African limited themselves too much to the motor and neurovegetative phenomena. . . . It was essential to change perspectives. . . . A leap had to be made, a conversion of values had to carried out. . . . A sociotherapy could only be possible to the extent one accounted for the social morphology and the forms of sociability. (Berthelier, 1979, p. 152)

These observations and conclusions, written a year after Fanon arrived at Blida, crystallized and defined the direction Fanon's clinical work would take. In his own words, Fanon henceforth "humbled himself" to the native culture and, rather than be arrogant or indifferent, became "timid and attentive." This Antillean who from birth was a hostage to European culture, history, and conceit had made a remarkable "leap" in *time, geography,* and *values* for a homecoming to the shores and cultures of Africa. Fanon subsequently undertook studies in ethnopsychiatry, writing on such topics as the attitudes of North Africans to madness, the sociology of perception and imagination, the psychocultural meaning of confession, and the search for effective clinical intervention in Third World countries.[2] The 1954 article of Fanon and Azoulay was clearly more than a clinical study on therapy outcome. It was in addition a theoretical and ideological attack on the French psychiatric establishment generally and the Algiers School of Psychiatry in particular.

---

[2]Some of these works are discussed in the Chapter 11. For a complete citation, see the bibliography of Fanon's works at the end of this volume.

Fanon's single-handed but relentless battle with the dominant psychiatric establishment whose views and treatment of the North African were thoroughly colonial and scandalous has not been sufficiently appreciated. In fact, few of Fanon's psychiatric writings fail to include, directly or implicitly, a critique of the dominant psychiatric establishment and its extension into the North African context. At issue for him were a series of theoretical, ideological, and clinical problems in approaching the North African patient, the community of which he is a member, and the role of psychiatry in the colonial social order.

It is important to note that the earliest and most persistent opposition to Fanon's reforms within Blida came from the European doctors and the colonial administration they represented. With the exception of Dr. Lacaton and a few interns, the European doctors at Blida were either openly hostile to or quietly resentful of Fanon. They opposed his efforts to change the *status quo* within the institution. Behind his back, as Geismer (1971, p. 68) pointed out, some of them even referred to him as the "Arab Doctor," which was their way of calling him the "Nigger Doctor." It would be a mistake to consider their resentment and opposition as only idiosyncratic reactions or interpersonal differences. Although no such doubt existed, there was also a more fundamental clash of perspectives, interests, and allegiance.

Blida-Joinville Hospital was actually a microcosm that reflected the larger colonial society of which it was a part. The inequities of privileges and power, the racial segregation of patients, and the differentials in salaries that for years characterized the institution were extensions of what prevailed in the larger colonial society. Indeed the patients were individuals who somehow could not cope or be coped with in that society. Their crises and certainly their incarceration were implicit, but poignant social and political commentary. The psychiatrists, too, employed by the state and themselves embedded in the sociocultural milieu, were by no means operating in a social vacuum or employing only their "technical expertise." They were the veritable representatives of the prevailing social order as their patients were the most obvious victims of it.

It was inevitable that Fanon's ideas and clinical reforms would constitute a challenge to the prevailing colonial framework and its Eurocentric values. The challenge first took root at Blida-Joinville Hospital, advanced further into a challenge of the larger psychiatric establishment, earlier skirmishes with it not sufficing, and then culminated in a direct, political, violent challenge of the social order itself. Thus Fanon's decision to join the liberation movement must perforce be viewed partly as a determination to liberate psyches he saw doomed to psychological death in Blida. His struggle against the European doctors in Blida, too, must be considered along with his persistent struggle against the Algiers School of Psychiatry and the larger French psychiatric establishment of which it was an extension.

Significantly, the founder of this influential school, Professor A. Porot, was also one of the founders of Blida-Joinville Hospital. Given that this was the largest psychiatric hospital in Algeria and that Porot elaborated his own medico-educational establishment, it would not be too farfetched to conclude that the European doctors in Blida were colleagues, students, or at least sympathizers of Porot and his school. Now what indeed was the Algiers School of Psychiatry about? Why did Fanon become its most formidable challenger and critic? And how did Fanon single-handedly effect a remarkable change in French psychiatric outlook?

FANON AND L'ÉCOLE D'ALGER

Berthelier (1979) has reviewed psychiatry in colonial Algeria and Fanon's revolutionary role in the raging battle of ideas within Algeria, that prized French colony. European psychiatry has had a relatively longer history in Algeria than in most African colonies. This had to do partly with the greater penetration of colonialism into Algeria, with French settlements effectively installed in Algeria, and partly with an earlier presence of Algerian immigrants in France. Moreover, as colonialism became established in Algeria and Algerian psyches, assimilation into French culture intensified to a point where efforts were made to assimilate Algerian madness into French madness. For at a very early date, many Algerians who suffered from mental disorders were sent to asylums in France for treatment.

French psychiatrists wrote little about the psychopathology of the Algerian before 1870. But writings about Algerian psychopathology increased as Algerians, in the throes of a psycho-cultural crisis, appeared in significant numbers in French asylums and as Algeria became an important colony of France. Among the early works of French psychiatrists, a few show a measure of a "culturalist approach" to the Algerian patient and of a wish to understand him in his social context. But the most persistent and dominant trend was that which asserted the genetic inferiority, unredeemable criminality, sexual perversion, and mental deficiency of the Algerian. The Algerian as a subhuman being, a bundle of perverse instincts, given to dangerous and uncontrollable impulses—such characterizations were used to justify colonial violence and subjugation. The historical function of these writings was to justify European conquest, scientifically, and more specifically, to fortify the Manichean psychology of French administrators, settlers, and citizens. The European as the embodiment of all that is good, rational, peaceful, and sublime was juxtaposed with the colonized native as the incarnation of evil, irrationality, impulsive violence, and beastly instincts.

Thus for instance, Meilhon concluded in 1915 that the Algerian, though less prone to suicide, has a greater susceptibility to alcoholism and sexual perversion and that his psyche was doomed to an irreversible degenerative process. One characteristic he emphasized was a dangerous impulsivity among Algerians: "It is a question of a sudden, instinctual, unconscious, blind action . . . it is the sign of a cerebral inferiority which is congenital, inherent to the race and found only among [European] patients who are inferior and degenerate" (Berthelier, 1979, p. 141). Earlier, Constance (1873) who had clinical charge of Algerian patients stated: "They are all so dangerous and violent patients that we are obliged to put them in the worst cells or cages to contain them; we have to treat them as wild and ferocious beasts" (Berthelier, 1979, p. 140).

This view of the Algerian as genetically inferior, dangerously impulsive, and incurably perverted became a widely accepted tenet in nineteenth-century French psychiatry and continued to be affirmed, reaffirmed, and embellished for nearly 80 years, from the conquest to the independence of Algeria. What is remarkable is how little the racism of French psychiatrists changed during these years and how the same claims, often made in the same words, have been reiterated with the aura of science and the zeal of a crusade. The most blatant expression of this racism is found in the influential remarks of Boigey (1908), a captain-physician, who wrote on the psychopathology of the Algerian and claimed that Muslims "never created any extraordinary things, never erected a capital, never built up any navy fleet, never studied deeply any science, never durably embellished [as did Europeans] any part of the world" (Berthelier, 1979, p. 42). He also characterized Muslims, and hence Algerians, as intellectually deficient, fanatic homosexuals, child molesters, masturbators and also unpredictable murderers, assassins, and terrorists. "In summary," Boigey concluded, "the mental state of the Muslim is a mixture of varied doses of craziness and tangle of delusions. . . . For those who go to the mosque, they are all violent, crazy persons who are in a state of somnambulence" (Berthelier, 1979, p. 143).

Boigey's falsified history and undisguised racism could well be dismissed as the ravings of a psychotic, bigoted man. One can easily surmise that his rabid racism was no doubt related to the fact that he was actively involved in the "pacification" of North Africa. But more significant and historic was the fact that Boigey's racism and crusade against Algerians and Muslims generally were to be reiterated for many years by French psychiatrists, most notably by A. Porot and his Algiers School of Psychiatry.

Writing about Algerian psychopathology in 1918, Porot characterized the Muslim as a liar, thief, and idiot, who was lazy, hysterical, and impulsively homicidal. In 1932, Porot elaborated on the murderous impulsivity of the Algerian native and identified the following causal factors: inherent mental debility, extreme credulity and suggestibility, perserveration, and weakness of affective as well as moral life. The Algerians were said to be infantile without the curiosity and questioning of European children, a horde driven by instinctual impulse toward murder and perversion. Porot gave scientific trappings to these claims when he asserted that "the native of North Africa, whose superior and cortical functions have hardly evolved, is a primitive creature whose life, primarily vegetative and instinctual, is mostly dominated by his diencephalon" (Berthelier, 1979, p. 147). Four years later, Porot reiterated the same conclusion in almost the same words: "The Algerian does not have a cerebral cortex or, to be more precise, he is under the dominance of the diencephalon as one would expect to find in any inferior vertebrae" (Berthelier, 1979, p. 147).

The gut racism of the ordinary European was not only given scientific respectability, but was also intensified by Porot. The scientific racism Porot institutionalized in Algeria was to remain dominant for nearly 40 years. Porot's students and contemporaries simply reasserted and embellished the notion that Algerians specifically and Muslims generally are inherently inferior. Any deviation from this ossified and sanctioned bigotry involved not a change in substance, but at best a touch of paternalism. Thus, for instance, Friboug-Blanc writing in 1927 about the North African middle class, concluded:

> These men, in one word, are big children. They have all the qualities and shortcomings but in extreme ways . . . Trustful, affectionate, generous, disinterested, full of touching spontaniety, unconcerned about past or future, they are also vain, liars, cowards, sometimes artful and thieves, but mostly emotional and suggestible to the highest degree. (Berthelier, 1979, p. 147)

Porot's stature and power grew as he developed in Algeria a medico-educational institute to justify the ruthless victimization of Algerians and, moreover, to institutionalize those to whom Europeans projected what they found unacceptable in themselves. What is remarkable is that Porot's assertions, years earlier, repeated many times subsequently, were again reiterated as late as 1960 in the work of Aubin, who was supervised by Porot himself:

> By lack of intellectual curiosity, credulity and suggestibility reached an extreme degree . . . the same fatalism aggravated the innate inappetence of the non-civilized for work, their abulia, their capriciousness and their impulsivity. (Berthelier, 1979, p. 148)

In short, as Berthelier summarized, the scientific racism French colonialism needed for justification was effectively "born around 1908 with Boigey's article, elaborated in 1918, completed in 1935, rediscovered in 1939 but also in 1947 in the thesis of Susini, in 1948 by Bardenat as well as in 1960 with Aubin's writings" (Berthelier, 1979, p. 148). The remarkable thing is that all this rubbish was written in the name of science and by otherwise rational, well-respected authorities. The characterization of the Algerian as an idiot, thief, liar, suggestible, and all such imaginable mud-slinging by Porot and his school was nowhere as influential as the theory that the North African was a born criminal. This latter claim was given a semblance of credibility when one looked at the high rate of homicide among colonized North Africans.

Fanon arrived in Algeria at a time when Porot's stature and influence were formidable, the scientific racisms he had elaborated were firmly established in psychiatric circles, and the school he founded was producing trainees who tended to echo his pronouncements. University students and particularly medical students had been taught these "scientific truths" about Algerians for well over 20 years when Fanon arrived in Algeria. The colonial administration and the settlers of course found Porot and his "scientific proofs" most congenial. Anyone who deviated from this beaten track or who questioned its tenets was thus suspect within the dominant psychiatric circle in Algeria and certainly insofar as the colonial administration was concerned. Fanon nonetheless stood his ground against this powerful psychiatric and colonial legacy.

We have seen the critique of Mannoni that Fanon had written long before he arrived in Algeria. Mannoni's racism and justification of colonialism were in fact more subtle and sophisticated than the rabid and crude racism elaborated by the Algiers School of Psychiatry. There seems little doubt that Fanon, now more experienced and committed than when he wrote *Black Skin, White Masks,* would sooner or later write a cogent critique of Porot and analyze the socio-historical function of his ideas. We have seen that the paper he wrote with Azoulay a year after he arrived in Algeria was an initial and somewhat mild critique of the French psychiatric establishment. If disappointment with Tosquellean reforms in Blida was not implied, the critique of Porot's emphasis on "motor and neuro-vegetative phenomena" was certainly unmistakable. Fanon came back to the same critique of the Algiers School of Psychiatry in subsequent works.

A paper Fanon presented before the First Congress of Negro Writers and Artists in Paris on September 1956 placed racist claims like those of Porot in a socio-historical perspective (Fanon, 1967b, pp. 31–44). He suggested that the racism of colonial intellectuals involved two stages as colonialism attained a measure of sophistication. First and in its crudest form, cultural anthropologists declared that the colonized had *no culture at all.* This was followed by the affirmation that all groups have culture, except there is a *hierarchy of cultures* whereby a given culture (of course European) is better or more advanced than another. Each of these claims correspond to the level of socioeconomic relations between the colonizers and the colonized. The psychiatrist's claim that there is no cortical integration in the colonized—more specifically Carother's depiction of the African as a "lobotomized European"— is simply an anatomical-physiological counterpart of the second stage. As the struggle for liberation intensifies, one begins to hear assertions of *cultural relativity*—an assertion that signals the emergence of reciprocal recognition between peoples.

A few years later in *The Wretched of the Earth,* Fanon returned to the same issue and directly focused on Porot and the Algiers School of Psychiatry. This latter critique is particularly important for at least two reasons: First, we see which of the numerous indictments of the Algerian Fanon chose to answer. Second and more importantly, we find a further elaboration of Fanon's explanation for the high rates of crime among the oppressed. Fanon's explanation of why there is high rate of intrafamilial violence and homicide among the oppressed is of particular significance in light of the data we presented in Chapter 8 and because other theories thus far offered in the literature are not as convincing.

Fanon began with a response to the common claim that the colonized is *lazy* or that his efficiency and work habits are deplorable. Violently protesting these stereotypes, some intellectuals among the colonized sought to show that blacks, Algerians, the colonized as a whole are indeed great and committed workers. Fanon argued that such a defensive reaction was unnecessary and in any case missed the point: "It is time to stop remonstrating and declaring that the nigger is a great worker and that the Arab is a first-rate at cleaning ground" (Fanon, 1968, p. 294). When the oppressed are lazy and inefficient at work, they are in fact sabotaging the oppressor's system and designs. At the biological level, these acts constitute a remarkable system of "autoprotection." Indeed under conditions of oppression, the exploited farmer or worker who is so intense at his work and refuses to rest is a *pathological* case. This laziness and inefficiency of the oppressed is a form of passive resistance—"a concrete manifestation of non-cooperation, or at least of minimum cooperation." They are indicative of a stage when the oppressed has not reached "maturity in political consciousness and decided to hurl back oppression." It is at this stage of passive resistance that the oppressed makes sure that any amount of labor and the "slightest gesture has to be torn out of him" (Berthelier, 1979, p. 148). One can see here how Fanon disagrees with Hegel on the meaning of work under conditions of oppression. For the former, the devoted labor the oppressor exploits is a sign of pathology; for the latter, it is the royal road to self-objectification and perhaps liberty.

According to Fanon, the oppressed also sabotage the prevailing laws, the payment of taxes, and the dominant morality. To obey the oppressor's laws, civil forms, and morality is to undermine oneself while to contravene them is a form of resistance, albeit an undeveloped one. Claims that the Algerian is a liar, a thief, a man never to be trusted were no doubt stereotypes the oppressor elaborated to fortify his Manichean psychology and to justify his violence. But also no honor, no dignity, no self-respect remained for the oppressed who actually are depersonalized individually and collectively. Honor, dignity, and self-respect are restored only in the framework of a national liberation struggle. Such a struggle mobilizes members for a common purpose, galvanizes them into a cohesive group, and integrates them into their own moral imperatives. Thus, as long as political consciousness is not attained and the oppressed remain in despair, it turns out that lies, thievery, and other forms of rudimentary resistance are rampant.

One aspect Fanon discussed in some detail concerns the claim of Porot and his school that the Algerian specifically and the North African generally is a born criminal who, prompted by diencephalic urges and brute instincts, kills frequently, savagely, and for no reason at all. These claims, Fanon emphasized, have been affirmed in various international conferences and told Algerian medical students for over 20 years. Fanon reviewed these claims not only to show their "poverty and absurdity," but also to clarify important theoretical and practical problems. That there had been a high rate of criminality among Algerians, Fanon conceded. But he showed that this high rate was historically and socially conditioned.

Fanon pointed out that, before the national liberation struggle, one noticed an appalling intensity and rate of crime among Algerians. Much of this crime occurred inside a "closed circle" of relatives, friends, neighbors, and acquaintances. It was an *intragroup* phenomenon; one Algerian victimized another Algerian. During this period of low socio-historical consciousness, the oppressed Algerian was unable to realize and face his "true protagonist." In fact because oppression permeated everyday living, the oppressed tended to serve each other as a "screen" and each hid from his neighbor their "national enemy." Each came to personify the oppressor, his image and reality; each served as a convenient, available target for his neighbor's pent-up anger and frustration. But the more often this occurred, the less the oppressed found the need to identify and face his "true protagonist."

Oppression frustrated all basic needs and made each Algerian the enemy of the other. Hunger brought intense competition for each loaf of bread. The obsession with food and the struggle to eke out a tenuous existence took priority over everything else, including morality and higher ideals. One looked not to history nor to the future but rather to the tyrannical demands of a famished belly, the heart-rending cries of a malnourished child, and the accusing glances of a wife with dried-up breasts. Under these circumstances, to steal is not a transgression of morality or of law, but rather a way of meeting basic needs and at the same time committing murder, at least symbolically.

The rage and violence engendered by such circumstances could of course not simply be wished away. One had to find some target for pent-up frustrations. Yet for the ordinary Algerian, the actual oppressors were practically and socially inaccessible. The police, laws, the threat of prison, and actual invasion by armies and tanks shielded the oppressors against the anger, frustration, and violence of the oppressed. Each Algerian therefore turned his rage at himself, his loved one, and his neighbor. Thus the exhausted and exploited laborer who came home discovered that the cries that denied him the rest he sorely needs were those of an Algerian child. The countless unemployed who competed for his job were Algerian. The grocer who refused him a loan and thereby kept poignant his hunger was an Algerian. The landlord who evicted him for failure to pay rent was an Algerian. The local judge and or the policeman who harrassed him to pay overdue taxes were Algerian. Everyday brought overwhelming feelings of rage, a profound self-hatred, an overpowering temptation to kill, and an Algerian who could serve as an immediate, convenient target. As each act was a murder, symbolically or actually, each murder was also a suicide.

Fanon asserted that the appalling rate of crime suddenly declined during the war of national liberation. As national consciousness and collective will for liberty took hold among the populace, as the true comrade and true enemy became differentiated, as the demarcation between a self that has every right to life in its own land and that of the other who ostensibly is alien and unjust was brought to the light of day, the smoldering rage became appropriately canalized and the rampant violence redirected to its logical target. In effect, the war of liberation "nationalized" all affective, cognitive, behavioral, and material resources. The oppressed who previously saw the enemy in himself and in his neighbor instead found a comrade in himself and in his neighbor. The oppressed who previously was an isolated individual obsessed with food and physical survival, which in any case eluded him, was later to show remarkable generosity and self-sacrifice.

In short, Fanon presented an incisive critique of Porot and the school he founded. He exposed the crude racism and justification of colonial oppression in their claims. Moreover, Fanon showed that the seemingly incomprehensible and reprehensible behaviors of the oppressed are meaningful and often justified reactions to oppression. The crimes of the oppressed cannot be explained by instinctual and diencephalic urges, but rather as *reactions* that, having lost purpose and an appropriate target, can be transformed into creative and liberative *actions*. The impact of Fanon's exposition on French psychiatric circles is suggested by Berthelier (1979, p. 153):

> What Porot was only able to keep secret, Fanon denounces, in the extreme, completely engaged in the struggle against colonial alienation. . . . It is for a good part, thanks to [Fanon], that a number among us have at this moment become aware that the Algerian and "bougnoule" were not necessarily synomymous, and that the colonized man was first an alienated man. . . . With Fanon will remain the merit of having clearly stated that the Western model was not an intangible dogma in psychiatry, that the pathology of the Algerian Moslem was inseparable from an analysis of the society which surrounds him and that an honest approach to mental illness emerges inevitably through the knowledge and understanding of the culture from which it emerges.

11

REVOLUTIONARY PSYCHIATRY OF FANON

I, the man of color, want only this: That the tool never possess the man. That the enslavement of man by man cease forever.
—Fanon, *Black Skin, White Masks*

It is never enough only to expose a human problem or even to offer conceptual paradigms exploring its structure and dynamics. The exposition and paradigms, to be authentic and valid, require *action* that puts the hypothetical against the actual and, above all, transforms what *is* to what *ought to be.* To commit oneself to the practice of healing and rehabilitating tormented psyches is no doubt a form of action—one that is always pregnant with heuristic and social import. Yet as we have already suggested, the action on behalf of the patient often turns out to be against the interest and well-being of the patient.

Questions that often present themselves to therapists working in situations of oppression can be posed thus: Is therapy really *for* this patient? If so, what should the therapist do with respect to the social forces that clearly undermine the well-being of his or her patient? And if one considers mental disorders also as a "pathology of liberty," is it possible to restore the well-being of the patient without at the same time endeavoring to restore his liberty?

This chapter looks at the contributions of Fanon toward a psychiatry of social and psychological liberation. It sketches the evolution of his clinical theory and practice to underscore the fact that a genuine endeavor to restore the health of the oppressed assumes a commitment to restore their liberty. As we have seen, the famous experiment at Blida forced Fanon to rethink clinical paradigms and techniques. This chapter highlights Fanon's attempt to delve into the experience of an oppressed people with a culture different from the one he had known. His own experience of oppression proved a critical bridge for comprehending "the truth" of others. Fanon's venture into ethnopsychiatry gradually led to an active challenge not only of establishment psychiatry, but also of the established social order. The chapter therefore shows Fanon's endeavor that the tool—in this case, psychiatry—never possess the man and that, with a bold application of it, enslavement cease wherever he found it.

EXPLORATION INTO ETHNOPSYCHIATRY

The Algiers School of Psychiatry represented one early predecessor of the subspecialty now called "ethnopsychiatry" or, more generally, "cross-cultural psychology." The views that the Algiers School propagated, and the historic function they served, were remarkably similar to those of behavioral scientists in other African colonies. Each colonial power, though relying primarily on military might, also had its own behavioral scientists whose task it was to explain and interpret the psyches and social behaviors of the colonized. All too frequently, however, the explanations and interpretations offered were substantively unoriginal, since these foreign scholars had simply given scientific trappings to the prevailing bigotry of Europeans.

Dr. Porto was thus the French counterpart of Dr. Carothers who, after 15 years of service to the British Empire, authoritatively asserted that the African was a "lobotomized Western European." Certainly, significant changes in psychological conceptions of the African have occurred since the 1960s—a fact illustrated by the changing conception of depression among Africans (Prince, 1967). A careful review of the literature in fact shows that changes in psychological conceptions correlate with changes in the sociopolitical domain. Hence the undisguised racism of the colonial era gave way to the subtle ethnocentism of the neo-colonial present (Bulhan, 1981a).

Fanon was of the generation that effectively called colonialism into question and effected its demise in Africa. Yet to have been one of the few black psychiatrists at the time—and a sociopolitically committed one at that—was no doubt a major challenge itself. There were countless misconceptions to be corrected, an undisguised racism to be combated, and alternatives to be thought out. Fanon traversed this route pretty much alone as a black psychiatrist, even though he worked in collaboration with Europeans who shared his outlook if not his commitment.

Writing and professional symposia offered a medium in which Fanon challenged distorted conceptions and presented some alternative formulations. Fanon wrote on topics ranging from the strictly biomedical to the sociopolitical. In addition to the work he collaborated on with Azoulay, four of his untranslated articles can be clearly grouped under ethnopsychiatry. Two of them, which we will discuss, illustrate his ethnopsychiatric thinking between 1954, when the historic experiment was reported, and 1956, when Fanon resigned from his job as *chef de service* at Blida to join the Algerian Freedom fighters.

In September 1955, a year after the famous experiment in therapy, Fanon and Dr. Lacaton presented to a congress of psychiatrists and neurologists their "Confession in North Africa." The presentation, though brief, is crucial for at least three reasons. First, we glean from it Fanon's evolving interest in ethnopsychiatry. Second, we again find his critique of establishment psychiatry, particularly the Algiers School. Third, it intimates a critique of domination and of the prevailing social order. Themes subtly suggested here later become elaborated clearly and passionately.

On the surface, the article cross-culturally explores the psychological and social meaning of confession for criminal acts. At a more fundamental level, it exposes some of the human problematics that arise when a situation of oppression is imposed on a community. For a situation of oppression pits one group against another and constantly tests the allegiance of each member to his group. It leads to failure of communication, mutual incomprehension, and ontological insularity between members belonging to the two coexisting, but opposing cultures. The dominant group imposes its ethico-legal precepts as it negates the validity and integrity of all that the oppressed uphold.

The oppressed on their part adopt a position of passive resistance, an autoprotective shield, which renders impossible any comprehension of their experience from the cultural perspective of the oppressor. The ontological insularity and mutual incomprehension come to play in court proceedings in which a member of the oppressed has allegedly committed a crime, which must be judged. Fanon and Lacaton examined the problems that arose when a psychiatrist was requested to serve as an expert witness for court proceedings in North Africa.

Ordinarily, the authors argued, confession for wrongdoing has both existential and social dimensions, a private as well as a public import. Existentially, confession implies a willingness to assume personal responsibility and, in so assuming, to affirm the meaning of one's being revealed through the act. Not to assume such responsibility for one's action or to falsely deny it is to experience a fundamental alienation of one's being, at least at that moment. Socially, confession indicates that an "auto-condemnation" has been provoked in the conscience, that the values and ethical precepts of the community, if not already internalized, are now reinstalled in the actor.

Thus the intent if not the consequence of the confession becomes for the actor "the ransom for his re-insertion into the group." Having confessed, the actor is reinstated as a member either then and there or after some sanction has been imposed and subjectively accepted. A realignment of existential and social imperatives thereby occurs and the collective once again opens the way for his membership in the group, with the rights and responsibilities this implies. But all of this of course assumes a "reciprocal recognition of the group by the individual and of the individual by the group."

Under these circumstances, the task of the psychiatrist requested to evaluate the mental condition under which the criminal act was committed is relatively straightforward. He examines the ideas, values, and motivations that prompted and attended the criminal act. His obligation is to delve deeply into the psychology of the actor, "find the truth of the act which will be the foundation of the truth of the actor," and to offer a meaningful interpretation to the court as well as to the community it represents. Since the judge, the actor, and the psychiatrist share the same ethico-legal and cultural universe, the judicial proceeding, the psychiatrist's interpretation, the rendering of justice, the subjective acceptance of the sanction by the guilty one, and the potential reinsertion of the norm-violater into the group is relatively comprehensible. But this is not so in a situation of oppression in which a member of the oppressed is being tried and evaluated in a colonial court.

Fanon and Lacaton underscored the complexity of confession in North Africa and the problem of rendering justice in colonial courts. A "native" who allegedly committed a grave crime like murder is brought to court along with an "eloquent dossier" prepared by the police. The dossier indicates that the accused has already confessed, having in addition revealed where the arms were hidden. It may also show that several witnesses swore that they have seen him perform the act. The confession and the witnesses having confirmed the guilt of the person, the judge subsequently requests a psychiatric evaluation to determine if such a grave crime had been committed when the accused was psychotic. The psychiatrist who takes his obligations seriously then proceeds to examine the "truth of the act," its motivation and meaning, in order to arrive at the "truth of the actor," his existential and social being. He relies on the diagnostic value of the confession and conducts a psychiatric interview, hoping to be able to offer appropriate explanation and measures to the court. Unfortunately, however, he finds this to be extremely difficult in cases involving North Africans.

To begin with, it often happens that the accused absolutely denies that he committed the act or that he ever confessed. If indeed he confessed to the police, he asserts that this was done under torture. Not infrequently, even the witnesses retract their declarations. What is more, the medico-legal expert finds that the accused, vehemently asserting his innocence, is actually a lucid and coherent person. The psychiatrist thus loses not only the diagnostic value of the confession, now reduced to a police frame-up, but finds himself in the presence of one without signs of pathology. All that is left for him are the eloquent dossier and the criminal act without an actor. Further rendering "criminological comprehension" impossible in the North African is the fact that the accused states his innocence but does little to prove his innocence actively. The accused takes an attitude of resignation, saying he accepts any judgment of the court in the name of Allah.

Typically, the European psychiatrist faced with this type of situation fell back to such common stereotypes of the North African as a lazy, no-good liar. Indeed, as we have seen, the Algiers School of Psychiatry had provided him ample "scientific proofs" that the North African is degenerate, untrustworthy, and phylogenetically defective. But Fanon and Lacaton assert that such a simplification only obstructs comprehension, detracts from a search of the "truth," and makes any rendering of justice defective. What is more (Fanon & Lacaton, 1955, p. 659),

> To affirm that the race is suffering from a propensity to lie or to voluntarily dissimulate the truth, or that the population is incapable of discerning the truth from the false, or even that it does not integrate certain givens of experience, particularly by virtue of phylogenetic defect, this is to explain away the problem without really resolving it.

To grasp the "truth" of the native and therefore to comprehend his ontological system require a fundamental shift in perspective. One must search for the condition under which confession is imbued with both existential and social validity, sanctions subjectively acceptable to the accused are imposed, and reinsertion into the group is possible. But how can confession have meaning when we have it only in a police dossier and the accused denies that he confessed to or committed the crime? Even if confession is obtained without torture, does it have any value in the absence of reciprocal recognition of the group by the individual and of the individual by the group? Can the verdict be just and rehabilitative if all we have is an act without an actor, an accused who is unwilling to appropriate the act and unwilling to accept the condemnation? And how could reinsertion of the individual into the group be possible when there was no insertion in the first place?

Obviously, these questions suggest much that is amiss in the system of justice and human communication in a situation of oppression. Fanon and Lacaton trace the problem to the coexistence of two opposed and mutually exclusive groups—one dominant, the other dominated. Each group binds its members with its own social contract and ethical universe. Each inculcates a distinct ontological system in its members and instills allegiance only to its own ethical precepts. The North African before a judge thus finds that his social contract with, and allegiance to, his group are challenged, that he is being tried not only for an *act*, but also for his very *being*. Little wonder then that he resists, so unshakably if passively, and subverts the European judicial process—confessing then denying, bearing witness then retracting, declaring his innocence then failing to prove it.

In effect, an accused who confesses his crime to the judge is at once disapproving his act and legitimizing the "eruption of the public into the private." By failing to appropriate the act, by denying and retracting, the North African is essentially refusing an eruption of an alien public into his private world. He may perforce submit to such sanctions as a jail term but this should not be confused with his being won over to believe in the legitimacy of the judge, his judgment, and the underlying alien social contract.

The article is actually less direct in its argument than our interpretation of it. Why Fanon and Lacaton chose to be less direct is indeed intriguing. Was it because a clear expression of their views entailed political risks at the time? Was it because of an academic and professional ambience that tended to dampen discussion of highly controversial and seemingly esoteric topics? Or was it because a clear political stand and an unambiguous commitment to the cause of justice had not yet crystallized in the authors? Our guess is that the choice of a subtle and less direct approach was tactical in view of the fact that at the time a clear exposition would entail political and professional risks.

In fact, both Fanon and Lacaton were by then considered the most radical psychiatrists at Blida-Joinville Hospital. Both had been alienated from their European colleagues at Blida for their ideas and practice, Fanon more than Lacaton. Both also ran a constant risk of police reprisal in the increasingly charged and dangerous atmosphere that then prevailed in Algeria. We will see later that Lacaton fell victim to police torture and humiliating physical abuse for his reformist outlook and that Fanon constantly ran the risk of a similar reprisal.

In 1956, Fanon in collaboration with Dr. Sanchez, a resident at Blida, wrote on the attitude of North African Muslims toward madness. The discussion here was less political and therefore less perilous than the one on confession. It nonetheless dealt with some misconceptions and aimed to restore respect to the North African approach to madness—an approach Europeans commonly considered primitive and senseless. In particular, Fanon and Sanchez refuted the view that North Africans look upon madness with absolute veneration and meaningless worship. Seeking to shed some light from the "inside" as psychiatrists in Blida, they first pointed out that establishments for treating the mad had been developed in the Muslim world before the Middle Ages, long before such institutions were introduced in Europe. This fact itself should suggest that a hasty condemnation of the North African attitude to madness is unwarranted and that perhaps something can be gained by a study of this attitude.

Fanon and Sanchez compared the attitude of Europeans toward madness to that of North Africans. They found differences in the human environment in which the mad find themselves in the two cultures, the marked difference of social stigma attached to madness, and the consequences these differences have to the psychology of the self in the afflicted. Implicit in the comparison was not only the desire to correct European misconceptions, but also the desire to find an appropriate psychiatric outlook relevant to the cultural and historical realities of the North African. We will see that this desire to be psychiatrically relevant, retaining the useful aspects in the indigenous society and introducing innovations found practical elsewhere, is a theme that remained with Fanon in subsequent years.

In comparing the two attitudes to madness, Fanon and Sanchez pointed out that Westerners believe that madness is a *disease* that alienates the victim from others and from himself. Yet Westerners tend to forget this in their interactions with the patient. They hold him responsible for his illness and actions. They feel a moral obligation to provide for his needs, but they also resent their "servitude." Viewing him as a "social parasite" who readily exploits his illness, Westerners counter his aggression with a veiled and sometimes open retaliation. His actions offend them as if he willfully intended malice and harm. Even the medical personnel and the relatives of the patient take offense and retaliate. Thus, for instance,

> an attendant feeling himself wounded by the arrogance of a megalomaniac might remain angry from it until the occasion arises wherein he could deprive the patient a snack or a walk. Then there is the mother who feels she was poorly welcomed by her son whom she has come to see in the hospital to visit and consequently leaves very bitter. (Fanon & Sanchez, 1956, p. 25)

All this is in striking contrast to the attitude of the North African toward persons afflicted with madness. Here the person is not held responsible for his illness. He is treated as an innocent victim of spirits (*genies*) over which he has no control. Since the affliction is an accidental occurrence, it could happen to anyone. If the afflicted acts aggressively, responsibility is imputed to spiritual forces that must collectively be appeased and confronted. But punishment, distrust, or exclusion of the afflicted rarely occurs. There is also no social stigma attached to madness and to those afflicted with it. The victim and relatives talk about the affliction openly and without embarrassment. One feels no need to conceal a condition for which he is not responsible and,

moreover, spirits are not passed on genetically in any case. This social acceptance of the afflicted, the explanation of madness in terms of external causation, and the collective efforts to seek resolution—all these enhance the possibility of the patient's recovery and his re-integration into the society.

In particular, the *affliction* is not confused with the *person*, since madness
is considered to affect "only the appearance never penetrating the underlying
self." The authors do not endorse all the indigenous approaches to madness.
They view therapeutic techniques as rudimentary, but they strongly recom-
mend the humanistic and holistic attitude of the North African to madness
(Fanon & Sanchez, 1956, p. 26):

> Resting solidly on cultural bases, the system is of great human value which does
> not confine itself only to the efficacy of the North African therapy. This natural
> method of assistance is imprinted with a profoundly holistic thought which keeps
> intact the image of the normal man, in spite of the existence of affliction. . . . [The
> North African] attitude is guided by a care of and respect to the person. It is not
> madness that creates the respect, the patience, the indulgence; it is rather the man
> affected by madness, attacked by spirits; it is man as such.

The attempt to place madness in its socio-historical and cultural perspective and to restore integrity to the indigenous conception was to Fanon analogous to the larger project of instituting political and social justice. The colonialism of Europe did not confine itself to economics or politics; it also
permeated psychiatric concepts and practices. Fanon therefore endeavored to
pioneer a psychiatry of liberation, at least within Blida-Joinville Hospital and
among his professional colleagues. His writings on ethnopsychiatry continued
not only to inform Westerners, but also to search for a psychiatry appropriate
to the needs and realities of his North African patients.

Fanon did not of course pioneer ethnopsychiatry. Others before him, including Emile Kraepelin, had long written on cross-cultural psychopathology.
Writings on the topic accumulated over the years and cross-cultural psychology is today a popular and respected subject. But what differentiates Fanon's
approach is this: His was a *radical* ethnopsychiatry that reached for the *roots*
of the subject.

Most of those who write on ethnopsychiatry tend to study remote and
non-Western societies with the aim of informing Westerners or of settling
academic debates in their societies. They gather endless data, exploit the cooperation of their "subjects" abroad, and take a hasty retreat with stories of their
exploits to their societies. Nothing comes back to the subjects and societies
they studied—not even a report of their findings. In contrast, Fanon's ethnopsychiatry was rooted in the very people he studied. Not only did he endeavor
to understand their world and serve their clinical needs, he also fully identified
with those he wrote about—learning their language, respecting their person as
well as their culture, and risking his life to help restore their human dignity.

PSYCHIATRY FOR SOCIAL LIBERATION

The year 1954 was not only a turning point for the direction Fanon's
psychiatric work was to take. It was also a historic watershed in Algerian

history. In that year, the Algerian struggle for liberty took a decisive turn as the various Algerian movements, previously divided and in disarray, forged the foundation for a united and frontal attack against colonialism. The ensuing war of liberation was to last nearly eight long and bloody years until 1962, when Algeria became an independent nation. The hemorrhage and psychic dislocation caused by the war was to be so massive that an ordinary psychiatric practice on isolated private problems became untenable if not dishonest.

Fanon's critical inquiry into psychiatric theory and practice was at first confined to an institutional context and professional circles. Reforms at Blida-Joinville Hospital and presentations at psychiatric conferences remained the foci of his endeavors. But as social unrest heightened among the Algerian populace and colonial administrators reacted with brutal repression, Blida-Joinville Hospital became less and less sheltered from the turmoil and reprisals that increasingly came to characterize life in Algeria. The psychiatric work at Blida and the critique of establishment psychiatry gradually led Fanon to conclusions similar to those others had arrived at by different means. In time, Fanon's critical inquiry into psychiatry merged with the highest and most practical critique of domination—namely, the popular struggle for liberation. The merger was gradual and perilous, but momentous when it was complete.

The Algerian struggle against colonialism did not of course begin in 1954. As exemplified by the early and popular uprising of Abdel Kader, resistance to colonial domination started in the 1830s when the French colonized Algeria. Abdel Kader's rebellion and the Kabylie insurrection of 1871 were defeated with superior arms, a better military organization, and the defections of tribal chiefs. The so-called "pacification of natives" subsequently opened the way for installing *colons*, European settlers, into Algerian soil.

The quest for political and social rights was thereafter met with brutal repression, on the one hand, and promises of reforms, on the other. This stick-and-carrot policy remained effective so long as a significant portion of the Algerian elite, led by the vascillating Ferhat Abbas, was convinced that assimilation into French society and the rights this implied were attainable. The vast majority of the Algerian population nonetheless clung to their Islamic tradition and Afro-Arab culture. The riots and rebellions that occurred before 1954 were sporadic and without lasting consequence. For decades, the Algerian populace tended to mark time and offered a passive but impermeable resistance with an underlying psychology that escaped European authorities.

The obstinacy of French colonialism in Algeria cannot be adequately realized without appreciating the special status Algeria held in the French imperial system. Algeria was a prized French colony not only for economic and strategic reasons, but also because there was a large and powerful settler community in that colony. Of all the colonies, Algeria in particular was considered an integral part of France. The expropriation of land and labor in Algeria, among the most intense of all the French colonies, began soon after conquest. Thus in 1840, Marshal Bugeaud, the conqueror of Algeria, advised the Chamber of Deputies: "Wherever good water and fertile land are found, settlers must be installed without questioning whose land it may be" (Davidson, 1978, p. 119).

Marshall Bugeaud's advice was taken and countless Algerians were displaced from their land or forced into temporary tenancy. By 1890, about 4 million acres of the best land fell into European ownership. European settlements gradually intensified and, by 1940, no less than 6 million acres, about one-third of the profitably cultivable land, came to be owned by about 2% of the whole population, mainly European settlers. The settlers were not all of French stock; an overwhelming majority of them were Southern Europeans of different nationalities. Algeria became a new frontier where land was grabbed without question and native labor exploited with impunity.

Much of the land expropriated was used for vineyards to make Algeria an "export enclave" of wine within the French imperial system. The irony was that most Algerians, professing the Muslim faith, did not drink wine and that the huge vineyards used land sorely needed for food production. It is estimated that, for instance, by the middle 1950s "cereal production stood at the same level as in the 1880s, although the population had tripled" (Davidson, 1978, p. 119). Thus hunger and disease increased among Algerians as the wealth and well-being of settlers soared. A Manichean psychology founded in this economics of inequity also became well entrenched. The system of governance too was devised to give European settlers absolute power. Establishment psychiatry generally and the Algiers School of Psychiatry particularly gave scientific trappings to the bigotry of settlers and justified the *status quo* of oppression.

The Algerian elite was for decades manipulated and kept under control with promises of reform and a policy of assimilation. Successive administrations in the colony espoused the policy of assimilation with the effect of dividing and hence ruling Algerians. But French administrators may not have been adverse to the assimilation of a small Algerian elite in *theory*, although such a notion itself was deeply abhorrent to European settlers. These settlers were violently opposed to any and all political concessions even to the moderate native elite, the so-called "évolués," who actually saw their destiny in assimilation into French culture. This deracinated and alienated petit bourgeoisie gradually realized that their colonial status was never temporary and that their hope for reform through peaceful means was futile. Any remaining illusions were dashed by such savage assaults as the Setif massacre of 1945, when riots, reprisals, and counter-reprisals left thousands dead and many more wounded.

In 1954 various Algerian movements, which previously had differed in ideology, tactics, and organization, began to unite around the *Comité Revolutionnaire pour l'Unité et l'Action* (CRUA). The CRUA grew out of and replaced the paramilitary and clandestine *Organisation Speciale* (OS) formed two years after the Setif massacre. The name was soon changed to the *Front de Liberation Nationale* (FLN). Gradually those who for decades sought assimilation into French society and the traditional nationalists joined forces in the FLN.

The Algerian War of Independence was dramatically inaugurated at dawn of All Saints Day, 1 November 1954, when the FLN staged a well-coordinated assault against French military installations, police headquarters, communication facilities, and public utilities throughout Algeria. The FLN and military wing subsequently initiated guerrilla warfare in rural as well as urban areas, focusing on key government facilities, settler farms, and collaborators with the colonial regime. Following each engagement, the guerrillas mixed with the population.

The colonial authorities and settlers responded with ruthless and increasingly indiscriminate retaliation. They held collectively responsible all villages and neighborhoods suspected of harboring FLN guerrillas. The settler vigilante groups in particular carried out wanton, widespread killings of Muslim Algerians in what they called "rat-hunts." Villages were bombed; many of their residents were resettled in poor and crowded areas where they could be easily monitored. Electrified barbed-wire fences were installed along parts of the border and in some urban areas to stem the mobility and growing strength of the FLN.

The repressed and festering violence of colonial Algeria suddenly erupted. By 1956, France had deployed well over 400,000 soldiers to Algeria, along with sophisticated air and naval forces. One interesting irony here is that the French General, Raoul Salan, who had personally decorated Fanon for heroic action during World War II, was assigned to command French forces in Algeria at a time when Fanon was already an active FLN member.

Nearly eight years of war brought an immense loss of lives. Estimates are that over 1 million Algerians and about 20,000 Europeans were killed. The ruthless way the war was conducted, the violence and counterviolence, and this immense human loss no doubt influenced Fanon's theory of violence. In reading about the struggle against colonialism in Algeria, one cannot help but be impressed by the stubborn refusal of the oppressors to acknowledge the humanity of the other, thereby engendering untold violence.

Vested interests and formed habits, always difficult to change, are even more difficult to modify in a situation of oppression. The last to make changes and amends are oppressors. They tend to learn little from history unless shocked into a rude awakening. It was in fact in 1954 that French colonialism suffered a humiliating defeat at Dien Bien Phu in Indochina. Yet it took nearly eight more years in Algeria and thousands of casualties before France came to acknowledge the Algerian people's right to self-determination. In any case, on July 3, 1962, after 132 years of French colonial rule, Algeria was declared an independent country.

Fanon's open support of the Algerian war of independence began in 1956 when he resigned his job as *chef de service* at Blida-Joinville Hospital. The decision to resign was both clinically and politically influenced. The reevaluation of Eurocentric psychiatry outlined in the 1954 article written in collaboration with Azoulay was followed by other works that, in retrospect, suggest that some form of confrontation with the colonial social order was in the making well before the resignation. For one thing, these works showed a growing interest in radical ethnopsychiatry—an interest itself of significant clinical and political import.

At the same time, the growing social ferment in Algeria and the brutal reprisals taken by the colonial administrators increasingly intruded into Fanon's clinical practice within Blida-Joinville Hospital. The social unrest and ruthless reprisals also underscored the fact that clinical and political problems could no longer be isolated and that a clinician's professional duties also entailed social responsibility. Indeed, periods of relative peace and stability tend to obscure this intimate relation between clinical and political concerns as between professional and social responsibility. But the Algeria of the 1950s made the connection starkly clear, particularly to a person like Fanon who asked himself if, by acting or failing to act, he contributed to the improvement or impoverishment of the human reality.

Fanon's radical outlook and his empathy toward Algerians preceded his arrival as *chef de service* in Algeria. But the practice at Blida and life in Algeria further radicalized his outlook and transformed his empathy into an unambiguous identification with the Algerians. How Fanon first made contact with the FLN and what services he provided it are documented by Geismar (1971). Fanon's initial work with the FLN involved a clandestine medical service for Algerian freedom fighters. Some of the captured freedom fighters were brought to Blida-Joinville Hospital after devastating torture by French authorities, as shown in the chapter, "Colonial Wars and Mental Disorders," in *The Wretched of the Earth* (1968). Others suffered war neuroses and came for treatment. But Fanon and the Algerian male nurses kept secret the political affiliations of these patients and the causes of their disorders.

Fanon's formal contact with the FLN was arranged by Pierre Chaulet, the son of a European settler who was an active collaborator with the FLN. The two men met in 1955 at Blida. Chaulet, himself a physician, was on a mission to establish a local unit of a supposedly charitable organization that was actually raising funds for FLN fighters and their families. Chaulet confided in Fanon his role in the work of the FLN and soon found in him a committed comrade. Fanon secretly committed himself to the struggle for national liberation while still the *chef de service* at Blida.

His life and work during this period reveal remarkable courage and personal stamina. He provided clandestine service to wounded FLN fighters at his home while regularly performing his "normal" duties at Blida, here also treating other freedom fighters, broken in torture or yet unapprehended. Some of the Algerian male nurses who worked with Fanon were themselves FLN members or sympathizers. It is said that Si Saddik, a top FLN administrator, was secretely treated by Fanon and hidden in his home until he recovered from severe nervous exhaustion. Simone de Beauvoir who, along with Sartre, had developed a personal friendship with Fanon reported some of his clandestine work with the freedom fighters for a year while still a *chef de service* at Blida. According to de Beauvoir (1965, p. 593), not only did he harbor guerrillas in his home or hospital, provide them sorely needed medicine, and teach them how to treat their wounded, but also:

> Eight assassination attempts out of ten were failing because the "terrorists," completely terrorized, were either getting discovered straight off or else bungling the

actual attack. "This just can't go on." They would have to train the *Fidayines*. With the consent of the leaders, he took the job on; he taught them to control their reactions when they were setting a bomb or throwing a grenade; and also what psychological and physical attitudes would enable them to resist torture. He would then leave these lessons to attend to a French police commissioner suffering from nervous exhaustion brought on by too many "interrogations."

As the intensity of the war increased, the rat-hunt for collaborators and sympathizers intruded into the hospital. A number of the staff at Blida were arrested, and some of them were tortured, while others disappeared forever. For instance, Dr. Lacaton, who worked for reform in the hospital and wrote with Fanon the article on confession, was arrested on suspicion of collaborating with the liberation movement. The "standard interrogation" of him led nowhere and therefore pushes and punches followed. These too failed to produce a self-incriminating confession or revelation of who else collaborated with the FLN, and the security police then subjected Dr. Lacaton to such "standard torture" as submersion in a bathtub, enemas of soapy water, and electrical shock to the genitals.

The authorities later decided that Dr. Lacaton was neither directly involved with the national liberation movement as suspected nor actively opposed to it as expected of a patriotic Frenchman. He was released, but in a most humiliating manner reserved for "ambiguous personalities." Half-conscious, Dr. Lacaton was taken to the farm of a European settler and dumped in a pigsty. This placed him in danger of being attacked by pigs and trampled on, itself a most obscene form of torture and execution. Fortunately, the doctor regained consciousness and escaped before the pigs could harm him. After a convalescence, Dr. Lacaton packed up and departed for France (Geismar, 1971, p. 77).

Fanon too constantly ran similar risks or worse. Yet he escaped arrest primarily because he was a "foreigner," neither an Algerian nor a European, and the authorities did not want to have word of their brutal torture leaked to the international community. This leniency was however only relative and quite circumscribed. Still, Fanon's commitment to the welfare of his patients superceded all other considerations. The length to which Fanon took his commitment is shown not only by his clandestine activities while at Blida but also by his bold complaints to authorities. For instance (Geismar, 1971, p. 79):

> There was an air force base close to the hospital. . . . Sometimes, throughout the night, jet bombers would come in and out of the base making a deafening roar over the wards. Fanon, along with the other doctors, knew that the planes were disturbing the patients' sleep and retarding their recovery; but only Fanon dared to complain . . . to the Chief of Staff of the air force in Algeria then to the Resident Minister's office.

Fanon's request to change the pattern of air flights was complied with for nearly a year. He also complained about the frequent and unexpected intrusion of authorities on the hospital grounds, arresting patients and staff alike.

> In 1955, because of Fanon, police were no longer permitted to carry loaded guns when they entered the hospital grounds. If possible they were to complete their business in the guardhouse at the gate of the institution. (Geismar, 1971, p. 80)

These small but significant changes could not of course forestall the tragic and devastating ravages of the war. There continued the brutal violence, the psychiatric casualties of both the freedom fighters and their torturers, both of whom Fanon treated, and the engulfing madness of a society at war. The moment fast approached for a decisive and unambiguous stand. Thus in 1956, Fanon resigned from his post as *chef de service* in Blida-Joinville Hospital. His letter of resignation, showing the integrity and courage of the man, was both a political act and a personal reaffirmation. In response, the Resident Minister ordered Fanon's departure from Algeria in 48 hours, or he would face imprisonment.

Following a short stay in France, Fanon moved to the FLN headquarters in Tunis. He served there as an editor and commentator for its most crucial periodical, *El Moudjahid*, and soon established himself as a key spokesman of the Algerian Revolution. He also served as an ambassador of the FLN, enlisting political and material support from Sub-Sahara Africa. Still, claims to the contrary, Fanon did not abandon psychiatry for politics. His clinical practice continued in Tunis, initially in the Psychiatric Hospital at Manouba and later in the Charles Nicolle Hospital. So did his work with FLN health centers and his professional writing on psychiatry.

At Manouba, Fanon attempted to introduce the reforms he brought to Blida. But conditions there were quite different from those at Blida. For one thing, he ran into conflict with the Tunisian director who was said to have been very touchy about bureaucratic hierarchy and formalities, neither of which was to Fanon's liking. His attempts to introduce reforms were resisted by the director, first on the grounds of limited budget. The conflict between the two men intensified as Fanon persisted in his reforms. When Fanon won the endorsement of the Tunisian Minister of Health, the director accused Fanon of being a Zionist and a spy of Israel, using as evidence his earlier writings against anti-Semitism and his association with Jewish doctors. The accusations however failed to discredit Fanon even in the charged climate of war and suspicion.

In fact, Fanon's revolutionary and professional credentials were by then well established within the FLN and increasingly recognized both in Tunis and abroad. Local and foreign interns sought to work with him. Once again, his closest professional allies were interns and indigenous nurses. In spite of the resistance to his reforms, Fanon was able to remove from his pavilion locked doors, straitjackets, and closed wards. He also introduced some aspects of milieu therapy. As in Blida, he fully committed himself to patient care and expected the same from his colleagues. Failure to meet these expectations brought harsh rebuke. His use of his own rare commitment and stamina as benchmarks for evaluating others often caused gnawing resentment. His belligerence and his readiness to take offense also made him a difficult person to work with, particularly when competence or commitment was in question. And once again doctors at Manouba, disagreeing with Fanon's views or joining the director's camp, called him "The Nigger" behind his back (Geismar, 1971, p. 138).

Psychiatry for Psychological Liberation

Fanon's active commitment to social liberation also entailed a commitment to psychological liberation. In spite of claims to the contrary, he never abandoned psychiatry for politics, nor did he neglect the relations between individual travails and the prevailing social order. It was indeed his ability to connect psychiatry to politics or private troubles to social problems and, having made the connection conceptually, to boldly *act* that made him a pioneer of radical psychiatry. It was certainly an important step to place the psychiatric institution at Blida and its demoralized patients within the larger colonial milieu. But more decisive was the conclusion that, if therapy aims at restoring integrity of mind and body, then the colonial order undermined that integrity in the first place and did not permit its restoration in the second place.

As he joined in the struggle for a social revolution that it was hoped would give birth to the "new man" and "new society," there still remained the immediate and serious predicament of those incarcerated within the walls of psychiatric institutions and by social exclusion. His work in the psychiatric hospital at Manouba and in the FLN Health Centers—where the anguish of dislocated Algerian refugees was particularly grave—further emphasized the fact that the project for psychological liberation had hardly begun. More and more, the centrality and urgency of liberty for psychiatric patients had become as obvious as it was for the colonized. And if madness is a pathology of liberty, as it was later defined, then the therapeutic task was primarily one of restoring liberty. Now how did Fanon endeavor to restore liberty for psychiatric patients? And what theoretical formulations guided this endeavor?

After his resignation from Blida-Joinville Hospital in 1956 to his death in 1961, Fanon wrote five psychiatric articles in addition to numerous sociopolitical works, most notably *A Dying Colonialism* (1967c) and *The Wretched of the Earth* (1968). The psychiatric articles, written alone or in collaboration with others, remain untranslated and relatively inaccessible. The neglect of these articles is unfortunate because some of them reveal a further and important evolution of Fanon's psychiatry. These works reveal his fundamental disillusionment with psychiatric hospitalization, his significant departure from Tosquellean approaches, his clear reformulation of madness as the pathology of liberty, and his firm conviction that therapy should, above all, restore freedom to patients. After several years of intensive application of the institutional therapy inspired by Tosquelles, Fanon concluded that therapy is most meaningful and effective within the dialectic of concrete, living society.

The article on agitation was written while Fanon was in Blida, although it was published on the very month he received the letter of expulsion and was forced to leave Algeria (Fanon & Asselah, 1957). This article is significant not only because it was written at a critical point in Fanon's psychiatric and political career, but also because, for the first time, we find in it an open critique of Tosquelles and of psychiatric hospitalization. Both critiques were elaborated in the subsequent articles on day hospitalization.[1]

---

[1]Earlier writers, including Gendzier (1973), have strangely ignored Fanon's critique of Tosquelles.

The article on agitation began with a distinction Tosquelles made between agitation of the "expressive type" and agitation of the "percepto-reactive type." Such a distinction implies generally the old *nature* versus *nurture* duality common in psychological conceptions and specifically the *instinct* versus *environment* opposition found in psychoanalytic thought. Fanon in any case argued that Tosquelles' distinction, although heuristically interesting, contained serious doctrinaire problems. In essence, he argued that the distinction was too simplistic, mechanistic, and clinically, not helpful.

In Fanon's view, the notion that one type of agitation is reactive and another nonreactive neglects the fact that agitation, like most other forms of psychopathology, emerges out of reciprocal relations, that it is provoked and maintained in human interaction, and that the sadomasochistic character of institutionalization exacerbates rather than ameliorates agitation. Fanon argued that, except in patients with severe organic defect, agitation is expressive *and* reactive. Since it emerges in reciprocal relations, agitation cannot be understood and effectively treated apart from the human context that initiates, maintains, and exploits it.

Instead of accepting Tosquelles' distinctions, Fanon argued that it is clinically more useful to distinguish agitation that is predominantly motor from predominantly verbal and verbo-motor agitations. In its pure state, according to Fanon, the motor type is most commonly observed among the severely retarded and the senile. Agitation that is predominantly verbal seems to be less neurologically based and more comprehensible, except in the stereotypic, archaic, and incoherent soliloquy of the organically defective. The verbo-motor type, best exemplified by mania, is the most studied because "precisely it restores the base melody of existing man." Thus in his view, agitation reveals a deeper existential and social meaning inasmuch as the human organism becomes comprehensible only by *saying* and *doing* in a temporo-spatial structure. Hence, "agitation is not only an enlargement, a 'psycho-motor' cancer. It is also and especially a modality of existence, a type of actualization, an expressive style" (Fanon & Asselah, 1957, p. 24).

Fanon's critique of his former teacher and his proposed alternative typology are interesting. But more substantive however is the dialectic of agitation he expounded from an interpersonal and institutional perspective. This dialectic, he argued, is most blatant in the psychiatric milieu that is supposedly a therapeutic instrument, but is in reality a repressive "second internment" with sadomasochistic aspects. The aggressivity and meanness observed in hospitalized patients are often provoked by this brutal internment. What is more, the internment provokes avoidable agitation and hallucinations.

Already rejected by society, the patient comes or is brought to the institution as a final refuge where at last he could be understood. In reality, according to Fanon, the institution "amputates and punishes" the patient. It rejects, excludes, and isolates him. In so doing, it confirms and legitimizes society's

---

This article and others show that, contrary to Gendzier, in particular, Fanon departed significantly from Tosquellean theory and practice.

attitudes toward the patient. The rejection, exclusion, and isolation also provoke more psychopathology and a vicious cycle in which the patient remains entrapped is begun. Isolated from real, living relations, the patient is forced into the unreal world of fantasy and hallucination. Rejection of his *symptoms*—provoked in or out of the institution—leads him to infer that what is rejected is his very *being*.

It was Fanon's view that agitation in particular and psychopathology in general test the degree of institutional resistance—its solidity and flexibility. A therapeutic milieu worthy of the name is, on the one hand, *solid* in structure to provide a base for psychologically uprooted patients and, on the other, *flexible* to permit the expression of human problems others could not tolerate. This dual character of solidity and flexibility thus forces us to comprehend and help the patient. Even when not induced by hospitalization, agitation tests the degree of institutional resistance, its solidity and flexibility. To reject the patient, to exclude and isolate him, is to compromise the therapeutic aim and to miss an opportunity for compassionate service.

Society has already rejected the patient, having earlier imposed requirements that are intolerably formal and somewhat monolithic. Yet the psychiatric institution has no organizational plan but to be repressive and punitive: "The lines of force which participate in the erection of the phenomenal field [in the institution] are of a disastrous poverty." The biological and emotional rhythm of the patient is disturbed, arrested, and forced into a second internment. The psychiatric personnel whose responsibility it is to understand and to heal become alarmed with signs of agitation and react in ways that further disrupt the fragile equilibrium of the patient.

Indeed one finds among the psychiatric staff a sadistic tendency as they hasten to subdue, threaten, and retaliate, producing a chain reaction. An attendant comes to the doctor and asserts: "Doctor, this patient has broken everything"; "Doctor, this patient has wounded three personnel"; "Therefore, Doctor, we have to restrain this patient." The straitjacket, the exclusion, and medication are quickly justified by the claim that all is to the interest of the patient. The patient thereby finds himself confronting a punitive doctor and his collaborators: "In effect, it is the service itself which is sadistic, repressive, rigid, non-socialized, with a catastrophic manifestation" (Fanon & Asselah, 1957, p. 22).

The patient already rejected by society finds his or her rejection further confirmed in the institutional milieu. Rejection by the real world and subsequent rejection by the psychiatric personnel foster the need for and the emergence of a pseudo-world with its novel relations and significations. For to isolate the patient is not only to confirm his rejection, but also to produce the metabolic and emotional conditions required for hallucination. In this sense, hallucination and agitation are fundamentally reactions, provoked conditions, and an experience integral to a disturbed social existence.

Disillusioned with the repressive and custodial character of psychiatric institutions, Fanon sought an alternative in day hospitalization. This mode of psychiatric management has three basic aims: (a) to reduce the incarcerative character of full hospitalization, (b) to provide psychiatric treatment with greater efficiency, and (c) to keep the patient in close contact with his own community. Historically, the first day hospital started in Moscow in 1932 out of such practical exigencies as a shortage of facilities rather than on theoretical or ideological grounds (Dzhagarov, 1944). Within the first four years of its service, this day hospital in Russia cared for 1,225 patients, most of whom were psychotic—a remarkable accomplishment given the dismal failure of traditional hospitalization. Almost independently, other countries subsequently introduced day hospitalization as an alternative to 24-hour, full hospitalization. Such hospitals for severely disturbed patients were established by the 1940s in England, Canada, and the United States.

Day hospitalization is today so common a component of psychiatric care in industrialized countries that it becomes difficult to sufficiently appreciate the significance of adopting it in Tunis during the 1950s. Africa was at the time undergoing a marked sociopolitical upheaval and the colonial powers that had stunted its development were under attack. In countries like Tunisia, in which independence was granted, the colonial powers, having developed a minimum infrastructure, left with the limited technology and expertise they brought, and in some cases vindictively destroyed what few facilities they had established. Tunisia had recently become independent and the national government was in dire economic and political need. It is, in fact, remarkable that its leaders had the will and courage to allow the experiment of day hospitalization—something most African countries have yet to attempt 20 years later.

When in 1958 the first day hospital was introduced in Tunis, partial hospitalization and the "open-door" policy in psychiatric care were largely confined to highly industrialized countries. Day hospitalization burgeoned mostly in the "Anglo-Saxon" countries of Western Europe and North America. A theoretical and methodological question, unanswered at the time, was if in fact day hospitalization could be introduced to treat severely disturbed patients, both chronic and acute, in a less developed country like Tunis. That Fanon and his colleagues provided an affirmative and empirical answer to this question was indeed significant. But more important in our view is the theoretical and moral justification Fanon presented for day hospitalization. Day hospitalization was first introduced elsewhere for varying reasons and exigencies, whereas day hospitalization was inaugurated in Tunis through a distinctly Fanonian perspective. This perspective had far-reaching implications for the conception and treatment of madness. It is unfortunate that Fanon did not live to refine and extend this perspective beyond the notion of day hospitalization.

There are two articles in which the work on day hospitalization in Tunis is discussed (Fanon & Geronimi, 1959, pp. 713–732). The first article was by Fanon alone and the second was written in collaboration with Dr. Geronimi, a former intern at Blida and a committed colleague in Tunis. The first article is primarily empirical, showing the impressive results achieved through day hospitalization in an underdeveloped country. The second is mainly theoretical, discussing the values and limits of day hospitalization. The first article is also a telling illustration of how rigorously empirical Fanon pursued problems when time and resources permitted. This point is important because his works that were translated in English do not reflect it and some, like Woddis (1972), have thereby concluded that Fanon was unempirical and a man given to wild speculation.

In the first article, Fanon reviewed the history and principles of the "open door" policy for psychiatric care. Traditional hospitalization removed the patient from his social milieu and hence his conflictual and necessary milieu. The institution promised to offer a "protective shield" to the patient from society, to the society from the patient, and to the patient from himself. But this proved to be a false protection in all three respects. Hospitalization became, in effect, a brutal internment characterized by repression, lethargy, and depersonalization. Day hospitalization was started in Tunis with the goals, first, of early diagnosis as well as early treatment and, second, of keeping the patient in maximal contact with his exterior social milieu.

Fanon pointed out that at the time they started day hospitalization in Tunis, there existed "at most twenty day hospitals in the world,'" all in highly industrialized countries, and "never an experience of day hospital was attempted in an underdeveloped country" (Fanon & Geronomi, p. 690). In reality, the total number of day hospitals then is subject to debate, but it is clear that Fanon was unaware of the interesting and pioneering work of Dr. Lambo in Nigeria.[2] Nonetheless, the questions Fanon posed were pertinent. From a methodological standpoint, can day hospitalization be viable and effective in an underdeveloped country like Tunis? From a doctrinal standpoint, can this type of service meet *all* the psychiatric demands of such a country?

Day hospital service in Tunis was started as a component of Charles Nicolle Hospital, a general hospital that had had a neuropsychiatric unit for more than 40 years. It had a different policy for admission than traditional asylums, but it relied on the same rigid, repressive, and punitive measures. Like asylums of the worst type, it used straitjackets, cells, bars, closed doors, and the other ugly tools of large establishments. The Tunisian Government wanted to expand its psychiatric facilities, but the futility of building the same old structures became obvious. A plan for a day hospital was therefore considered and eventually implemented within the Charles Nicolle Hospital. It was agreed that the new day hospital remain of small capacity so that its "therapeutic efficacy could be rationally studied and augmented."

How the plan was implemented and the role given to patients are themselves noteworthy. The Ministry of Health having boldly endorsed the plan, a team of patients was put to work to demolish the prison-like cells. The bars, the straitjackets, the handcuffs, and all the instruments of incarceration and repression were removed. The building was renovated and refurbished. The new center was limited to 80 beds: 40 men and 40 women. Six small beds were, in addition, reserved for children in the women's section.

The old staff who, accustomed to the sadomasochistic relations of the old institution, looked at the patient not as "the most important part of the ser-

[2]T. A. Lambo (1956) started an innovative day hospital at Aro Hospital in Nigeria.

vice" but rather as the veritable "enemies of the personnel's tranquility," was transferred. A new, better educated staff was employed and rigorously trained, with high premium placed on competence and a "welcoming attitude" toward patients. Each member was in charge of no more than six to eight patients with whom he or she worked every day and throughout the period of their hospitalization. The quality and efficiency of communication between patients and personnel, between relatives and personnel, and between staff and doctors in charge were particularly emphasized. There was regular psychological and medical surveillance. Patients' dreams, anxieties, relations with family members, sleeping habits, and behavior in the center were carefully recorded. New crises or relapses were immediately attended to and monitored.

Alone or accompanied by relatives, patients arrived at the Neuro-psychiatric Day Center at 7:00 A.M. and stayed there until 5:30 P.M. The center closed its doors by 6:00, when all the patients left for home. Except on Sundays, the center provided daily services. On arrival in the center, each patient was received by the assigned staff member who, after breakfast was served, reviewed the patient's medical and psychological regimen. Therapeutic activities were carefully planned for maximal effect and tailored to the needs of each patient. These included psychotherapy, sleep and relaxation therapy, insulin therapy, electroshock therapy, and chemotherapy. Some of these techniques are today considered archaic and even brutal. That Fanon used them shows how much he was rooted in his own time, even as he endeavored to question and transcend it.

Of particular interest is the form of psychotherapy Fanon employed. His approach to psychotherapeutic technique was what today may be called "eclectic." He employed psychoanalytic psychotherapy, behavioral therapy, and existentialist-oriented psychotherapy. In particular, Fanon adopted Sandro Ferenczi's psychoanalytic techniques in which the therapist takes an *active* and *involved* role in therapy.[3] The behavioral techniques he utilized were based on the Pavlovian theory of Second Signal System.[4] Along with individual and group therapy, he used socio-drama for which the content, significantly, was *biographical* rather than *fictional*. Patients were encouraged to recount their personal experiences to the group who, in turn, gave their opinion, criticism, support, and the opportunity for feedback as in "identification through mirror." Each patient was encouraged to confront himself and others through verbalization, explication, and taking a stand. But attacking a patient's *conscience* or *being* was at all times avoided. Patients did not pay the doctor—a

---

[3]Sandor Ferenczi, a Hungarian psychoanalyst and a close disciple of Freud, is best known for his innovations in therapeutic technique. He emphasized the need for shortening therapy through greater *activity* and *involvement* on the part of the analyst— a perspective that served to alienate him from other analysts of his time, including Freud, but that was later gradually assimilated in psychoanalysis. For details, see Paul Roazen (1974, pp. 363–371).

[4]Ivan Pavolov had used mainly dogs, later monkeys and gorillas, for his pioneering work on conditioning. But as his interest shifted to human neurophysiology, he postulated the Theory of Second Signal System to take into account the human capacity for language and complex associations as in speech and writing.

fact that was carefully taken into account because it modified the quality of transference and countertransference.

A major portion of the article empirically describes the demographic and diagnostic characteristics of the patients seen during the first 18 months of the center's existence. Data for 1958 and 1959 are compared and contrasted, and some changes and remarkable accomplishments are shown for that period. During the last seven months of 1958, 345 patients were admitted to the center. The volume of admissions almost doubled in the next 11 months, to a total of 670 patients. Thus, during the 18 months considered, over 1,000 patients were admitted of whom fewer than 0.88 percent required full hospitalization. In 20 months, more than 1,200 were admitted *and* treated with the average duration of stay shortened to 25 days. No suicide, homicide, or violence of medico-legal import occurred during this period.

This level of efficiency and efficacy is particularly remarkable when one considers that during the first year there was only one *chef de service* who, in the absence of interns, "assumed all therapeutic" needs of the 80 patients. We are not informed who that clinical director was, although one suspects it may have been Fanon himself. In a footnote to the second article on day hospitalization, written in collaboration with Dr. Geronimi, another intriguing point is made, that one of the two doctors had started the first day hospital in Algeria. If in fact it was Fanon who started the first day hospital in Algeria, more research is needed on his work at Blida.

The impressive results of the first article are actually exceeded by the poignant theoretical and humanistic articulations of the second article. The latter focuses on considerations of doctrine and the values and limits of day hospitalization. Fanon and Geronimi pointed out that two characteristics distinguish their neuropsychiatric day center from other psychiatric establishments in Tunis: First was its attachment to a general hospital and second its "formula of hospitalization." Given the social stigma and isolation of traditional asylums, the authors emphasized the need for integrating psychiatric care in the professional and material infrastructure of a general hospital. Such an integration makes possible effective utilization of the services of internists, radiologists, surgeons, and others who can immensely contribute to patient care. It can also rehabilitate the psychiatrist in the eyes of his colleagues, since his isolation in closed asylums confers on him a "mysterious and, taken together, disquieting" character. But most of all, in the eyes of the patient, the psychiatrist becomes a doctor among other doctors and the mental patient comes to be viewed only as a "sick person" like other sick persons.

More fundamental than their endorsement of the medical model is the theoretical and moral justification they offer for day hospitalization. They argue that day hospitalization breaks away from the brutal practice of coercion as well as confinement and most of all that it aims to restore the *freedom* of the patient. The liberty day hospitalization confers is, they regretfully admit, never real and complete. For it is indeed relative and limited. What is more, there is often the temptation of doctors to oppose the exit of an obviously very ill patient who would rather have his freedom than be hospitalized. The doctors in the center sometimes succumbed to this temptation, but very rarely.

The authors nonetheless emphasized that their experience amply demonstrates that partial hospitalization that permits patients to go to their homes and immerse themselves in their world of relations is more acceptable to them and therapeutically more effective. Day hospitalization, they pointed out, minimizes the dialectic of the *master–slave* or *prisoner–jailer* relationship that characterizes traditional approaches. The sadomasochistic relations engendered by confinement and isolation are also attenuated. The doctor–patient relationship regains a "sense of normalcy." Their encounter becomes more and more the meeting of "two free people [which] is necessary in all therapy, and more so in psychiatry " (Fanon & Geronimi, 1959, p. 717). The patient comes without coercion, he also leaves without feeling an unrealistic gratitude to a doctor who allowed it. Confinement disarms the patient, forces him to give himself up completely; it is a battle between unequals, a submission to the doctor's every whim. "Day hospitalization, on the other hand, offers a passive support, a momentary freedom, a reinforcement of the personality, like a prolonged and therapeutic visit" (Fanon & Geronimi, 1959, p. 715).

Basic to the doctrine enunciated is a particular conception of psychopathology, a firm commitment to the being of the patient, and a therapeutic approach aiming to restore freedom in the very society in which it was lost. Madness comes to be defined as a pathology of liberty. The patient's liberty is constantly undermined psychologically—by anxieties, obsessions, inhibitions, contradictions—and socially—by victimization, rejection, coercion, and confinement. Denied his right of liberty by forces within and without, the patient is condemned to exercise his liberty in the unreal world of phantoms.

Traditional psychiatry simply reinforces and legitimizes this brutal reality even as it ostensibly claims to have the interest of the patient at heart. It is from this perspective that one can appreciate "the attitude of revolt" against hospitalization found among patients who are least disorganized—those who still retain a measure of an *active self* and have not yet renounced their *world of relations.* Although day hospitalization is accepted by such patients, those who have an inactive self and have renounced life in the real world prefer complete hospitalization. These are the ones who have totally succumbed to the pathology of liberty. The therapist must understand and reinforce this attitude of revolt as he combats this tendency to surrender liberty.

Fanon and Geronimi emphasized that the real context for sociotherapy is the dynamic and living society itself. No genuine healing or restoration of liberty can be effected apart from it. In fact, their disillusionment with the institutional therapy that Tosquelles pioneered is clear, although they concede its advantages in large and dehumanizing asylums. They pointed out that in such establishments the "neo-society" of institutional therapy was an important advance because it counteracted the regressive tendencies of patients as it offered them a modicum of social contact and tasks in the closed asylum. It also helped the therapists to understand what could have "happened outside," while fruitfully studying mechanisms like identification, projection, and instinctual inhibition. But then comes their incisive critique (Fanon & Geronimi, 1959, pp. 719–721).

> It must always be remembered that with institutional therapy we create frozen institutions, strict and rigid rules, schemes which rapidly become stereotypical. In the neo-society, there is no invention, no creative dynamism, no newness. There seem to be no veritable dislocation, no crises. The institution remains that "cadaveric foundation" of which Mauss speaks. . . . [Moreover] the inert character of the pseudo-society, its strict spatial limitation, the restricted number of movements and, why hide it, the actual experience of confinement-imprisonment, considerably limit the curative and rehabilitative value of its sociotherapy.
>
> That is why we believe today that the true milieu for sociotherapy is concrete society itself.

Day hospitalization keeps the patient in the social and familial milieu out of which his problems arose and in which he must take his rightful place. The therapist every day confronts a living person having active relations with the living world: This patient has not "cut antenna," so to speak. At night and whenever the patient choses, he returns to his family and friends. On his way to and from the center, he rides the bus or train with others whom he knows in his neighborhood and place of work. One took special care to avoid disengagement of others from the patient and of the patient from others. At all times, his world of relations retains its reality and density.

The therapist therefore faced, on the one hand, a personality in crisis at the very heart of its environment and, on the other, a real, dynamic, and active society in the very heart of the patient. It is from this perspective that one clearly observes the rupture in the "synthetic unity" of the person to his milieu and seeks to restore that unity. Symptoms and troubled affectivity are no longer abstracted or isolated from their source. They are offered dialectically and the therapist thinks and acts dialectically. One is forced to abandon the symbolic and imaginary games of institutional therapy and becomes immersed in society itself, not its caricature.

This orientation to a dynamic and living reality forces a rethinking of conceptions and techniques. The reification of descriptive semiology and nosology gives way to an existential approach that takes into account the activities, assaults, and vulnerabilities of the self in a dynamic social milieu. It is in this psychosocial dialectic that the therapist decides the time, place, and type of his intervention. At the center, the patient is provided his own space, his privacy is respected, and no demand is made upon his liberty or immediate appearance. He wears and brings what he wants. What is questioned is not "the form of his being," but rather "the form of his existence."

Fanon and Geronimi concluded that day hospitalization is inappropriate in cases in which "the organic participation in the illness" is massive and dominant, therefore requiring constant medical surveillance. However, they added that even for such cases, thanks to chemotherapy, the period of complete hospitalization could be reduced, and early transfer to day hospitalization becomes possible. The other categories they thought inappropriate for day hospitalization are patients who present clear danger to others or to themselves and of course those in police custody. They further emphasized that each center be small and "avoid at all cost the creation of those monsters which are classical psychiatric hospitals." Significantly, they urged stronger legislation for patients' rights and appropriate consideration to those who live in distant or rural areas. Their last sentence is most noteworthy:

> In summary, a very strict legislation should be established, guaranteeing to the *maximum the liberty* of the patient in getting rid of every incarcerative and coercive aspect of internment. (Fanon, 1967b, pp. 53–55)

This was Fanon's psychiatry until his death at the age of 36. The noble project of restoring liberty to captives of colonialism and of the psychiatric establishment had only begun when he died. There have been some advances made here and there, but that project still awaits realization. Liberty continues to elude the majority—whether colonized or neo-colonized, incarcerated or overdrugged. A small elite, sham and corrupt, has usurped what many have fought, bled, and dreamed for in those colonies that Europe underdeveloped to develop itself. The mental health profession too has betrayed its declared goals of prevention and healing once it joined in the rampage for profit, power, and control. It caters willingly to those who can afford it, at the same time neglecting or abusing those victims for whom hope of liberty remains frustrated.

Fanon presents an alternative for those who desire that the tool never possess the man and that enslavement cease, if not forever, at least in their own personal and professional life. The letter of resignation he wrote while in Blida (Fanon, 1967c, pp. 53–54) is a moving and principled document rare in psychological literature. It summarizes the revolutionary and humanistic thrust of his psychiatry.

> If psychiatry is the medical technique that aims to enable man no longer to be a stranger to his environment, I owe it to myself to affirm that the [colonized and, we may add, the patient], permanently an alien in his own country, lives in a state of absolute depersonalization. . . .
> The function of a social structure is to set up institutions to serve man's needs. A society that drives its members to desperate solutions is a non-viable society, a society to be replaced.
> It is the duty of the citizen to say this. No professional morality, no class solidarity, no desire to wash the family linen in private, can have a prior claim. No pseudo-national mystification can prevail against the requirement of reason.

12

TOWARD A PSYCHOLOGY OF LIBERATION

For Europe, for ourselves, and for humanity . . . we must work out new concepts, and try to set afoot a new man.
—Fanon, *The Wretched of the Earth*

These are the last words in Fanon's last book. He intended them for people of color, the oppressed—those who for too long looked to Europe for inspiration, models, and guidance. But the oppressed are everywhere and Fanon's urging to fashion new concepts and to set afoot a new *person* should speak to everyone— or almost everyone. It is in this chapter that I conclude the intellectual excursion we made into the rugged landscape of oppression—into the distant past, reviewing the violence of slavery, into the recent past, recalling the fire and fury with which colonization proceeded, and into the present, sketching the plight of blacks penned in ghettoes and multiple forms of death.

I attempted to place these developments within a broader historical perspective, hoping to show that underlying much of the violence that exploded to an unprecedented scale in the world was a greed for profit, a boundless wish for self-aggrandizement, and a sedimented Manichean psychology. Underscored was the fact that amnesia for the painful past may be a convenient defense but never a reliable foundation for programs of amelioration and development. Thus focusing on racism, I reviewed recurrent pronouncements of scholars, discussed the role of psychology and medicine in oppression, examined different manifestations of violence, ventured into the sociogeny of madness, and explored various paradigms that seemed pertinent to the psychology of oppression.

The guide and inspiration for this difficult, but I hope worthwhile sojourn was Frantz Fanon whose thought, practice, and person I set out to interpret and clarify. Although a great deal has been written on Fanon, it seemed to me necessary to present a comprehensive discussion of his psychological contributions and to offer data that support his seminal ideas. I did so not only to familiarize others with his little-known psychological contributions, but also to affirm Fanon's historical and intellectual significance for oppressed people of color.

Of course, Fanon was by no means infallible nor was his analysis without

251

problems. For to claim otherwise is simply to wade in dogma and the cult of personality. In addition to Fanon's controversial assertions on violence and social classes, one could very well show that serious problems arose because of his overreliance on the medical model. Fanon's unqualified endorsement of violence in *The Wretched of the Earth* confounds the humanistic kernel of his overall thought and contradicts his own clinical illustrations of how violence begets further violence, as well as other unanticipated complications in the lives of the survivors. It seems to me that the same Fanonian thesis on violence could be offered to analyze the process of decolonization without a hysterical celebration of counterviolence in *all* conditions of oppression. Moreover, his contention that madness is the result of a sociohistorical predicament, but his reliance on medical means of diagnosis and treatment, pose fundamental problems unexplored by him and his contemporaries.[1] Nonetheless, I decided to emphasize his positive contributions partly because this seemed a necessary first step and partly to salvage valuable and seminal insights from the ravaging critiques—better, the "wrecking operation"—of those who would have us seek no personal models or theoretical paradigms but those that are Eurocentric and theirs.[2]

What Fanon committed himself to was not a search for elegance in paradigms shorn of lived experiences nor the sterile monologues of intellectuals cut off from the travails, aspirations, and struggles of people. Rather, his was a commitment to *living beings* and to any action—clinical practice, writing, and revolutionary violence—that restored the integrity of people and basic human values. It so happens that those who attack his person and ideas forget that there is a violent history to be reckoned with, that generations have been denied an authentic biography and history, and that this attack on Fanon is not unrelated to that historical violence on people of color.

For when Europe unleashed its avarice upon the rest of the world, it globalized human bondage and drastically changed the character of oppression. Europe's encroachment and self-aggrandizement brought forth slavery, colonialism, apartheid, racism, and, in Fanon's words, "an avalanche of murders." Through plunder of land and labor, with bayonets and the Bible, Europe developed itself and simultaneously underdeveloped people of color. Europe's stubborn wish to own and control transformed various peoples into the owned and controlled. Europe's greed to have *more* also forced many into being *less*.

[1]Macro-analysis at the national level but micro-interventions at the individual level also leave out such critical mediating institutions as the family and the web of interpersonal relations to which *identified patients* belong. One danger in this shift between macro-analysis and micro-intervention is to forget the significant ways family and intimate relations intensify or buffer against assaults of oppression, and, hence, to declare that oppressed peoples are inevitably pathological or, conversely, that social revolutions complete cure all psychological disturbances. In reality, all social revolutions are incomplete, at least from a psychological standpoint, and more remarkable than the psychological vulnerabilities of the oppressed is their seemingly inexhaustible resilience. I explore these themes in a work in progress.
[2]An example of this is the diatribe of Jack Woddis (1972) and the unfair critique in Gendzier's writings, particularly those following her book *Frantz Fanon: A Critical Study* (1973). I discuss these issues in *Frantz Fanon Revisited: A Case of Benign Neglect or Selective Distortion*, unpublished.

The victims of this violence span eras and continents. The bloated belly of an African child in a refugee camp or the tormented resident of Soweto controlled with awesome power today bears testimony to the same victimization as does the dejected look of a black American in a prison, a mental institution, or a decrepit housing project. The millions of slaves lost in the Middle Passage, the ravages of tribal wars instigated to divide and rule, the ruthless exploitation of every human and material resource—all these still remain sedimented in social existence and in the deeper recesses of the psyche. There are also many victims whose plight is hardly heard or seen. These include Native Americans, Australian aborigines, and the Maoris of New Zealand. In other words, the human wreckage of Europe's avarice and violence is strewn everywhere. No ecology, no culture, no psyche remains untarnished.

It has been said that those who do not know the past are doomed to repeat it. Ideally, it should be possible to know and write about our infamous past without blaming contemporaries for it. Each of us should be judged, held accountable, and confronted, not for crimes of past generations but for the actions he or she takes in *our* time and with respect to the living. To inspire feelings of guilt for the inhumanity of one's predecessors or of shame for the dehumanization of one's ancestors has not been my aim. But if neither can be helped in reviewing that past, I believe guilt and shame can be used constructively as lessons for the future and the impetus for proactive, preventive action.

Indeed the familiar distinctions between victims and villains, development and underdevelopment, civility and barbarity, sanity and madness are becoming increasingly blurred. There are, no doubt, those who still profit from and deliberately carry on the historic violence. Yet for most persons, white or black, the bankrupt legacy infused with a Manichean psychology exacts its toll, directly or indirectly. That we are born into that legacy or socialized at a tender age in one or the other camp of the Manichean world is beyond our choice and responsibility. To live it uncritically and be outlived by that legacy without taking part in an effort to change it is however a matter of *personal* choice and responsibility.

The focus of this work has been clearly on the historic violence of Europe on people of color. However, to infer from this conclusion an inherent criminality or defect in Europeans or their descendants amounts to sheer racism and is contrary to my (and Fanon's) aims. Certainly violence is not a monopoly of Europe or of its descendants; some African governments such as the one over which Idi Amin once presided have also afflicted oppression and wanton murders on their own people. This fact should serve as a sobering antidote to anti-white racism. A reversal of Manichean psychology where blacks hurl insults, stones, or steel on whites is a nonviable solution and no amount of blaming others can justify an evasion of responsibility to change what *is*. There are certainly many whites who themselves have been victims of that historic violence discussed in this work and many blacks who willingly served in complicity with oppression—including slavery, colonialism, and apartheid. In other words, skin color is not a badge of criminality or innocence, but rather the personal stand taken is evidence of one or the other.

During the past two decades, one talked about neocolonialism that indeed was real and pervasive. Today however there is accumulating evidence that "autocolonialism," the highest phase of social oppression, has emerged under the leadership of homebred tyrants. Callous and inept dictators like the ones currently reigning over many African countries are of course not new in human history. Now and then, one found "village dictators" who, obsessed with a need for abject loyalty and with continuing their ineptitude, knew little else but to rule by terror tactics and summary executions. But the African tyrants of today, many of them products of colonial servitude, rule with lethal arms sent as "aid" by more "developed countries" in a manner reminiscent of the way firearms and gunpowder were shipped to Africa during the slave trade.[3]

We said earlier that the oppressed, denied individual biography and collective history, are made appendages to the biographies and history of others. In a very real sense, Europe's assault on people of color brought forth a legacy of self-expansion and entitlement, on the one hand, and self-diminution and deprivation, on the other. This legacy has become so integral to everyday living and prevailing consciousness that one takes it for granted almost as one does the rising and setting of the sun or the blossom and foliage of the seasons. Earlier chapters discussed the multiple forms of death and the immense loss of "person-years" this historic violence has entailed for blacks. Psychologists would certainly do well never to mask this fact with postulates of "aggressive instinct," innate and fixed, that make *everyone* and in the end *none* responsible.

To this day, it is the Europeans and their descendants who are competing for world dominance. The two superpowers are poised for a nuclear holocaust, an absolute catastrophe for all, if one or the other cannot have its way and impose its whims. The earth has been voraciously disemboweled of its resources and its inhabitants used as objects and disposed of at will. Indeed, with the doomsday clock moved to a just few minutes before "midnight" to emphasize current perils of nuclear war, the historical self-aggrandizement and avarice for control have now reached extremely dangerous heights, the ultimate of *antisocial* and *self-destructive* madness. It is obviously in everyone's interest to no longer acquiesce for fear of losing the security of the herd. The competition for dominance and self-aggrandizement is now spilling over to outer space, while the immense toll for the reckless adventure begun a few centuries earlier is taking its toll through the air we breathe, the water we drink, the environment we inhabit, the carcinogens we cannot avoid, the neighbor we learned to distrust, the lethal arms buildup in many corners of the world, and the anxiety of imminent destruction we try to repress.

[3]Two intriguing aspects of social, interpersonal, and personal life concern, on the one hand, how the past survives in the present and, on the other, how anticipated outcomes determine behaviors in the present. Thinking of oppression in *linear* terms is actually simplistic and even misleading. A better way of studying oppression is one based on the concept of *circular* causation, whereby perpetrator and victim, subject and object, actor and acted upon form components of the same, self-perpetuating *system*. The current relations of African governments to their people and to dominant powers are better understood in these terms.

Those in the so-called underdeveloped countries who have decided to catch up with the "developed countries" need to rethink what it is they want to catch up with, which genuine contributions of Europe they must adopt, and what of their own they would do well to retain. There is no necessary correlation between the development of *things* and the advancement of *people*. And if such a correlation were to hold, Euro-America has yet to exemplify it with the certainty that a superficial look or a self-conceit may suggest. One has only to visit a "nursing home" into which the elderly are dumped, a psychiatric institution in which overdrugged zombies move aimlessly and with blank stares, a ghetto where many sleep hungry or homeless amidst plenty, and even the home of a well-to-do family whose members daily pop pills to find the calm, not to mention the serenity, that eludes *homo consumen*.

On the contrary, it seems that those who turned into forming and molding things have come to dominate nature and rule the world, all the while dehumanizing others and themselves. Those who turned to people, elaborating a human-centered culture in which even things were imputed with anthropomorphic attributes, have become defenseless victims to the predation of the former and to such natural disasters as drought and disease. Is this pattern really inevitable or is it possible to have a world in which the worth and relations of people are not compromised while nature is "creatively" transformed to fulfill human needs? Can psychologists, inasmuch as it is their vocation to search for solutions to human problems by human means, contribute to changing our shared legacy of violence and the contemporary dilemma?

It is obvious that history is made and group identities reclaimed not on account of psychologists and their theories, but as a result of the organized and willed actions of social groups. Equally obvious is that human suffering, known from time immemorial and in every society, finds no panacea in "modern psychotherapy," which only has a history of about a hundred years. In reality, modern psychotherapy is thus far limited to only a few societies and, for that matter, mainly to a few social classes within those societies. What is more, behavioral scientists who study social oppression concur that psychology has traditionally served the function of *social control* rather than of *social change* and that "modern psychotherapy," if made available to and accepted by the oppressed, tends to emphasize self-compromised *adjustment*, not self-liberating *revolt* to an intolerable *status quo* of oppression.

Yet to leave matters there adds nothing but another note of pessimism in a domain of human relations in which, because of oppression, pessimism and cynicism are rife. There is certainly little to be gained by throwing out the baby (in this case, psychology) with the bath water (i.e., psychology's history of race, class, and sex bias). For however niggardly its traditional guardians may have appeared to the oppressed, psychology can contribute immensely to the struggle of the oppressed. But this cannot happen in the absence of fundamental change in the parochial values and limited priorities of establishment psychology.

There are indications that Euro-American psychologists are gradually "desegregating" their theories as well as their practices. Various constructive critiques of traditional tenets and practice have increasingly emerged within psychology during the past two decades, exposing unrecognized cultural, class, and sex biases of psychologists. People of color have also joined the field in steady but growing numbers since Fanon's death, bringing with them different experiences and alternative formulations. As classrooms and neighborhoods increasingly desegregate to reflect the diversity of races and cultures, so too will the intellectual tenets and social doctrines inevitably become less Euro-centric and hegemonic. Such a diversification in theory and practice should be celebrated rather than lamented. For psychology will be enriched to the extent that it incorporates diverse cultural experiences; it will merit claims to "human science" to the degree it is suffused with different value orientations; it will also make significant strides in social responsibility inasmuch as its gates are open to various clientele.

This work, as its title shows, has been concerned primarily with the psychology of oppression and with the contributions of one psychologist—namely, Frantz Fanon. To write on the psychology of liberation was not its aim because, as pointed out earlier, there was first a need to clearly define the problems, placing them in historical as well as conceptual perspective. What I therefore present in these last pages is only the broad outline for a psychology of liberation. I will address here only questions of priorities and perspective, but defer issues of technique and tactics. A degree of oversimplification of the major socio-historical developments and elaborate psychological traditions seems inevitable in any brief discussion, though I hope that the following suggestions offered stimulate thought.

The essential points I will discuss can be summarized thus: (a) Underlying much of prevailing psychological theory and practice are the ethic of indi-vidualism, the ideal of individual autonomy, a particular conception of basic human needs, as well as an exclusive emphasis on individual change, which together reflect fundamental cultural as well as class biases, and (b) one essen-tial precondition for a psychology of liberation is to reformulate the psycholog-ical outlook, basic human needs, and foci of change in ways that take into account the priorities and frustrations of the oppressed.

FROM INDIVIDUALISM TO COLLECTIVE WELL-BEING

Inasmuch as it concerns itself with human realities of a given era and a particular social group, psychology inevitably remains integral to the historical and cultural current of its time and place. For instance, looming large in psy-chological literature is the emphasis on individualism. Informing most therapeutic interventions is also the ideal of "individual liberty." Thus the various personality theories and indeed the pivotal role of "personality" in psychology show this emphasis on individuals as the unit of analysis and primary concern. Diagnostic classifications are also about individuals or, more specifically, about symptoms and traits of individuals commonly shorn of their dynamic and relational essence. Therapeutic goals are equally about the attainment or restoration of adjustment, adaptation, equilibrium, competence and/or autonomy in individuals. This emphasis on individualism and the ideal of individual autonomy has deep historical roots in the cultural and economic evolution of Europe and North America. To attempt here even a modest discourse on these socio-historical developments and their psychoaffective consequences would surely take us far beyond our intent. But several points should be emphasized.[4]

Philosophical debates on "individual liberty" had gained increasing currency from the seventeenth century on in countries in which capitalism burgeoned. The capitalist mode of production and its ethic of maximizing profit conditioned a rapid erosion of traditional bonds and social values. Production in these countries required, on the one hand, the attenuation of all socio-legal obstacles to the accumulation of profit for the bourgeoisie and, on the other, the isolation and reduced resistance of workers who, as *individuals*, could enter into contractual relations to sell their labor. Thus almost from the start, the ethic of individualism and the ideal of individual liberty were Janus-faced: On the one hand, they implied freedom of unfettered development and privatization of social privileges to the interest of those with capital; on the other hand, they entailed a weakening of resistance among workers by reducing them into socially defenseless individuals who privatize their collective victimization.

By the twentieth century, the ethic of individualism and idealization of individual liberty reached their zenith in North America and Western Europe. Associated with these were also the cult of individual privacy and the assumption of necessary conflict between the individual and society. From the perspective of those who enjoyed economic and political privileges, it was a question of enjoying, without interference, privileges that had become "rights," extending these privileges into every aspect of their life, and most certainly barring any infringement of them by "society"—more particularly the amorphous mass of have-nots. The imperatives of capital development, combined with rapid migration, urbanization, technological advances, and new patterns of industrial production that together provided the material impetus for individualism and compartmentalization of life, were stimulated. Everyday living gradually became more atomized, leaving most persons only tenuous and shifting social anchors. A markedly self-centered and schizoid orientation toward life and others became institutionalized and "normalized." Moreover, *having* became the measure of *being*, time a commodity to be gained or lost, and relations with others a matter to be justified in the balance sheet of economic assets and liabilities.

The discipline of psychology emerged in this socio-historical and cultural context. The ethic of individualism and the ideal of individual autonomy were thus inevitably incorporated into its theories and techniques. Indeed psychology in the generic sense we have been using (hence, it includes psychiatry)

---

[4]See, for instance, I. Meszaros (1970) for a detailed discussion of individualism in Euro-American culture.

flourished and gained "currency" through its efforts to deal with the psychological problems spawned by rapid social change, intensifying class conflict at home, and raging wars abroad. Whether these dealings have served the function of rehabilitation and amelioration or of social control and reification is a matter still hotly contested.[5]

The crucial point to emphasize here is that psychology has been embedded in the socio-historical and cultural context that gave it life and relevance. Developing in a social environment that extolled the ethic of individualism and an ideal of individual autonomy, it was axiomatic and expected that psychology too would incorporate this ethic and ideal in its theories and practice. Without such embeddedness in or consonance with the values and needs of its community, psychology would have little relevance to those who primarily seek its services, fund its research, and share its promises. But fundamental problems arise when this psychology—its underlying ethic and ideals—are readily assumed to reflect the values and priorities of people everywhere.

To be sure, individuality and the ideal of individual autonomy are not inherently negative or problematic. Rather, their salience and actual realization depend on where one is situated in the social order. The well-to-do can extol the ethic of individuality and search for individual autonomy because their *collective liberty* is already realized. Their clamor for "individual rights" is but a wish to further extend and refine that collective freedom. What is more, their collective freedom and individual rights essentially boil down to an "absence of restraint" from the full enjoyment of privileges and possibilities that too frequently amounts to an absence of restraint from imposing their will and interest on others. In short, their collective liberty was obtained through violence and their individual rights are but condensed social violence.

The oppressed, in contrast, can hardly speak of "individual rights" so long as their collective liberty is usurped and denied. The liberty they seek is "a recognition and fulfillment of necessity" inasmuch as their basic human needs are frustrated and their humanity stunted. It is therefore the attainment of collective liberty that takes precedence, since without it any extension or refinement of individual rights is impossible. Indeed the adoption of individualism leaves the oppressed defenseless, divided, and highly prone to capitulation. The aim of personal salvation when one's group is oppressed is often a chimera and, if attained, involves one or another form of alienation and sometimes even outright self and/or collective betrayal.

The contrast of predicaments can be underscored by the realities of the well-to-do and the poor in urban America. Thus for instance, one finds elaborate legal and social safeguards for the property, person, and even privacy of the former group. The privileges they enjoy in society—favorable conditions for accumulation of surplus value, highly profitable tax loopholes, better educational opportunities, access to the best legal defense, lenient measures in case of criminal acts—these are carried into the interpersonal domain and family life. Their home is like the proverbial "castle" protected by laws and well-built

[5]See, for instance, D. Ingleby (1980).

structures. Each member of the family claims his or her part in the family privileges and seeks to give full expression to individuality. Each acts as a majority of one, particularly in encounters with the oppressed. The family boundary and the relations within it remain relatively sacrosanct with little interference by the state and its machinery of control unless there is a major and noticeable disaster.

The poor, in contrast, have little or no properties to protect; their bodily and psychological integrity are constantly violated; their space and density permit little privacy. Educational opportunities, working conditions, tax laws, the administration of justice—all these and more work against them. The frequent comings and goings of landlords, police officers, social workers, and a host of others render their homes more like an inescapable and disarming "trap" than a protective and protected "castle." The provision of state aid to meet basic needs of nutrition and shelter entails state interference in family life. Who lives there, who relates to whom, and what happens in the family is scrutinized by officials, mental health workers, and representatives of the Welfare Department. In many instances, to be a father and unemployed means to forfeit membership in one's family, leaving behind morsels and tribulations for the rest. The penetration of the state and public agencies into the family are equally underscored by frequent court proceedings regarding custody of children, including their placement in institutions on the recommendations of mental health workers but against the desperate objections of parents. In short, the material and socio-legal order in society work against the oppressed, even though claims abound that they have (theoretically, of course) equal rights.

Psychological theory and practice, permeated by prevailing inequities and ideology, do not therefore necessarily reflect the priorities of the oppressed. A psychology tailored to the needs of the oppressed would give primacy to the attainment of "collective liberty" and, since such liberty is attained only by collectives, would emphasize how best to further the consciousness and organized action of the collective. It is crucial to emphasize that individualism is not the natural order of life and that there is no necessary or immutable conflict between personal well-being and social welfare. Rather than extolling individualism, an ethic that in any case is culture bound, it seems more tenable to first assert that *sociality* is fundamental and definitional to human living. Otherwise, to speak a language, hence communicate and bond with others, would not be of such pivotal importance in human existence. Without language and sociality, even the elaboration of civilizations would be inconceivable. Moreover, to assume a necessary antagonism between the individual and society is to forget that the development of self and even of life itself would be impossible without other people's recognition, nurturance, and cooperation.

In asserting these basic facts, one need not of course deny that individual differences in reaction and threshold do exist; that aspiring to individuality is not necessarily an aberration; that development involves differentiation and integration in function as in form; that conflict in individuals, between individuals, and among groups occur; and that the relation between individual and society is by no means always harmonious. The point instead is that sociality, human interdependence, and intersubjectivity offer a more fundamental initial ground for the psychology of liberation than the assumption of individualism as the natural order of life or of a belief in a necessary conflict between the individual and society. In short, to begin with how sociality is internalized, expressed, modified, and breached in different conditions promises a reliable and realistic foundation for developing a psychology of liberation.

Psychology actually is not only embedded in its class and cultural context, but it also remains enmeshed in the problems of that context. Some of the ironies establishment psychology has yet to escape include the theoretical fragmentation of human existence under socioeconomic conditions that atomize reality (thus posing difficulties in elaborating a comprehensive and unified psychology), the commoditization of therapy and friendship in accordance with the laws of supply and demand (thereby fostering a professional preference to cater and "cozy up" to those who can most afford but least need help), the overreliance on the metaphor of the machine to describe *human* problems in a highly mechanized world (hence confusing people with machines and machines with people), and the assumption of necessary conflict between individual and society (when in reality the conflict is socio-historically conditioned).

In earlier chapters it was argued that the theoretical and methodological preoccupation to control and predict, although undoubtedly leading to fruitful scientific discoveries, has been coterminous with an enduring and bloody history of conquest and domination. The high premium placed by Euro-Americans on mastering nature and hence changing the environment to meet human needs also entailed the elaboration of a world in which some were masters and others slaves. Evidently, in struggling to control nature, there has been a confusion as to what really constitutes "nature" and who indeed qualifies as "human." Our historical highlights have shown that the oppressed were often reduced to objects among other objects of nature and, along with nature, controlled, exploited, and predicted.

One may very well thus wonder: How much of psychology is universal and how much Euro- and class-specific? By what standards and comparisons could such a determination be made when studies of non-Western peoples or the oppressed are seen through the prism of Euro-American and middle-class biases? How can one be certain that prevailing conclusions about, say, the so-called instincts have universal relevance to people everywhere or that they rather are the alienated revelations of an alienated social existence? And if mainstream psychology is biased to the ruling group, what orientation and postulates can one derive from the experiences and psychology of the oppressed?

FROM INSTINCTS TO HUMAN NEEDS

Psychologists have written extensively on the nature as well as the vicissitudes of "instincts" and "needs." Freud's postulate of dual instincts— namely, sex and aggression—are perhaps the best known and most closely integrated in psychological theory and practice. But there have also been other theorists and clinicians who proposed different motives for human behavior. To emphasize that there is by no means an unanimity of views on what constitutes the most basic instincts or needs of people, one need not detail, for instance, McDougall's (1908) cataloguing of a battery of instincts (including what he called the "instinct of submission," which he associated with blacks), or Henry Murray's (1962) listing of thirty-nine human needs, or Maslow's (1970) delineation of five essential needs.

It is worth noting that 60 years ago Bernard (1924) had counted some 14,000 instincts postulated in the literature, with many others suggested since then, and that Gordon Allport (1961) aptly pointed out: "It is easy to invent instincts according to one's needs."[6] Instincts and needs are both theoretical constructs used to explain the why and what of behavior—its underlying goals, regularity, and potentiality. They are a convenient fiction—better said, hypotheses—that may or may not help to describe, explain, and/or predict behavior.

The notion of instincts, though still retained in psychoanalysis, has gradually been found problematic in psychology and many replaced it with the concept of needs, following Murray's (1962) formulations. The notion of fixed traits, which, on the one hand, downplays the salience of context and, on the other, limits human possibilities has also been increasingly recognized as untenable. This becomes most obvious when one considers the claims of sociobiologists that aggression, xenophobia, and selfishness are innate and dominant features of people when in reality these claims are but rationalizations for the historical violence, schizoid orientation, and self-centered behavior of a ruling group.[7]

I do not intend to carefully evaluate postulated instincts or needs, but I do want to emphasize that the particular instincts or needs one postulates reveals one's conception of human nature, one's views of limits or possibilities, and one's priorities for change. Moreover, postulated instincts and needs, inasmuch as they have been conceived in a particular social and cultural context, have tended to be biased to the realities of certain groups. It is therefore important to reconsider the question of basic human needs in developing a psychology of liberation and reformulate it in ways that take into account not only the frustrations of, but also the possibilities for the oppressed.[8]

To begin with, one very basic but often ignored fact is that the struggle for food (and water in many parts of the world) can no longer be assumed irrelevant to human psychology. The psychology governing the acquisition of food, its distribution, and conditions of shortage loses importance only in social and

[6]Cited in A. Thomas and S. Sillen (1974, p. 15).

[7]A highly informative exposition on sociobiology and its services as rationalizing bulwark for xenophobia, racism, and selfishness is presented by Martin Baker (1981).

[8]The following discussion on "needs" is offered not in order to present a complete and final catalogue of human attributes, but rather to underscore the need for an alternative perspective and priorities to those prevailing in psychological thought. One must, in all cases, be careful not to assume fixed traits or encase people in a narrow view of "human nature."

historical conditions under which starvation and malnutrition are hardly known, neither as facts of everyday life nor as ever-present threats. Yet famine, drought, and hunger occur all too frequently in many parts of the world. The folklore, myths, and rituals elaborated in many cultures with respect to food and food shortage show the salience of satiation and hunger to human psychology.

Considering further the amount of time and energy most people spend in cultivating, acquiring, exchanging, and worrying about food, one realizes that the everyday realities of a large sector in the world's population have yet to receive attention in psychological circles. Indeed contact with the poor and powerless majority in the world underscores that shortage of food—its physical sequelae, resulting psychological insults, attendant social or interpersonal conflicts, and associated fantasies—dominates and informs human psychology. Thus any attempt to grapple with the psychology of oppression is incomplete without taking into account the incessant struggle for food.

Using experiences from situations of oppression suggests the following basic needs and/or powers of people: (a) biological needs of which the need for food is most basic, (b) sociability and rootedness, (c) clarity and integrity of self, (d) longevity and symbolic immortality, (e) self-reproduction in praxis, and (f) maximum self-determination.

Significantly, these basic attributes refer, on the one hand, to essential human *needs* and, on the other, to essential human *powers*. Each asserts itself as a need to be gratified and turns into a power once gratified. As needs, they are actualities to be overcome; as powers, they are potentialities to be realized. But since in reality none of them is absolutely frustrated or completely fulfilled, they simultaneously exist as needs inasmuch as they are partially frustrated and as powers insofar as they are partially gratified.

Without detailing the dynamics and relationships of these basic human attributes, it is important to stress a few crucial points. Following other theorists, I prefer to consider these attributes, in need–power terms rather than instincts. Although there is some justification to posit instincts to show that people are part of nature, indications are that an instinctualist orientation poses more problems than it resolves. For one thing, the sole emphasis on man's unity with nature (including animals) ignores that, on the one hand, the most determining and, on the other, the most deadly challenge each of us confronts is his own fellowmen.

Moreover, although listed in some order, these basic attributes are best considered together in their organic and dialectical relations rather than in isolation or in terms of a "hierarchy" of importance. These basic attributes exist in all people at all times, the ones most frustrated being those most manifest and pressing in a given temporal or social condition. The schematic ordering of needs into a pyramid, as in Maslow's "hierarchy of needs," only betrays an elitist outlook, unwittingly mirroring the existing hierarchy of social classes. Also untenable is the implication that only the rich have the possibility or monopoly of "self-actualization."

The desire for the maximum satisfaction of such biological needs as food, sex, and shelter seem too obvious to require exposition. The desire for sociality and rootness, as we have already suggested, is equally fundamental, being no less critical than fulfilling biological needs. Sociality is not peculiar to human beings alone. Animals, too, are social beings, although their behavior is guided and dominated by "instincts." Even then, what are instincts but the stored, sedimented "wisdom" of the species, acquired by the collective and aimed at the perpetuation as well as the enhancement of the collective? Animals may live primarily by instincts, but human beings, to remain human, rely on and live within *culture*. And at the foundation of culture is sociality. For to acquire culture presupposes not only a remarkable power of learning and teaching, but also an enduring capacity for interdependence and intersubjectivity. Not only the development of our higher powers of cognition and affect, but also the development of our basic senses rest on the fact that we are social beings.

In a sense, an infant at birth is a bundle of possibilities, a living candidate to many but not infinite alternatives, awaiting a series of social "re-births" and self-realizations. If failure to satisfy biological needs leads to disease and physical death, then denial of human contact, communication, and affirmation (even opposition of others) leads to a social and psychological "starvation" or "death" no less devastating than, and conditioning, physical death. We take this fact for granted precisely because we are so embedded in our social world, realizing the deadly effects of social isolation in such examples as "voodoo death" and concentration camp experiences. We earlier suggested how, during the Middle Passage, countless African slaves, suffering from "fixed melancholy," a condition of utter shock and grief, remained unmoved by threat or punishment. Despondent and stripped of their natural bonding, they squatted down with their chins on their knees, their arms around their legs, and died one after another at a remarkable and alarming rate.

Psychologists have written extensively on "self-psychology" from various perspectives. It would of course take us far beyond our intent to review the contributions from psychoanalytic, existential, phenomenological, neo-Piagetian, or cognitive behavioral writings on the self—its definition, development, and dialectic with the environment.[9] Suffice it to point out that self-psychology has recently attracted the interest of various schools of thought all of which, to different degrees and from different perspectives, emphasize that the self—whether considered as the whole person of the individual, a psychic organization, a meaning–making system, or otherwise—is invariably embedded and formed in a social world. In other words, the self is a *social self*, having its origin, affirmation, and transformation in sociality.

---

[9]For a psychoanalytic perspective to the self, see, for instance, Edith Jacobson (1980) and Ornstein (1978), the latter presenting a selection of Heinz Kohut's works; see also Dillon (1978) for a phenomenological perspective in the tradition of Merleau-Ponty; Ferguson (1980) presents a Meadian discussion of the self, whereas Kegan (1983) offers a fascinating neo-Piagetian elaboration. Moreover, Suls (1982) brings together various psychological perspectives to the study of self, including that of the cognitive behaviorists.

An infant is born with a body, but not with a self. The latter emerges only after birth, following simultaneous processes of maturation (in which perceptual ability and coordinated motility are acquired) and reciprocal interaction with others in an ever-expanding social context. Selfhood can only exist within a body, but it is more than the body inasmuch as it incorporates aspects of its environment, extends into objects of possession, and represents the human capacity of meaning-making. The pursuit of self-clarity is thus intimately bound with the clarity developed first about one's body, the body's boundary and attributes, and later one's larger world. This pursuit of clarity has survival, developmental, and organizing value. It entails both a differentiation from as well as an integration with others and with one's past. Without some clarity of the self, however tentative and tenuous, there can be no meaningful relating with others, no expression of inherent human potentials, no gratification of essential needs—in short, no life as we know it.

But this process of self-clarity, ending only when the body dies, requires a fundamental respect of one's self-integrity, with a minimal insult to one's being as to one's body. When assaults on one's being are experienced at critical developmental periods or with certain regularity, self-clarity is hardly attainable or is at best rendered incomplete and negative. The experiences of the oppressed show not only the centrality of this need for clarity and integrity of the self, but also how structural and formal constraints of oppression result in painful ambiguities and constrictions of the self.

Despite the best of medical technology, our bodies are sooner or later assailed by disease and death. However much we deny it, physical death awaits each of us. The denial is universal but always incomplete since, consciously or unconsciously, our inevitable death informs how and for what we live. It is thus never whether or not but rather how or when, under what conditions and for what ends, we shall meet our death. The desire to prolong life is so deeply ingrained in us that we do remarkable things to postpone or at least deny our death. But since our physical death and the consciousness of it haunt us, we relentlessly endeavor to die later rather than sooner and take recourse to avenues of symbolic immortality through our children, social relations, cultural elaborations, theological convictions, and/or other modes of "transcendence."

As Lifton (1983) has clearly shown, images of death reduce to basic feelings of separation, disintegration, and stasis, whereas images of life entail social connectedness, bodily integrity, and experiences of vitality. Earlier we saw that the oppressed have far higher rates of morbidity and mortality than their oppressors and, what is more, the expropriation of their space, time, energy, mobility, bonding, and identity results in both psychological and social death. It is significant that the satisfaction of only biological needs cannot by itself maintain human life and that human history and individual biographies bear ample testimony that under certain conditions people do forego physical life rather than accept psychological or social death.

The pursuit of longevity and symbolic immortality is hardly attainable and meaningful without some form of purposive engagement through praxis, which, by definition, is imbued with consciousness and intentionality. By *praxis* we refer to one crucial aspect of what psychologists broadly call "behavior." To be sure, no equivalence of the two terms is intended. *Behavior* refers generally to any and all observable human as well as animal activity. It is a measurable unit of activity, and its conceptualization commonly lacks relational and intentional import. In meaning and import, praxis is different in at least two ways. First, it refers only to *human* activity. Second, praxis does not refer to *all* human activity. *Praxis* underscores goal-directed and socially meaningful activities that render people active agents in a world they transform; and they in turn are transformed by it. There are various forms of praxis (Vazquez, 1977). Productive labor is however praxis *par excellence,* since it is by means of labor that people elaborate social relationships and satisfy their human needs. Unalienated labor is also one effective means through which people, individually, unveil their implicit identity, objectify it, and, collectively, build a civilization.

It is thus through praxis that people re-produce themselves in the objective world, make explicit their personality, and validate themselves as well as their knowledge. The pursuit of self-reproduction through praxis makes possible the acquisition of food on which to live, the realization of social grounding, and the actualization of individuality and potentials. In acting upon and transforming our world, what matters is not only the product of one's praxis, but also the very process and fact of active engagement with others and one's context that dialectically happens to be an engagement with one's self as well. That is why experiences of alienated labor or forced unemployment, both of which are rampant among the oppressed, entails not only a frustration of biological and social needs, but also an ontological impasse and existential stagnation.

The fulfillment of these needs is possible only when there exists a measure of self-determination. The quest and struggle for self-determination is as fundamental and definitional to people as are the other needs previously outlined. Little wonder that the right of self-determination is one of the fundamental principles enshrined in the United Nations Charter and forms the kernel of constitutions of governance defining human rights as well as responsibilities. *Self-determination* refers to the process and capacity to choose among alternatives, to determine one's behavior, and to affect one's destiny. As such, self-determination assumes a consciousness of human possibilities, an awareness of necessary constraints, and a willed, self-motivated engagement with one's world.

Self-determination is intimately bound with the notion and experience of freedom. It is important to emphasize that we are not as free as we wish to be, since structural and historical constraints do exist, and we are not as externally determined as we fear we are, since we do possess a measure of choice, influence, or control in what happens to us or in what we make happen. History and social conditions presents alternatives but also constraints. We can choose to act or not to act. But even when we lack alternatives in the world as we find it, we do possess the capacity to interpret and reinterpret, to adopt one attitude and not another. Without the right of self-determination, we are reduced to rigid and automatic behaviors, to a life and destiny shorn of human will and freedom[10]

Self-determination is also both a means of fulfilling other human needs and an end unto itself. We know for sure that, under certain conditions and historical moments, people do take up arms and risk physical death to retain or reclaim their right of self-determination. To overlook this fact, as psychologists unfortunately tend to do, is to omit a crucial human dimension and a critical motive of history. To emphasize only the significance of unconscious inner promptings or mechanistic environmental determinism, underplaying the importance of conscious and organized human agency, is equally to forget that willed change in persons and predicaments is impossible without the right and capacity of self-determination. The powerful influence of the unconscious and of the environment need not of course be denied or underestimated in order to underscore the fact that the pervasive clamor for self-determination among the oppressed reflects one universal aspect of human essence, a persistent project for which all is risked.

These basic needs are in reality not fully or equally fulfilled. In a world of scarcity, governed by dialectical laws, conflicts exist among needs, between needs and resources, between technology and the environment, and certainly among people. The needs themselves can reappear in different guises and intensity at any given moment. What appear to be "natural needs" here and now could be supplanted by "artificial needs" there and then. The satisfaction of biological needs could turn to its obverse—namely, avoidance of pain and injury. Sociability may lose ground to narcissistic and self-centered preoccupations. The quest for clarity and integrity of self may degenerate to the adoption of a Manichean view of self-other with the violent consequences previously illustrated. The wish for longevity and symbolic immortality may be reduced to an obsession with death and hence losing ground and joy in *being* here or *living* now. The pursuit of self-reproduction through praxis may be supplanted by the thoughtless destruction of the environment and the hoarding of material goods. The endeavor for extending self-determination may amount to only the conquest and domination of the other—that is, the denial of self-determination for others.

From Adjustment to Empowerment

Frustration of the needs listed previously is what makes a given condition of life oppressive, dehumanizing, and sooner or later, resisted at the risk of physical death. A central question that often arises concerns the process and means of effecting change in people as well as in circumstances in order that these needs are met and human potentials realized. One common but very specific means of seeking change is psychotherapy, which ordinarily focuses on the individual.

---

[10]In this respect, Edward Deci's book (1980) is worthy of note.

Psychotherapy is a planned, purposive, and confiding interaction between a trained, socially sanctioned "healer" and an identified "sufferer" (Frank, 1982). The focus may be broadened to include groups and family members, but the *raison d'être* and emphasis in psychotherapy is that *someone* has been a problem to himself and/or to others. There is now a growing realization, though not fully acted upon, that the identified "patient" is part of a larger problem (conventionally narrowed to nuclear family dynamics) and that this person is as much a problem to others as others are to him.

We leave aside the debate on whether one form of psychotherapy is better than another or if a given approach changes subjective states, symptoms, behavior, or total personality. Generally speaking, such debates are important and the huge resources devoted to psychotherapy outcome studies necessary. In reality, however, these debates over similarities and differences between approaches lose their salience when one is considering the oppressed who, in any case, have thus far least profited from the debate, research, and clinical practice. It should of course be noted that even those who focus on relieving subjective symptoms alone often argue that change in this domain will have behavioral and social consequences.

Another common approach to change is that which aims to directly transform social institutions and systems by organizing and mobilizing people. This approach may or may not have explicit goals of changing persons, but it usually is guided more or less by an articulated world view, a conception of what calls for change, and goals to be realized through social intervention. It so happens that both approaches—namely, psychotherapy and social change—have different relevance and urgency to people not simply because of personality differences but more importantly because of where a group is situated in the prevailing social order.

The fact that establishment psychologists focus only on the first—that is, changing symptoms, behaviors, and personalities but not institutions and social structures—shows in part their own class position and allegiance. However, those psychologists who work with the oppressed find that they must work to change pathogenic social conditions as well as persons. And here is the rub. For indeed psychotherapy aims toward change and stabilization of an identified victim. There are immediate and personal difficulties to be resolved, pain and torment to be relieved, and the personal interests of the "patient" to be given priority. Frequency and duration of contact are however limited, usually to about one hour a week and often no more than a dozen sessions.

Now assuming that a member of the oppressed seeks psychotherapy and it is provided, that appointments are kept, and that therapy proceeds as planned, what realistic changes can be expected? Is it not a worthy accomplishment if at least the anguish of symptoms and a self-defeating pattern of behavior have been changed through psychotherapy? At the same time, however, was a concession made to the prevailing social order by effecting *adjustment* to it? Is it reasonable to state that psychotherapy may be appropriate and necessary for *this* patient, but essentially conservative with respect to the *status quo* of oppression? Is psychotherapy therefore basically an instrument of social control, not social change? If so, are there ways of helping this victim with his immediate, specific, and pressing problems but not by compromising the goals of the collective?

These critical questions become salient in working with the oppressed. It is of course unconscionable to deny anyone the right of therapy in order to ensure the realization of a "revolution" in the uncertain future. Yet questions of changing causes and not only symptoms, of preventing and not only treating casualties, of empowering victims to solve their problems and not keeping them dependent and powerless, of fostering a collective action and not a self-defeating privatization of difficulties—these issues must be squarely confronted in situations of oppression.

Of course one can learn many things from establishment psychology in working with individual casualties. These include, to cite only a few, understanding the power and dynamics of the unconscious, an appreciation of childhood experiences with attending formative scripts for the self and relation with others, manipulating environmental conditions to change behavior, and acquiring skills for hermenuetic as well as methodological rigor. But the crucial frontiers that remain unexplored include how victims of oppression can be empowered to act in a coordinated way to change themselves, their social conditions, and historical predicaments. Herein lies one of Fanon's pioneering contributions.

Interventions in conditions of oppression typically run into two major pitfalls that recur with remarkable frequency and hence require careful consideration. One common pitfall is that those who undertake psychotherapy among the oppressed focus on the immediate and "private" distress of individuals, but lose sight of the shared victimization and the necessity for social transformation. They fail to act upon the pathogenic social reality and in the end merely sanction it. Their intervention, if sought by the oppressed and when successful, is therefore doomed to an essentially "bandaging operation" on a few casualties who nonetheless return to the same, unaltered conditions of oppression. Sooner or later, it is realized that the labor of a psychotherapist with the oppressed is akin to the labor of Sisyphus. For some, the resulting pessimism becomes an excuse to join those who long ago threw their lot in the more lucrative pasture of private practice, working with those who can afford it. A few persist undaunted, as some must, with their bandaging operation, settling for less—both in impact and remuneration.

Another equally common pitfall is that those who work toward social and community transformation forget that it is above all *people* who are the subjects of history. Either they conceive of change abstractly, fixated on grand structures lacking human content, or they seek to make visible impacts on material objects, using real and living persons as fodder for their grand ambitions. In consequence, even the very people in whose name everything is ostensibly justified are compromised, betrayed, and sacrificed. Such reformers fail to recognize the hypocrisy of talking about remote goals of social justice while abusing and stunting real and living persons around them.[11]

[11]The hollow promises of change and the frequent miscarriages of justice are best illustrated by

In reality, both pitfalls reflect a failure to adopt a dialectical perspective. In the first, one focuses only on identified victims and their immediate problems without engaging in their concrete and lived socio-historical context. This amounts to an attempt to rehabilitate biographies without any grounding in history. The result is usually either a minimalist view of change or, worse, a conservative outlook that blames the victim. In the second, an account of the larger context and remote goals is taken while the reformer is disengaged from, and subsequently disengages, the very persons on whose behalf the change is ostensibly sought and justified. This amounts to a way of making history without actualized biographies, save that of self-styled activists and leaders. The result is at best an imposition of change from "the top," a paternalistic attitude toward the oppressed and a veiled tyranny in practice.

Some critiques of psychotherapy are admittedly so sweeping and categorical that they amount to a therapeutic nihilism. One must appreciate that therapy, the traditional or even interminable type, does provide a service to certain categories of people. The search for a unitary, fixed, and universally relevant mode of psychotherapy is indeed futile. It is more prudent, as Strupp (1982, p. 53) pointed out, to ask "Which constellation of patient characteristics and problems are most amenable to which techniques conducted by which type of therapist in what type of setting?" Implementing such a therapeutic program is certainly easier said than done, but Strupp's remark underscores that no mode or technique of intervention, however sophisticated in theory or buttressed by professional respectability, can have equal relevance to different people, in different social predicaments, as practiced by different therapists.

Freud himself warned against viewing psychoanalysis as a panacea, even for the type of patient for whom, and from whose experiences, his therapeutic modality was developed. Indeed his modest goal of helping these patients learn substitution of "ordinary human unhappiness for neurotic misery" is contrary to present-day claims of psychotherapeutic omnipotence. There is a common tendency to claim that a given modality or technique that has shown efficacy for some persons and/or for some problems has equal relevance for all persons and for all problems. There is also the opposing tendency according to which a given modality or technique is considered absolutely irrelevant for all if it does not meet the needs of the group to which one feels committed. The first tendency illustrates therapeutic imperialism and the second therapeutic nihilism.

Each social group, if determined to forge or reclaim its authentic biographies and history, must define its own problems, seek its own solutions, and choose its own means. It can of course learn from the experiences, insights, and errors of others. But it cannot appropriate—lock, stock, and barrel—problems or solutions of others in order to forge authentic biographies and history. This is so in therapy as in other areas of life. What works for white, middle-class neurotics cannot equally meet the needs and priorities of the poor, the powerless, and/or the culturally different. To assume that it can or must—an

---

the loudly declared "revolutionary" aims and "socialist" pronouncements of the ruthless military juntas who today reign over Africa.

assumption made all too frequently—is not only to misappropriate and misapply, but also to commit the ethnocentrism and solipsism discussed earlier. The well-documented rejection and failure of prevailing psychotherapy practice with a majority of the oppressed has many causes. I will mention only a few to underscore the need for alternatives.[12]

As indicated earlier, not only are few clinical services offered the oppressed, despite alarming reports of need, but also what little is offered is generally low in quality. Numerous studies show patients from low socioeconomic groups are not readily accepted for psychotherapy; that they are more usually insitutionalized and overmedicated; that they have high dropout rates in outpatient treatment, but are institutionalized longer as inpatients; and that they are more often assigned inexperienced therapists.

Of the many barriers to therapeutic efficacy with people of color, the racial and class impediments to therapeutic alliance loom large. Griffith (1977) has shown the multiple problems plaguing the encounter of white therapists and black patients. These include problems that both therapist and patient bring to the encounter by virtue of their class and color. The therapist may assume that all blacks are inextricably locked into a psychology of oppression, hence taking for granted an immutable "mark of oppression," or he may succumb to his own anxiety and guilt and thus avoid any mention of racism, thereby giving "the illusion of color blindness." Another set of problems poses a threat to therapeutic alliance in the encounter of a black therapist and a black patient. Significantly, these problems center on the question of identity. The black therapist may have his own unresolved conflicts about being black and therefore may adopt a counterproductive "denial of identification" or he may take a posture of overinvolvement, blunting therapeutic objectivity and engagement, by succumbing to "overidentification." Even if the therapist experiences no problems with his blackness, his class position and values are potential sources of mutual distrust and misunderstanding.

Also to be noted is that the prevailing psychotherapy is often constrained by the time-worn dichotomy of *subject* and *object* and the underlying epistemological reductionism that has long characterized Western thought. One set of treatment modalities gives primacy to cognitive and subjective states (harking back to the *idealist* outlook), whereas the other assumes the supremacy of external and environmental forces (consistent with *empiricism*). The first emphasizes "insight" into and "reliving" of experiences, thereby giving priority to internal changes and to the subject. The second, which favors the object, focuses on behavioral contingencies and their manipulation in the belief that changes in external objects will necessarily engender internal changes. Most treatment modalities derive from one or the other reductionist approaches, with a few attempting integration of the two essential approaches.[13]

Yet the dichotomy between subject and object, the separation of change

---

[12]The preceding chapters already suggested other problems of traditional psychotherapy with the oppressed.

[13]See, for instance, Sampson (1981).

within from change *without,* and the fact that both approaches spring from Eurocentric and class-specific values pose fundamental barriers to the development of a liberative psychology. The dichotomy of subject/object evades or at best only partially addresses the simultaneous task of the oppressed to transform themselves and their social conditions. What is more, psychotherapists of both orientations have been known to fall far short of their competencies when "treating" black patients. Those who favor internal change often succumb to a well-rehearsed stereotype that blacks and the poor are impervious to "insight." Those who focus on external domains usually limit themselves to modifying only the behavior of the person, but undertake no program to change his pathogenic social conditions. The first implicitly arrives at a verdict that little or nothing can be done to change the patient's predicament; the second installs more vigorous social controls and hence sanctions the *status quo* of oppression.

The lessons of the "community mental health movement" in the United States also show that vested professional interests, the politics of funding, and hardened biases outweigh fleeting concerns about social justice and the plight of the oppressed. The history and consequences of the community mental health movement cannot be justly summarized in a few words. One must nonetheless mention that the social unrest of the sixties brought an allocation of resources to forgotten populations. The availability of funds, impressive structures, and exciting possibilities came to lure many professionals who otherwise would hardly have ventured into ghettoes and ghettoized racial feelings. Professional attitudes began to change, traditional tenets were reexamined, and some innovative practices were introduced.

But the clamor for "community" and "prevention" became a whimper and was almost muted as federal funding dried up and a conservative mood overtook the nation. Mental health professionals once again flocked away from the poor and the slums to wherever funds could be had—private practice, the defense establishment, and sundry other lucrative ventures. To this political and economic reality, research and practice were adeptly adjusted. Notions of community and prevention, more speculatively talked about than seriously acted upon, lost their appeal and urgency. And the more the poor and the oppressed were quieted and pacified, the more they were once again cast into a familiar oblivion.

One lesson from this brief moment of reform and its essential failure is that the oppressed cannot rely on others for solutions. Another is that no amount of external funding, no measure of professional *mea culpa,* and no flood of promises by well-meaning reformers can substitute for self-empowerment and social activism by the oppressed. Great disappointments await the oppressed who leave their destiny or the fulfillment of their frustrated needs to professional or bureaucratic elites whose actual allegiance is to the *status quo.* The litany of pseudoscientific justifications for oppression aside, this elite remembers the oppressed only when "the natives" are restive and violence is in the air, when smoldering rage and fire can no longer be contained within the bodies and neighborhoods of the oppressed. It is then that they rush like firemen to put out or contain what threatens the prevailing structure of privilege and dominance. But once the oppressed are "pacified" with violence, the threat of violence, drugs, or some reforms, this elite, with the exception of a few whose concern with social justice is genuine, rushes back to its accustomed comforts and amnesia.

What is needed in situations of oppression is a mode of intervention that bridges the separation of insight and action, internal and external, individual and collective. The oppressed are economically and socially too pressed to wait indefinitely for an insight apart from lived realities. For how could one engage in endless monologues while swamped by demands on one's time, space, energy, mobility, and bonding? Can one arrive at internal harmony while faced with threats of eviction, the tyranny of an employer or unemployment, life on borrowed time, restricted movements, and relations rendered objectively conflictual? By what justification can reality be kept in abeyance while there are so few options but to either simply drown or barely keep afloat in turbulent social currents with a minimum of self-determination? Would it not be possible to gain insight while acting on real problems, treating not only through words but in deeds, emphasizing not how one is unlike but like others, and helping forge new bonds nurtured in a collective struggle?

Indeed the very structure and medium of therapeutic intervention itself requires critical reevaluation and supercession. For how can an intervention liberate the patient from social oppression when the "therapist–patient" relation itself is suffused with the inequities, nonreciprocity, elitism, and sado-masochism of the oppressive social order? Can there be realistic grounds for changing self-defeating behaviors and a negative self-concept in a context in which only the "doctor" initiates and the "patient" accommodates, where one is powerful and the other powerless, where one exudes omnipotence and the other is locked into impotence, where one remains, confident and all-knowing, in the comfort of his office and values while the other reaches out, alone and helpless, to an alien context and a friendship for sale? By what conjurer's tricks could one effect fundamental changes in the personality, relation with others, and social conditions of the oppressed when presumably the "healing" relation itself is a microcosm of the *status quo* of oppression? Is it therefore surprising that the oppressed have not come in droves to seek help from mental health professionals and, if a few of them turn to "therapy" as a last resort, that they soon drop out and return to their old travails?

Psychologists have studied the myriad aspects of madness. Remarkably, however, the obvious and immediate have been neglected for the obscure and remote. The relation of madness to oppression, the denial and/or abdication of liberty, which is an essential characteristic of both, the uncritical reenactment in "therapy" of the inequities and power relations prevalent in society—these fundamental aspects have been neglected for elusive causes and cures. For whatever contributions may derive from accumulating biomedical and traditional psychological research, and there are undoubtedly many, the problem of madness and oppression will nonetheless continue to elude us so long as the questions of *inequity*, *power* and *liberty* are evaded.

One can easily show that society tends to react more reflexively when it is a question of those who somehow come to be identified as "abnormal." The group often reacts with an anxiety of epidemic proportion and an organic sense of threat. It matters little if the putative "patient" is actually harmless to himself or to others. The diagnosis that he is mad, therefore wild and dangerous, is irrevocably taken for granted. Hence the group undertakes swift and violent measures to protect itself from a peril it conjures up, creates, or exaggerates. The community feels safe once it kills the identified deviant, performs on him brutal psychosurgery, keeps him in chains, locks him up, or forces his compliance with potent medications. It is remarkable how often the mysteries of madness, including its "cure," were sought in the attributes and constitution of the identified patient without considering seriously the psychosocial dialectic of those who feel the compulsion to classify, ghettoize, and persecute some of its members. Of course, scientific advances have been made over the years and ostensibly brutal measures of control have been humanized. Yet as often happens, the more things change, the more they remain the same.

If madness reflects something about the putative patient and the social milieu to which he or she belongs, racism is, psychologically speaking, a projection of a "blackness within" on a safe object. Mannoni who analyzed the psyche of the colonizer pointed out that, in the final analysis, "the Negro . . . is the white man's fear of himself" (Mannoni, 1964, p. 200). The more white people externalize their unacceptable "blackness within" to safe objects whose skin color is "black," the more they find comfort in who they are. The more blacks are kept in ghettoes, the more unacceptable impulses are ghettoized. The more whites scapegoat blacks, conjuring up a shared threat, the more they find grounds for an otherwise unlikely alliance.

Winthrop D. Jordan (1970, p. 134) made the observation that through slavery Americans "may in fact have found enhanced fluidity of the American social structure above the racial line" and that "the firmness of Negro exclusion may have served as a bedrock . . . permitting the revolutionary social mobility among whites without the crippling apprehensiveness that proper social ordering was entirely by the board." It is ironic that the nation that came into existence with the solemn assertion that "all men are equal" was at the same time dependent on the enslavement of blacks and that Jefferson who drafted its constitution was himself a slaveowner. One wonders what the character and destiny of the United States would have been without slavery and without the projective screen blacks continue to provide.

The point here is less about speculations of what may have been than what in reality happens to be. Blacks not only served the economic needs of whites, they also have been made a unifying scapegoat, an anchor for shared identity, and the human receptacles into which are dumped unseemly and misanthropic proclivities. Without the presence of an exploited and scapegoated mass of blacks, North America may have turned out to be a continent of warring nations, a new battleground for descendants of those who could not live together in Europe, dragging countless others into at least two world wars. In a sense, beyond the obvious causative role of objective oppression, the multiple death and alienation rampant among blacks in the United States serve a psychosocial and prophylactic function for whites. If nothing else, the belief that there exist blacks who live under worse conditions than one's group, that they represent what one never wishes to be, or that they even exemplify the dangerous "Wild Man" against whom the group should band together—such beliefs do serve psychologically and socially integrative functions for whites. The question is, however, will blacks continue in this double jeopardy of objective oppression and psychological cannibalism? And what can psychologists do to help change their predicament?

Much has no doubt changed in the attitude of whites and behavior of blacks during the past decades in the United States. Yet there still remain vestiges of old stereotypes and exclusionary practices; one also continues to find some blacks who willy-nilly live out such imposed images as that of the Wild Man, Caliban, Sambo, or Uncle Tom.[14] Indeed as in other conditions of oppression, blacks in America are to this day caught in a narrow and perilous balancing between a socio-syntonic affirmation of the self and an ego-syntonic conforming to the prevailing social norms in society. Since their being is often apprehended through the haze of racial stereotypes, their socio-syntonic behaviors may probably be ego-dystonic, whereas actions that to them are ego-syntonic may be to others socio-dystonic.

Thus the elaborated stereotypes and institutional practices entail a vicious cycle. To embody the stereotypes and adhere to the norms is to validate the status quo of oppression and hence to subvert the interests of the self and group. To reject and resist them is to invite confrontation with forces seeking to enforce and perpetuate the status quo. Thus a black person who openly resists living out the images of Sambo or Uncle Tom risks a diagnosis of "antisocial personality" or even "paranoid schizophrenia." The person who meekly submits to these stereotypes and controls risks not only self-estrangement and betrayal of group interests, but also the psychoaffective rupture both entail. In this sense, then, the difference between the criminal justice system and the mental health industry is one of form, whereas, from the perspective of the oppressed, the difference between "crime" and "insanity" is partly one of degree in personal complicity. The oppressed who is a "criminal" is revolting alone without consciousness and even conscience whereas the oppressed who is "insane" has capitulated to such a crushing degree as to be a battleground of seething contradictions.

Given this higher potential of being either a "criminal" or "insane," the oppressed cannot attain liberty by individual means and without consciousness. To revolt against or even to capitulate to a status quo of oppression without risking criminality or insanity, one must therefore be anchored in a collective that helps bridge the socio-syntonic and ego-syntonic. And no program of amelioration, no plan of rehabilitation, and no intervention with the best of intentions can have lasting and redemptive consequences without the empowerment of the collective and active engagement of victims. Powerlessness and demoralization characterize the oppressed—whether they

---

[14]In *Capitalism and Cannibalism*, now in preparation, I discuss the archeology of racism and madness as well as the historical and symbolic import of these stereotypes.

are locked in mental institutions, penned in slums. or kept in check by internalized but ego-dystonic social norms. In therapy as in all interventions with the oppressed, the paramount significance of collective goals and social praxis needs to be recognized.

As Vazquez (1977) amply demonstrated, the ruling group in society and the ruling ideas they espouse have historically stigmatized praxis and those on whom they forced the chores of cheap labor and servitude. Leaving to slaves and workers the job of tilling the land, of fighting wars, of erecting buildings, and of toiling in factories, they kept for themselves the luxury and prestige of contemplation and intellectual endeavors. Thus except for activities related to political governance, scholarly endeavors, or artistic work, most other forms of praxis and those social groups laboring for others have remained stigmatized.

Psychology too tended to favor cognition and affect over praxis when, in reality, only purposive, organized, and socialized activity is the foundation for psychological transformation, for validation of knowledge, and for the elaboration of civilization. Undoubtedly, the transition from the old introspectionism to behaviorism marked a watershed in the history of psychology. The redefinition of psychology as the scientific study of behavior led to many advances in theory, research, and practice. The pitfalls of "introspectionism" and the problems derived from purely subjective claims are too well known. At the same time however, the tendency to emphasize discrete behaviors stripped of relational and intentional content rather than organized and willed human activity has its own pitalls. Not only does such an approach serve to decontextualize human activity, it also leads to a neglect of human agency as well as the consciousness it entails. Praxis requires a measure of antecedent consciousness and motivation, which in turn transform as a result of praxis.

Therefore a break from the ahistorical, decontextualized, and desocialized consideration of "behavior," a return to an emphasis on praxis that reconnects people through organized actions toward common goals, restores their lost attributes as subjects, and helps them regain rights they have been denied is very much needed. The transition to what I would call *psycho-praxis* should be not only in theory, but also in interventions. Intellectualization of experience in therapy sessions and shedding tears in the privacy of a consulting room may indeed result in some insight and some relief from immediate pain. But the goal of changing persons and circumstances requires more—above all socialized praxis. Change should be sought not only *in* the person, but also of the social milieu.

As Fanon clearly indicated, to lock up a person in a cell, left to his fantasies and hurts, is simply to sanction and intensify the very "pathology" to be cured. It is also to reenact, in the name of science and care, the very sadomasochism, rejection, and violence prevalent in his social life. Moreover, it is not enough to search for a "cure" by conjuring up imaginary roles and concocting artificial groups when *real* aspects of the person and his social milieu can be engaged, confronted, and changed in the *real* society.

The oppressed—whether incarcerated in institutions or made captives by a prevailing social "normalcy"—can rehabilitate themselves and change their predicament only inasmuch as they rehabilitate and disalienate their praxis.

Their space, time, energy, mobility, bonding, and identity cannot be restored by inaction. Physical, social, or psychological death is too heavy a price for an accustomed passivity, a corrosive apathy, self-defeating individualism, and predictability of stagnation. Psychological work with the oppressed must give priority to organized and collective activity to regain power and liberty. One critical focus of intervention has to do with unraveling, through active involvement and demonstrations in the social world, the self-defeating patterns of relating, the tendency toward betrayal of the self and/or others, the internalized script for failure and disaster, as well as the conditioned fear of taking a stand or even fear of freedom—all of which derive from a contrived system of socialization, an elaborate formula to produce willing victims. Another crucial focus is the comprehension and refinement of strategies as well as tactics for regaining power and liberty.

Saul Alinsky(1972,p. 13) made the point that "men *speak* of moral principles but *act* on power principles." We may add that, in acting on power principles, there are those who have power and those who do not—the oppressors and the oppressed—with the moral principles often justifying this state of affairs. Psychological work with the oppressed that is not about disalienation of praxis and regaining of power tends to produce morally entrapped and compromised *objects*, not liberated and creative *subjects*.

It is by acting toward, with, and/or against others that our wishes become revealed, our knowledge develops, our personality is objectified, and a change in people, as well as of circumstances, is effected. It is also by reinserting the individual into the group through actions with and on behalf of a collective that even a paranoia once privatized and pathological could find collectively shared and hence nonpathological appropriation. One cannot but marvel at the many belief systems that if declared only by one individual qualify for "madness," but when espoused by a collective are extolled as "religion" or justified on grounds of "national security."

Power and liberty are of course never given; they are demanded, taken, and assumed. For if and when "given," they are at best conditional, often superficial, and readily "taken away." The struggle for power and liberty, the forging of authentic biography and history, at once entail a struggle against a force poised to maintain the *status quo* and a struggle to eject internalized controls and images. In most situations of oppression, this dual struggle cannot realize its goal within the narrow confines of prevailing legality, proselytized religious precepts, enforced institutional regulations, and ordinary social etiquette. Which of these aspects constitute genuine human values worth retaining and which constitute only mechanisms of domination always need critical evaluation. There comes the time when a demand of the oppressed for the same rights enjoyed by others is quickly condemned as an illegal act, a sacrilege, a defiance, or simply rude behavior. The oppressed can advance only if conscious and convinced of higher laws and morality than those which ensnare them in servitude.

Organized, conscious, and collective action is an antidote to alienation in its various forms. It canalizes psychic energies for constructive ends, binds members who otherwise turn against each other, and remains the most reliable means to self-determination. In *Dying Colonialism*, based on his observations during the Algerian struggle for liberty, Fanon demonstrated how a radicalized and activated community, determined to take control of its destiny, frees up its hidden reservoir of energy and creativity. Biographies become enriched as the group sets out to make its own history. People who for a long time suffered abuses in silence or privatized their troubles took up the cause of liberty with remarkable courage and a sense of belonging. Dead and ritualized elements of the indigenous culture regained new life and dynamism. As history was being reclaimed, as fixed traditions were regaining dynamism, so too were individual biographies being restored to their natural course of *becoming*.

The relation between people—between men and women, husband and wife, parent and child, leader and led—also underwent drastic changes. The imperatives of the nation and of forging collective destiny superseded the rigid roles of family life, paternal authority, traditional roles, and old conventions, including sexual behavior. Significantly, as Fanon affirmed, once a dominated group takes control of its history, it assimilates at a remarkable speed but in its *own terms* alien ideas and technology that previously were rejected outright or accepted with organic ambivalence. This is so because under conditions of oppression, when reciprocity and equality are negated, one tends to resist the influences of the other. If and when such influences are assimilated, what is assimilated is often distorted and self-defeating. This fact is amply demonstrated by the adoption of even Western medicine under conditions of oppression.

In short, the psychology of oppression is a topic of pivotal significance to which Fanon made seminal and pioneering contributions. At the kernel of this psychology are the facts of pervasive violence, a Manichean view of the world, an ambiguity of the self, and various forms of death. If in fact recorded history is the history of the victor, establishment psychology is also an elaborated system of rationalizations for the *status quo* and a refined instrument of social control. We have seen how much violence is unleashed in the name of scholarship, science, and healing. A psychology of liberation would give primacy to the empowerment of the oppressed through organized and socialized activity with the aim of restoring individual biographies and a collective history derailed, stunted, and/or made appendage to those of others. Life indeed takes on morbid qualities and sanity becomes tenuous so long as one's space, time, energy, mobility, bonding, and identity are usurped by dint of violence.

To transform a situation of oppression requires at once a relentless confrontation of oppressors *without*, who are often impervious to appeals to reason or compassion, and an equally determined confrontation of the oppressor *within*, whose violence can unleash a vicious cycle of autodestruction to the self as well as to the group. For without this dual confrontation, the search for personal harmony remains illusive, madness becomes rampant even through sanctioned normalcy, interpersonal violence persists even among loved ones, and death in its various forms remains pervasive. Apart from a conscious and determined struggle, there is no quick fix, no mental exorcism, no struggle for private salvation that can herald a restoration of usurped biography and history. The struggle for justice through violence must, of course, be a last resort not only because such means exact untold miseries for all involved, particularly the oppressed, but also because they leave behind a legacy of wrecked psyches and antidemocratic tendencies. Yet, consideration of these dangers should not justify inaction or imply that lost rights can be reclaimed without a persistent *demand*.

The organized activity and the organized institutions of the oppressor must be countered with the reorganized activity and the reorganized institutions of the oppressed. Goals must be defined, programs to fulfill them developed, and the oppressed shaken to organized action within a structure of human values imbued with a clarity of what truly is "prosocial" from the "antisocial" and of what constitute *human* needs apart from *superficial* needs. The true meaning of violence, crime, accountability, and liberty are deliberately so confounded by the oppressor that the oppressed are readily ensnared in a web of confusions and internalized prohibitions that are as defeating as the array of external controls. We have seen how, in consequence, the oppressed are made captives to a vicious cycle of social, psychological, and physical death.

Psychologists who take seriously their concern for the oppressed must foster, teach, and perfect what Pinderhughes (1972) called "confrontation tactics" and Pierce (1970) "offensive mechanisms." Fanon (1968) was making essentially the same point, but in its extremes because the particular oppressive condition of which he wrote and sought to transform was brutally violent and proved impervious to all but counterviolence. The particular confrontation tactics or offensive mechanisms taken of course depend on the type of oppressor one faces, the resources at hand, and the timing that is most opportune. But whether by peaceful or violent means, it is only through organized struggle that the oppressed can change themselves *and* their predicament. Few put this as aptly as did Frederick Douglass (Fonder, 1968, p. 61):

> If there is no struggle, there is no progress. Those who profess to favor freedom, and yet depreciate agitation, are men who want crops without plowing up the ground. They want rain without thunder and lightning. They want the ocean without the awful roar of its many waters. This struggle may be a moral one; or it may be a physical one; or it may be both moral and physical; but it must be a struggle. Power concedes nothing without a demand. It never did, and it never will. Find out just what people will submit to, and you have found out the exact amount of injustice and wrong which will be imposed upon them; and these will continue till they are resisted with either words or blows, or with both. The limits of tyrants are proscribed by the endurance of those whom they oppress.

SELECT REFERENCES

Abate, Y. (1978). African population growth and politics. *Issue: A Quarterly Journal of Opinion,* 7(4), 14–19.

Adam, H. M. (1974). *The social and political thought of Frantz Fanon.* Doctoral thesis, Department of Government, Harvard University, Cambridge, MA.

Adams, P. L. (1970). The social psychiatry of Frantz Fanon. *American Journal of Psychiatry, 127*(6), 809–814.

Adebimpe, V. R. (1981). Overview: White norms and psychiatric diagnosis of black patients. *American Journal of Psychiatry, 138*(3), 279–285.

Adler, A. (1956). *Understanding human nature.* New York: Fawcett.

Akinkugbe, O. S., & Betrand, E. (Eds.) (1976). *Hypertension in Africa.* Lagos, Nigeria: Literamed.

Alinsky, S. D. (1972). *Rules for radicals,* New York: Vintage Books.

Allport, G. W. (1961). *Pattern and growth of personality,* New York: Holt, Rinehart & Winston.

Apel, K.-O. (1972). Communications and the foundations of the humanities. *Acta Sociologica, 15,* 7–27.

Aptheker, H. (1974). *American negro slave revolts.* New York: International Publishers.

Arendt, H. (1970). *On violence.* New York: Harcourt, Brace, & World.

Baldwin, B. A., Floyd, H. H., & McSeveny, D. R. (1975). Status inconsistency psychiatric diagnosis: A structural approach to labeling theory. *Journal of Health Social Behavior, 16,* 257–261.

Baldwin, J. A. (1975). Theory and research concerning the notion of black self-hatred: A review and reinterpretation. *Journal of Black Psychology, 5*(2), 51–78.

Banks, W. C. (1976). White preference in blacks: A paradigm in search of a phenomenon. *Psychological Bulletin, 83*(6), 1179–1186.

Barker, M. (1981). *The new racism,* Frederick, MD: Altheia Books.

Bateson, G. (1959). Cultural problems posed by a study of schizophrenic process. In A. Auerback (Ed.), *Schizophrenia: An integrated approach.* New York: Roland Press.

Bateson, G. (1960). Minimal requirement for a theory of schizophrenia. *Archives of General Psychiatry, 2,* 477–491.

Bensing, R., & Schoeder, O. (1960). *Homicide in an urban community.* Springfield, IL.: C. C. Thomas.

Bernal, J. D. (1977). *Science in History* (Vols. 1–4). Cambridge, MA: MIT Press.

Bernard, L. L. (1924). *Instincts: A study in social psychology.* New York: Holt.

Berthelier, R. (1979, January–March). Psychiatres et psychiatrie devant le musulman algerien. *L'Évolution Psychiatrique, 44*(1), 139–160.

Binitie, A. (1975). A factor-analytic study of depression across cultures (African and European). *British Journal of Psychiatry, 127,* 559–563.

Blake, W. (1973). The influence of race on diagnosis. *Smith College Studies of Social Work, 43,* 182–192.

Blassingame, J. W. (1972). *The slave community: Plantation life in the Ante-Bellum South.* New York: Oxford University Press.

Block, R., & Zimring, F. (1973). Homicide in Chicago: 1965–70. *Journal of Research in Crime and Delinquency, 10,* 1–12.

Bradshaw, E., & Harington, J. C. (1982). A comparison of cancer mortality rates in South Africa with those in other countries. *South African Medical Journal, 61,* 943–946.

Brattle, V. M., & Lyons, C. H. (1970). *Essays in the history of African education.* New York: Teachers College Press.

Brenner, M. H. (1973). *Mental illness and the economy.* Cambridge, MA: Harvard University Press.

Brenner, M. H. (1977, May–June). Personal stability and economic security. *Social Policy, 8,* 2–4.

Breslin, R. W. (1983). Cross-cultural research in psychology. *Annual Review of Psychology, 34,* 363–400.

Brody, B. (1970). Freud's caseloads. *Psychotherapy: Theory, research, and practice, 7*(1), 8–12.

Brown, R. M. (1975). *Strain of violence: Historical studies of American violence and vigilantism.* New York: Oxford University Press.

Bulhan, H. A. (1979). Black psyches in captivity and crises. *Race and Class, 20*(3), 243–261.

Bulhan, H. A. (1980a). Frantz Fanon: The revolutionary psychiatrist. *Race and Class, 21*(3), 252–271.

Bulhan, H. A. (1980b). The revolutionary psychology of Frantz Fanon and notes on his theory of violence. *Fanon Center Journal 1*(1), 51–71.

Bulhan, H. A. (1980c). Dynamics of cultural in-betweenity: An empirical study. *International Journal of Psychology, 15,* 105–121.

Bulhan, H. A. (1981a). Psychological research in Africa: Genesis and function. *Race and Class, 23*(1), 25–41.

Bulhan, H. A. (1981b). Psychological research in Africa: Genesis and function. *Présence Africaine, 116,* 20.

Bullock, H. A. (1955). Urban homicide in theory and fact. *Journal of Criminal Law and Criminal Political Science,* 565–575.

Burns, A. (1948). *Color Prejudice: With particular reference to the relationship between whites and negroes.* London: Allen and Unwin.

Cabral, A. (1973). *Return to the source: Selected speeches.* New York: Monthly Review Press.

Carlson, D. G. (1977). African fever, prophylactic quinine and statistical analysis: Factors in the European penetration of hostile African environment. *Bulletin of the History of Medicine, 51*(3), 386–396.

Carmichael, S., & Hamilton, C. V. (1967). *Black Power: Politics of liberation in America.* New York: Vintage Books.

Carothers, J. C. (1951). Frontal lobe function and the African. *Journal of Mental Science, 97,* 12–48.

Carothers, J. C. (1953). *The African mind in health disease.* Geneva: World Health Organization, 1953.

Castantino, J., Kuller, L., Perper, J., & Cypress, R. An epidemiologic study of homicide in Allegheny County, Pennsylvania. *American Journal of Epidemiology, 106,* 314–324.

Caute, D. (1970). *Frantz Fanon.* New York: Viking Press.

Chase, A. (1977). *The legacy of Malthus: The social cost of the new scientific racism.* New York: Knopf.

Chassan, J. (1963). Race, age and sex in discharge probabilities of first admissions to a psychiatric hospital. *Psychiatry, 26,* 391–393.

Chavkin, S. (1978). *The mind stealers: Psychosurgery and mind control.* Westport, CT.: Lawrence Hill.

Chinweizu, (1975). *The West and the rest of us: White predators, black slaves and the African elite.* New York: Vintage Books.

Clark, K. B. (1965). *Dark ghetto.* New York: Harper & Row.

Cohen, D. (1977). *Psychologists on psychology.* New York: Taplinger.

Cohen, B. M., et al. (1934). Statistical contributions in the Eastern Health District. *Human Biology, 11,* 112–29.

Cole, J., & Pilisuk, M. (1976). Differences in the provision of mental health service by race. *American Journal of Orthopsychiatry, 46,* 510–525.

Cooper, R., et al. (1981). Improved mortality among U.S. Blacks, 1968–1978: The role of anti-racist struggles. *International Journal of Health Services, 11*(4), 511–522.

Davidson, B. (1978). *Let freedom come: Africa in modern history.* Boston: Little, Brown.

Davis, M. (1977, August). Occupational hazards and black workers. *Urban Health*, 6(5), 16–18.

Davis, R. (1981). Demographic analysis of suicide. In L. E. Gary (Ed.), *Black men* (pp. 179–195). Beverly Hills, CA: Sage Publications.

de Beauvoir, S. (1965, 1977). *Force of circumstance* (Vol. II). New York: Harper & Row.

Deci, E. (1980). *The psychology of self-determination*, Lexington, MA: Lexington Books.

Deragotis, L., *et al.* (1971). Social class and race as mediator variables in neurotic symptomatology. *Archives of General Psychiatry*, 25, 31–40.

Derogatis, L. R., Yevzeroff, H., & Wittelsberger, B. (1975). Social class, psychological disorder, and the nature of the psychopathological indicator. *Journal of Consulting and Clinical Psychology*, 43, 183–191.

Dillon, M. C. (1978). Merleau-Ponty and the psychology of the self. *Journal of Phenomenological Psychology*, 9, 84–98.

Dixon, V. J .(1976). World view and research methodology. In L. M. King, *et al.* (Eds.), *African philosophy: Assumptions and paradigms for research on black persons* (pp. 51–100). Los Angelos: Fanon Center Publication.

Dohrenwend, B. P. (1975). Sociocultural and sociopsychological factors in the genesis of mental disorders. *Journal of Health and Social Behavior*, 16, 365–392.

Dohrenwend, B. P., & Dohrenwend, B. S. (1969). *Social status and psychological disorders: A causal inquiry.* New York: Wiley.

Dohrenwend, B P., & Dohrenwend, B. S. (1974). *Stressful life events: Their nature and effects.* New York: Wiley.

Dougall, J. W. C. (1932). *Characteristics of African thought.* London: Oxford University Press.

Douglass, F. (1969). *My bondage and my freedom.* New York: Dover.

Draguns, J. G. (1974). Values reflected in psychopathology: The case of the Protestant Ethic. *Ethos*, 2(1), 115–136.

Draguns, J. G. (1980). Psychological disorders of clinical severity. In H. C. Triandis & J. G. Draguns (Eds.), *Handbook of cross-cultural psychology* (Vol. 6, 99–174). Boston: Allyn & Bacon.

Dugard, J. (1978). *Human rights and the South African legal order.* Princeton, NJ: Princeton University Press.

Dumont, R. (1966) *False start in Africa.* London: Sphere Books.

Dzhagarov, M. A. (1944). *Day hospitalization and the mentally ill*, Moscow.

Eckholm, E. .(1982). Human wants and misused lands. *Natural History*, 9(1), 33–48.

Ehrenreich, J. (Ed.) (1978). *The cultural crisis of modern medicine.* New York: Monthly Review Press.

Ellenberger, H. (1970). *The discovery of the unconscious: The history and evolution of dynamic psychiatry.* New York: Basic Books.

Erikson, E. H. (1965). *Childhood and society.* New York: Norton.

Erikson, E. H. (1968). *Identity, youth, and crisis.* New York: Norton.

Evans, R. I. (1975). *Konrad Lorenze: The man and his ideas.* New York: Harcourt, Brace, Jovanovich.

Fanon, F. (1951, May). L'Expérience véçu du noir. *Espirit*, Paris.

Fanon, F. (1959). L'hospitalisation de jour en psychiatrie, valeur et limites. I. Introduction générale. *La Tunisie Médicale*, 38(10).

Fanon, F. (1967a). *Black skin, white masks.* New York: Grove Press.

Fanon, F. (1967b). *A dying colonialism.* New York: Grove Press.

Fanon, F. (1967c). *Toward the African revolution.* New York: Grove Press.

Fanon, F. (1968). *The wretched of the earth.* New York: Grove Press.

Fanon, F., & Asselah, S. (1957, January). Le phénomène de l'agitation en milieu psychiatrique. Considerations générales—signification psychopathologique. *Maroc Medical.*

Fanon, F., & Azoulay, J. (1954). La socialthérapie dans un service d'hommes musulmans, difficultés méthodique. *L'Information Psychiatrique*, 30(9).

Fanon, F., & Geronimi, C. (1959). L'hospitalisation de jour en psychiatrie, valeur et limites. II. Considérations doctrinales. *La Tunisie Medicale*, 38(10).

Fanon, F., & Lacaton, R. (1955). *Conduites d'aveu en Afrique du Nord.* Congrès des médicins aliénistes et neurologues de France et des pays de langue française. 53rd session, Nice, 5–11 September.

Fanon, F., & Sanchez, F. (1956). Attitude de musulman maghrebin devant la folie (with F. Sanchez). *Revue pratique de psychologie de la vie sociale et d'hygiene mentale*, No. 1.

Fanon, F. *et al.* (1955). Aspect actuels de l'assistance mental en Algérie. *L'Information Psychiatrique*, 31(11), 689–732.

Fanon, J. (1982, February). Pour Frantz, pour notre mère. *Sans Frontiere*, 5–11.

Faris, R. E. L., & Dunham, H. W. (1939). Mental disorders in urban areas: An ecological study of schizophrenia and other psychoses. Chicago: University of Chicago Press.

Ferguson, K. E. (1980). *Self, society, and womankind: The dialectic of liberation*. Westport, CT: Greenwood Press.

Finkelman, D. (1978). Science and psychology. *American Journal of Psychology*, 9(2), 179–199.

Fireside, H. (1979). *Soviet psychoprisons*. New York: Norton.

Fischer, J. (1969). Negroes and whites and rates of mental illness: Reconsideration of a myth. *Psychiatry*, 32, 428–446.

Fonder, P. S. (Ed.) (1968). *Selections from the writings of Frederick Douglass*. New York: International Publishers.

Foucault, M. (1965). *Madness and civilization: A history of insanity in the age of reason*. New York: New American Library.

Frank, J. D. (1982). Therapeutic components shared by all psychotherapies. In J. H. Harvey & M. J. Parks (Eds.), *Psychotherapy research and behavior change* (Vol. 1, pp. 7–37). Washington, DC: American Psychological Association.

Frazier, F. F. (1957). *The black bourgeoisie*, Glencoe, IL.: The Free Press.

Frederickson, G. M. (1971). *The black image in the white mind: The debate on Afro-American character and destiny 1817–1914*. New York: Harper & Row.

Fredrickson, G. M. (1981). *White supremacy: A comparative study in American and South African History*. Oxford: Oxford University Press.

Freire, P. (1971). *Pedagogy of the oppressed*, New York: Herder and Herder.

Freud, S. (1938). *The basic writings of Sigmund Freud* (A. A. Brill, Trans.). New York: Modern Library.

Freud, S. (1953). *A general introduction to psychoanalysis*, New York: Permabooks.

Freud, S. (1961). *Civilization and its discontents*, New York: Norton.

Fried, M. (1969). Social differences in mental health. In J. Kosa, A. Antonovsky, & I. K. Zola (Eds.). *Poverty and health: A sociological analysis*. Cambridge, MA: Harvard University Press.

Garfinkel, H. (1967). Inter- and intra-racial homicide. In M. E. Wolfgang (Ed.), *Studies in homicide*. New York: Harper & Row.

Gary, L. E. (Ed.) (1981). *Black men*. Beverly Hills, CA: Sage.

Geismar, P. (1969, 1971). *Fanon: The revolutionary as prophet*. New York: Grove Press.

Gelles, R. J., & Straus, M. E. (1979). Determinants of violence in the family: Toward a theoretical investigation. In Burr *et al.* (Eds.). *Contemporary theories about the family* (pp. 549–581). New York: The Free Press.

Gendzier, I. L. (1973). *Frantz Fanon: A critical study*. New York: Pantheon.

Gendzier, I. L. (1976). Psychology and colonialism: Some observations. *The Middle East Journal*, 30(4), 501–515.

Gershon, E. M. (1967). The social character of illness: Deviance or politics? *Social Science and Medicine*, 10, 219–224.

Geyer, R. F. (1972, 1974). *Bibliography Alienation*, Amsterdam: Netherlands Universities' Joint Social Research Centre.

Gibby, R. G., *et al.* (1953). Prediction of duration of therapy from the Rorschach test. *Journal of Consulting Psychology*, 17, 348–354.

Gil, D. G. (1981). The social context of domestic violence: Implications for prevention. *Vermont Law Review*, 6(2), 339–340.

Goffman, E. (1961). *Asylums*. New York: Doubleday-Anchor.

Goin, M. K. (1965). Therapy congruent with class-linked expectations. *Archives of General Psychiatry*, 13, 133–137.

Grier, W. H., & Cobbs, P. M. (1969). *Black rage*. New York: Bantam Books.

Griffith, M. S. (1977). The influence of race on the psychotherapeutic relationship. *Psychiatry*, 40, 27–40.

Guellal, C. (1971, August). Frantz Fanon: Prophet of revolution. *The Washington Post*.

Guthrie, R. (1976). *Even the rat was white*. New York: Harper & Row.

Guttmacher, M. (1967). The normal and the sociopathic murderer. In M. E. Wolfgang (Ed.), *Studies in homicide* (pp. 114–133). New York: Harper & Row.

Haase, W. (1964). The role of socio-economic class in examiner bias. In R. Reisman, *et al* (Eds.), *Mental health of the poor*. New York: Free Press.

Hagnell, O. (1966). *A prospective study of the incidence of mental disorder*. Stockholm: Svenska Bokforlarget Norsteds-Bonniers.

Haller, J. S. (1970a). The physician versus the Negro: Medical and anthropological concepts of race in the late nineteenth century. *Bulletin of the History of Medicine, 44*, 154–167.

Haller, J. S. (1970b). Race, mortality, and life expectancy: Negro vital statistics in the late nineteenth century. *Journal of the History of Medicine and Allied Sciences, 25*(3), 247–261.

Haller, J. D. (1970c). Concepts of race inferiority in nineteenth-century anthropology. *Journal of the History of Medicine, 25*, 40–51.

Hammon-Tooks, W. (1975). African world view and its relevance for Psychiatry. *Psychologica Africana, 16*, 25–32.

Harper, F. D. (1976a). *Alcohol abuse and Black America*. Washington, DC: Howard University Press.

Harper, F. D. (Ed.) (1976b). *Alcohol abuse and the black community*. Alexandria, VA: Douglass Publishers.

Harsch, E. (1980). *South Africa: White rule, black revolt*, New York: Monad Press.

Harvey, J. H., & Parks, M. M. (1981). *Psychotherapy research and behavior change, The Master Lecture Series* (Vol. I). Washington, DC: American Psychological Association.

Haward, L. R. C., & Roland, W. A. (1954). Some inter-cultural differences on the Draw-A-Person Test: Part I, Goodenough scores. *Man, 54*, 86–88.

Haward, L. R. C., & Roland, W. A. (1955). Some inter-cultural differences on the Draw-A-Person Test: Part II, Machover series. *Man, 55*, 27–29.

Hearnshaw, L. S. (1981). *Cyril Burt: Psychologist*. New York, Vintage Books.

Hegel, G. W. F. (1966). *The phenomenology of mind*. London: Allen and Unwin.

Hepple, A. (1967). *Verwoerd*. Baltimore, MD: Penguin.

Heston, L. L. (1966). Psychiatric disorders in foster home reared children of schizophrenic mothers. *British Journal of Psychiatry, 112*, 819–825.

Hirsh, C. S., *et al*. (1973). Homicide and suicide in a metropolitan county. *Journal of the American Medical Association, 223*, 900–905.

Hoffman, F. L. (1896). Race traits and tendencies of the American Negro. *American Economic Association, 11*, 6–9.

Hollingshead, A. B., & Redlich, F. C. (1958). *Social class and mental illness*. New York: Wiley.

Hope, R. O. (1979). *Racial strife in the U.S. Military*. New York: Praeger.

Hurley, R. (1969). *Poverty and mental retardation: A causal relationship*. New York: Wiley.

Ingleby, D. (Ed.) (1980). *The politics of mental health*, New York: Pantheon Books.

Jacobson, E. (1980). *The self and the object world*, New York: International Universities Press.

Jahoda, M. (1958). *Current concepts of positive mental health*. New York: Basic Books.

Jones, E. (1974). Social class and psychotherapy: A critical review of research. *Psychiatry, 37*, 307–320.

Jones, H. (1981). *Bad blood: The Tuskegee Syphilis Experiment*. New York: Free Press.

Jones, M. (1953). *The therapeutic community*. New York: Basic Books.

Jordan, W. D. (1969). *White over Black: American attitudes toward the Negro 1550–1812*. Baltimore, MD: Penguin.

Jung, C. G. (1930). Your Negroid and Indian behavior. *Forum, 83*, 193–199.

Kamin, L. J. (1974). *The science and politics of I.Q.* New York: Wiley.

Kaplan, A. (1964). *The conduct of inquiry: The methodology for behavioral sciences*. Scranton, PA: Chandler.

Kaplan, H. B., & Warheit, G. J. (1975). Introduction to recent developments in the sociology of mental illness. *Journal of Health and Social Behavior, 16*, 343–346.

Kardiner, A., & Oversey, L. (1951). *The mark of oppression*. New York: Norton.

Keat, R., & Urry, J. (1975). *Social theory as science*. London: Routledge & Kegan Paul.

Kegan, R. (1982). *The evolving self: Problem and process in human development*. Cambridge, MA: Harvard University Press.

Kelly, G. A. (1972). Notes on Hegel's "Lordship and Bondage." In A. MacIntyre (Ed.), *Hegel: A collection of critical essays* (pp. 189–217). Notre Dame, IN: University of Notre Dame Press.

King, L. M. (1978). Social and cultural influences on psychopathology. *Annual Review of Psychology, 29*, 405–433.

King, L. M. (1982). Alcoholism studies regarding Black Americans. In *Alcohol and Health Monograph* (Vol. 4, 385–407). Washington, DC: ADMHA Document.

Klebba, A. M. (1975). Homicide trends in the United States. *Public Health Reports, 90*(3), 195–204.

Kleiner, R., *et al.* (1960). Mental disorders and status based on race. *Psychiatry, 23*, 271–274.

Kluckhohn, C. & Murray, H. (Eds.). (1948). *Personality in nature, society, culture*. New York: Knopf.

Kluckhohn, F., & Strodtbeck, F. (1961). *Variations in value orientation*. New York: Row, Peterson.

Kojeve, A. (1969). *Introduction to the reading of Hegel*. New York: Basic Books.

Kovel, J. (1971). *White racism: A psychohistory*. New York: Pantheon.

Kramer, M. *et al.* (1973). Definition and distribution of mental disorders in a racist society. In C. Willie, *et al.* (Eds.), *Racism and mental health*. Pittsburgh, PA: University of Pittsburgh Press.

Kroeber, A. L. (1920). "Totem and Taboo": An ethnological psychoanalysis. *American Anthropologist, 22*, 48–55.

Kroeber, A. L. (1920). "Totem and Taboo" in retrospect. *American Journal of Sociology, 45*, 446–457.

Lambo, T. A. (1956). Neuropsychiatric observations in the Western Region of Nigeria. *British Medical Journal, 15*, 1388–1394.

Leighton, A. H., *et al.* (1963a). *The Character of danger: Psychiatric symptoms in selected communities*. New York: Basic Books.

Leighton, A. H., *et al.* (1963b). *Psychiatric disorders among the Yoruba*. Ithaca, NY: Cornell University Press.

Lemkau, P., Tietze, C., & Cooper, M. (1942). Mental hygiene problems in an urban district. *Mental Hygiene, 26*, 100–119.

Lifton, R. J. (1983). *The broken connection: On death and the continuing of life*. New York: Basic Books.

Lloyd, J. W. (1971). Long-term mortality study of steelworkers. *Journal of Occupational Medicine, 13*, 53–60.

Lorrion, R. P. (1973). Socioeconomic status and traditional treatment approaches reconsidered. *Psychological Bulletin, 79*, 263–270.

Lorrion, R. P. (1974). Patient and therapist variables in the treatment of low income patients. *Psychological Bulletin, 81*, 344–354.

Lorrion, R. P. (1978). Research on psychotherapy and behavior change with the disadvantaged: Past, present, and future directions. In L. Garfield & A. E. Bergin (Eds.), *Handbook of psychotherapy and behavior change: An emperical analysis* (pp. 903–938). New York: Wiley.

Luborsky, I., *et al.* (1971). Factors influencing the outcome to psychotherapy. *Psychological Bulletin, 75*, 145–185.

MacDougall, W. (1908). *Social psychology*. New York: Luce.

Malzberg, B. (1959). Mental disease among negroes: An analysis of first admissions in New York State, 1949–51. *Mental Hygiene, 43*, 422–459.

Mannix, D. P. (1962). *Black cargoes: A history of the Atlantic slave trade*. New York: Viking Press.

Mannoni, O. (1962). *Prospero and Caliban: The psychology of colonization*. New York: Praeger.

Marx, K. (1964, 1973). *The Economic and Philosophic Manuscript of 1844*. New York: International Publishers.

Maslow, A. H. (1970). *Motivation and personality*. New York: Harper & Row.

McGhee, J. D. (1983). The changing demographics in Black America. In *The state of Black America*. New York: National Urban League.

Mears, F., & Gatchel, R. J. (1979). *Foundations of abnormal psychology*. Chicago: Rand McNally.

Memmi, A. (1965). *The colonizer and the colonized*. New York: Orien Press.

Memmi, A. (1968). *Dominated man*. Boston: Beacon Press.

Meszaros, I. (1970). *Marx's theory of alienation*. New York: Harper & Row.

Mischel, W. (1968). *Personality and assessment.* New York: Wiley.

Mishler, E. (1979). Skinnerism: Materialism minus the dialectic. *Journal for the Theory of Social Behavior, 6,* 21–47.

Morel, E. D. (1969). *The black man's burden,* New York: Monthly Review Press.

Morton, S. G. (1839). *Crania Americana or a Comparative View of the Skulls of Various Abroginal Natives of North and South America.* Philadelphia: John Pennigton.

Murphy, G., & Kovach, J. E. (1972). *Historical introduction to modern psychology.* New York: Harcourt, Brace, Jovanovich.

Murphy, J. M. (1973) Sociocultural change and psychiatric disorder among Rural Yoruba in Nigeria. *Ethos, 1,* 239–262.

Murray, H. A. (1962). *Explorations in personality.,* New York: Science Editions.

Myers, J. (1981). The social context of occupational disease: Asbestos and South Africa. *International Journal of Health Service, 11,*(2), 227–245.

Newman, G. (1979). *Understand violence.* New York: Lippincot.

Nghe, N. (1963, February). Fanon et les problems de l'independence. *La Pensée,* 23–36.

Norton, S. M. (1966). Homicide in Baltimore. *Maryland State Medical Journal,* 55–66.

Ofosu-Appiah, L. H. (1971). *People in bondage: African slavery in the modern era.* Minneapolis, MN: Lerner.

Ornstein, P. H. (Ed.) (1978). *The search for the self: Selected writings of Heinz Kohut* (Vols. 1 & 2). New York: International Universities Press.

Parin, P., & Morgenthaler, F. (1970). Character analysis based on the behavior pattern of "primitive Africans." In W. Muensterberger (Ed.), *Man and his culture: Psychoanalytic anthropology after "Totem and Taboo"* (pp. 187–210). New York: Taplinger.

Passamanick, B. (1963a). Some misconceptions concerning differences in the racial prevalence of mental disease. *American Journal of Orthopsychiatry, 33,* 72–86.

Passamanick, B. (1963b). A survey of mental disease in an urban population: An approach to total prevalence by race. *American Journal of Psychiatry, 119,* 299–305.

Patterson, O. (1982). *Slavery and social death: A comparative study.* Cambridge, MA: Harvard University Press.

Paul, J. A. (1978). Medicine and imperialism. In J. Erehreich (Ed.), *The cultural crisis of medicine* (pp. 271–286). New York: Monthly Review Press.

Paxton, R. O. (1975). *Europe in the twentieth century.* New York: Harcourt, Brace, Jovanovich.

Pettigrew, T. F. (1964). *A profile of the Negro American.* Princeton, NJ: Van Nostrand.

Pinderhughes, C. A. (1972). Managing paranoia in violent relationships. In G. Usdin (Ed.), *Perspectives on violence* (pp. 111–139). New York: Brunner/Mazel.

Pokorny, A., & Overall, J. (1970). Relationship of psychopathology to age, sex, ethnicity, education, and marital status in state hospital patients. *Journal of Psychiatric Research, 7*(3), 143–152.

Poussaint, A. F. (1983). The mental health status of blacks. *The state of Black America* (pp. 187–239). New York: National Urban League.

Prince, R. (1967). The changing picture of depressive syndromes in Africa. *Canadian Journal of African Studies, 1*(2), 177–192.

Pugh, T., & MacMahon, B. (1962). *Epidemiologic findings in the United States mental health hospital data.* Boston: Little, Brown.

Rabkin, J. G., & Struening, E. L. (1976). *Ethnicity, social class, and mental illness.* New York: Institute of Pluralism and Group Identity.

Riegel, K. F. (1975). From traits and equilibrium toward developmental dialectics. In W. W. Arnold (Ed.), *Nebraska symposium on motivation* (Vol. 23, pp. 349–408). Lincoln: University of Nebraska Press.

Ritchie, J. F. (1943). *The African as suckling and as adult.* Livingstone: Rhodes Livingstone Paper No. 9.

Roazen, P. (1974). *Freud and his followers.* New York: New American Library.

Robin, G. (1963). Justifiable homicide by police. *Journal of Criminal Law, Criminology, and Police Science, 54,* 225–231.

Rodney, W. (1974). *How Europe underdeveloped Africa,* Washington, DC: Howard University Press.

Roheim, G. (1943). *The origin and function of culture.* Nervous and Mental Disease Monograph. New York: Johnson Reprint Corp.

Roheim, G. (1943, 1944). War and the covenant. *Journal of Criminal Psychopathology, 4, 5,* 842–53.

Rome, H. P. (1974). Depressive illness: Its sociopsychiatric implications. *Psychiatric Annals, 4,* 54–68.

Rose, H. M. *Black homicide and the urban environment.* Bethesda, MD: National Institute of Mental Health.

Rosenoff, A. J. (1917). Survey of mental disorders in Nassau County, New York. *Psychiatric Bulletin, 2,* 109–131.

Rosenthal, D., & Frank, J. (1958). Fate of psychiatric clinic outpatients assigned to psychotherapy. *Journal of Nervous and Mental Diseases, 127,* 330–343.

Roux, E. (1966). *Time longer than rope: A history of the Black Man's struggle for freedom in South Africa.* Madison/Milwaukee: The University of Wisconsin Press.

Rushforth, N. B. *et al.* (1977). Violent death in a metropolitan county: Changing patterns in homicide, 1958–74. *New England Journal of Medicine, 297*(10), 531–538.

Sachs, A. (1969). *South Africa: The violence of Apartheid.* London: International Defence and Aid Fund.

Sampson, E. E. (1981). Cognitive psychology as ideology. *American Psychologist, 36*(7), 730–743.

Sarbin, T. R., & Mancuso, J. C. (1982). *Schizophrenia: Medical diagnosis or moral verdict.* New York: Pergamon Press.

Sartre, J.-P. (1968). *Anti-Semite and Jew,* New York, Schocken Books.

Schaffer, L., & Myers, J. K. (1954). Psychoptherapy and social stratification. *Psychiatry, 17,* 83–88.

Schexnider, A. J. (1983). Blacks in the military. *State of Black America* (pp. 241–269). New York: National Urban League.

Schwab, J. *et al.* (1973). Social psychiatric impairment: Racial comparisons. *American Journal of Psychiatry, 130,* 183–186.

Seedat, Y. K., Seedat, M. A., & Nkomo, M. N. (1978). The prevalence of hypertension in the urban Zulu. *South African Medical Journal, 53,* 923–927.

Seeman, M. (1959). On the meaning of alienation. *American Sociological Review, 24,* 783–791.

Seeman, M. (1975). Alienation studies. *Annual Review of Sociology, 1,* 91–123.

Seiden, R. H., & Frietas, R. P. (1980). Shifting patterns of deadly violence. *Suicide and life-threatening behavior, 10*(4), 195–209.

Senghor, L. S. (Ed.) (1948). *Anthologie de la nouvelle poésie negre et malgache de langue franccaise.* Paris: Presses Universitaries de France.

Sharpley, R. H. *Treatment issues: Foreign medical graduates and black patient population.* Cambridge, MA: Solomon Fuller Institute.

Sikakane, J. (1977). *A window on Soweto.* London: International Defence and Aid Fund.

Sjoberg, G. (1967). *Ethics, politics, and social research.* Cambridge, MA: Schenkman.

Skinner, B. F. (1953). *Science and human behavior.* New York: Free Press.

Sorel, G. (1970). *Reflections on violence.* London: Collier Books.

Sow, I. (1980). *Anthropological structures of madness in Black Africa.* New York: International Universities Press, 1980.

Srole, L., Langer, T. S., Michael, S. T. *et al.* (1962). *Mental health in the metropolis: The Midtown Manhattan Study.* New York: McGraw-Hill.

Stampp, K. (1956). *The peculiar institution.* New York: Vintage Books.

Steinmetz, S. & Strauss, M. A. (1974). *Violence in the family.* New York: Harper & Row.

Strupp, H. H. (1982). The outcome problem in psychotherapy: Contemporary perspectives. In J. H. Harvey & M. M. Parks (Eds.), *Psychotherapy research and behavior change* (Vol. 1, pp. 43–71). Washington, DC: American Psychological Association.

Suls, J. (1982). *Psychological perspectives on the self* (Vol. 1). Hillsdale, NJ: Erlbaum.

Susser, M., & Cherry, V. P. (1982). Health and health care under Apartheid. *Journal of Public Health Policy, 3*(4), 455–475.

Swinton, D. H. (1983). The economic status of the black population. *The state of Black America* (pp. 45–105). New York: National Urban League.

Szasz, T. S. (1970). *The manufacture of madness: A comparative study of the inquisition and the mental health movement.* New York: Harper & Row.

Szasz, T. S. (1974). *The myth of mental illness: Foundations of a theory of personal conduct.* New York: Harper & Row.

Takagi, P. (1979). Death by police intervention. In R. Brenner & H. Kravitz (Eds.), *A community concern: Police use of deadly force.* Washington, DC: National Institute of Law Enforcement and Criminal Justice.

Task Panel Reports submitted to the President's Commission on Mental Health (Vol. 3) 1978, see particularly, the report "Mental health of Black Americans" (pp. 822–873).

Thomas, A. & Sillen, S. (1974). *Racism and psychiatry.* Secaucus, NJ: Citadel Press.

Torrey, E. F. (1973). Schizophrenia universal?: An open question. *Schizophrenia Bulletin, 7,* 53–59.

Tosquelles, F., & Fanon, F. (1953). *Congrès de medicins alienistes et neurologues de France et des pays de lange française,* 51st session, Pau, July 20–26.

Townsey, R. D. (1981). The incarceration of black men. In L. E. Gary (Ed.), *Black Men* (pp. 229–256). Beverly Hills, CA: Sage Publications.

Triandis, H. C., & Draguns, J. G. (1980). *Handbook of cross-cultural psychology: Psychopathology* (Vol. 6). Boston: Allyn and Bacon.

Usdin, G. (Ed.). (1972). *Perspectives on violence.* New York: Brunner/Mazel.

U.S. Department of Health and Human Services (1980). *Health United States* (DHHS Publication No. PHS 81–1232, prepublication copy). Hyattsville, MD: National Center for Health Statistics.

Vaughn, J. P., & Miall, W. E. (1979). A comparison of cardiovascular measurements in Gambia, Jamaica, and the United Republic of Tanzania. *Bulletin of the World Health Organization, 57,* 281–289.

Vazquez, A. S. (1977). *The Philosophy of praxis,* London: Merlin Press.

Warheit, G. J., Holzer, C. E., & Arey, S. A. (1975). Race and mental illness: An epidemiologic update. *Journal of Health and Social Behavior, 16,* 243–256.

Weber, M. (1958). *The Protestant Ethic and the Spirit of Capitalism.* New York: Scribner's.

Weis, N. S. (1976). Recent trends in violent deaths among young adults in the United States. *American Journal of Epidemiology, 103,* 416–422.

Welsing, F. C. (1974, May). Cress theory of color confrontation. *Black Scholar,* 32–40.

Wilkinson, G. S. (1975). Patient-audience social status and the social construction of psychiatric disorders. *Journal of Health and Social Behavior, 26,* 28–38.

Williams, C. (1976). *The destruction of black civilization: Great issues of a race from 4500 B.C. to 2000 A.D.,* Chicago: Third World Press.

Williams, E. (1966). *Capitalism and Slavery,* New York: Capricorn Books.

Willie, C. V., Kramer, B. M., & Brown, B. S. (1973). *Racism and mental health.* Pittsburgh, PA: University of Pittsburgh.

Wilson, E. O. (1978). *Sociobiology: The new synthesis.* Cambridge, MA: Harvard University Press.

Woddis, J. (1972). *New theories of revolution.* New York: International Publishers.

Wolfers M. (1974). *Black Man's Burden revisited.* London: Allison & Busby.

Wolfgang, M. (1958). *Patterns in criminal homicide.* New York: Wiley.

Wolfgang, M. (1967). *Studies in homicide.* New York: Harper & Row.

Wolfgang, M. (1976). Family violence and criminal behavior. *Bulletin of the American Academy of Psychiatry and Law 4*(4), 316–327.

World Health Organization (1977, March). Apartheid and mental health (Vol. 22). Geneva: WHO.

Wyndham, C. H. (1981a). Economically active manpower in the various population of the RSA, Part I. Leading causes of death: Health strategies for reducing mortality. *South African Medical Journal, 60,* 411–419.

Wyndham, C. H. (1981b). The loss from premature deaths of economically active manpower in the various populations of the RSA. Part II. Man-years of economically active life lost from premature death. *South African Medical Journal, 60,* 5458–5462.

Wyndham, C. H., & Irwig, L. M. (1979). A comparison of the mortality rates of various population groups in the Republic of South Africa. *South African Medical Journal, 55,* 796–802.

Yamamoto, J., & Goin, M. K. (1966). Social factors relevant for psychiatric treatment. *Journal of Nervous and Mental Disorders, 142,* 332–339.

Yamamoto, J., *et al.* (1967). Racial factors in patient selection. *American Journal of Psychiatry, 124,* 630–636.

Zahar, R. (1974). *Frantz Fanon: Colonialism and alienation.* New York: Monthly Review Press.

Zubin, J., & Spring, B. (1977). Vulnerability—a new view of schizophrenia. *Journal of Abnormal Psychology, 86*(2), 103–126.

SELECT BIBLIOGRAPHY

BOOKS BY FANON

Fanon, F. (1967a). *Black skin, white masks* (Chales Lam Markmann, Trans.). New York: Grove Press.

Fanon, F. (1967b). *A dying colonialism* (Haakon Chevalier, Trans.). New York: Grove Press.

Frantz, F. (1967c). *Toward the African Revolution* (Haakon Chevalier, Trans.). New York: Grove Press.

Fanon, F. (1968). *The wretched of the earth* (Constance Farrington, Trans.). New York: Grove Press.

PUBLISHED ARTICLES[1]

Fanon, F. (1951, May). "L'Experience vecu du noir. *L'Espirit*, Paris.

Fanon, F., & Tosquelles, F. (1953). *Sur quelques cas traités par la méthode de Bini.* Congrès des médicins aliénistes et neurologues de France et des pays de langue française, 51st session, Pau, 20–26 July.

Fanon, F., & Tosquelles, F. (1953). *Sur un essai de réadaptation chez une malade avec épilepsie morphéique et troubles de caractère grave* (with F. Tosquelles, Saint Albans). Congrès des médicins aliénistes et neurologues de France et des pays de langue française, 51st session, Pau, 20–26 July.

Fanon, F., & Toquelles, F. (1953). *Indication de thérapeutique de Bini dal le cadre des thérapeutiques institutionelles.* Congrès des médicins aliénistes et neurologues de France et des pays de langue française. 51st session, Pau, 20–26 July.

Fanon, F., Despinoy, M., & Zenner, W. (1953). *Note sur les techniques de cures de sommeil avec conditionnement et contrôle électroencéphalographique.* Congrès des médicins aliénistes et neurologues de France et des pays de langue française. 51st session, Pau, 20–26 July.

Fanon, F., & Despinoy, M. (1953, June). A propos de syndrome de Cotard avec balancement psychosomatique. *Les Annales Médico-Psychologiques*, 2.

Fanon, F., & Azoulay, J. (1954). La socialthérapie dans un service d'hommes musulmans, difficultés méthodologieque. *L'Information Psychiatrique, 30*(9).

Fanon, F., Azoulay, J., & Sanchez, F. (1954/55). *Introduction aux troubles de la sexualité chez les Nord-Africains.* Unpublished manuscript.

Fanon, F. (1955). Réflexions sur la ethnopsychiatrie. *Conscience Maghrebine*, 3.

---

[1]Dr. Ntongela Masilela, in *The Fanon Center Journal* (Vol. 1, no. 1, 1980), compiled a most comprehensive bibliography of works by and on Frantz Fanon. Geismar (1971), Gendzier (1973), and Zahar (1976) also provide bibiliography of works by Fanon.

Fanon, F., Dequeker, J., Lacaton, R., Micucci, M., & Ramee, F. (1955). Aspect actuels de l'assistance mental en Algérie. *L'Information Psychiatrique 31*(1).

Fanon, F., & Lacaton, R. (1955). *Conduites d'aveu en Afrique du Nord.* Congrès des médicins aliénistes et neurologues de France et des pays de langue française, 53rd session, Nice, 5–11 September.

Fanon, F., & Sanchez, F. (1956). Attitude de musulman maghrebin devant la folie. *Revue pratique de psychologie de la vie sociale et d'hygiene mentale,* 1.

Fanon, F., & Geromini, C. (1956). *Le T.A.T. chez la femme musulmane. Sociologie de la perceptions et de l'imagination.* Congrès des médicins aliénistes et neurologues de France et des pays de langue française, 54th session. Bordeaux, August 30–September 4.

Fanon, F. (1957, January). Le Phénomène de l'agitation en milieu psychiatrique. Considérations générales—signification psychopathologique (with Asselah). *Maroc Médical.*

Fanon, F., & Levy, L. (1958). A propos d'un cas de spasme de torsion. *La Tunisie Médicale, 36* (9).

Fanon, F., & Levy, L. (1959). Premiers essais de méprobamate injectable dans les états hypocondriaque. *La Tunisie Médicale 37*(10).

Fanon, F., & Geromini, C. (1959). "L'Hospitalisation de jour en psychiatrie, valeur et limites. I. Introduction générale; II. Considérations doctrinales" (Part II with C. Geronomi). *La Tunisie Médicale 37*(10).

Works on Fanon

Bouvier, P. (1971). *Fanon,* Paris: Editions Universitaires.

Caute, D. (1970). *Frantz Fanon.* New York: Viking; London: Collins Fontana.

Geismar, P. (1971). *Fanon: The revolutionary as prophet.* New York: Grove Press.

Genzier, I. L. (1973). *Frantz Fanon: A critical study.* New York: Pantheon.

Hansen, E. (1977). *Frantz Fanon: Social and political thought.* Columbus, OH: Ohio State University Press.

Zahar, R. (1974). *Frantz Fanon: Colonialism and alienation* (W. F. Feuser, trans.). New York: Monthly Review Press.

INDEX